Psychiatry: Breaking the ICE

Introductions, Common Tasks and Emergencies for Trainees

Psychiatry: Breaking the ICE

Introductions, Common Tasks and Emergencies for Trainees

EDITORS

Sarah Stringer

Independent Section 12 Approved Doctor
Extreme Psychiatry Course Lead and Honorary Lecturer, King's College London, UK

Juliet Hurn

Consultant Psychiatrist, North-West Southwark Support and Recovery Team (Community team), South London and Maudsley NHS Foundation Trust, UK

Anna M Burnside

Consultant Liaison Psychiatrist and RAID Clinical Lead, East London NHS Foundation Trust, UK

WILEY Blackwell

This edition first published 2016 © 2016 by John Wiley and Sons Ltd

Registered office: John Wiley & Sons, Ltd, The Atrium, Southern Gate, Chichester, West Sussex, PO19 8SQ, UK

Editorial offices: 9600 Garsington Road, Oxford, OX4 2DQ, UK
   The Atrium, Southern Gate, Chichester, West Sussex, PO19 8SQ, UK
   111 River Street, Hoboken, NJ 07030-5774, USA

For details of our global editorial offices, for customer services and for information about how to apply for permission to reuse the copyright material in this book please see our website at www.wiley.com/wiley-blackwell

Library of Congress Cataloging-in-Publication Data

Psychiatry (Stringer)
  Psychiatry : breaking the ICE : introductions, common tasks, emergencies for trainees / [edited by] Sarah L. Stringer, Juliet Hurn, Mujtaba Husain.
    p. ; cm.
  Includes bibliographical references and index.
  ISBN 978-1-118-55726-6 (pbk. : alk. paper)
  I. Stringer, Sarah, editor. II. Hurn, Juliet, editor. III. Husain, Mujtaba, editor. IV. Title.
  [DNLM: 1. Physician's Role–Handbooks. 2. Psychiatry–Handbooks. 3. Physician-Patient Relations–Handbooks. WM 34]
  RC454
  616.89 – dc23
                         2015016163

A catalogue record for this book is available from the British Library.

Wiley also publishes its books in a variety of electronic formats. Some content that appears in print may not be available in electronic books.

Cover image: gettyimages-182861610/Smashed Ice copyright David Venon

Set in 9/11pt, MeridienLTStd by SPi Global, Chennai, India.

1   2016

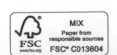

Contents

WARD

ON-CALL

Appendices

Contributors

Christina Barras
ST6 General Adult Psychiatry, South West London & St George's Mental Health NHS Trust, London, England

Katherine Beck
Academic Clinical Fellow, Kings College London and Core Trainee, London, England
South London and Maudsley NHS Foundation Trust, London, England

Penelope Brown
Consultant in Forensic Psychiatry, South London and Maudsley NHS Foundation Trust, London, England
Clinical Research Fellow in Forensic Psychiatry, Department of Forensic and Neurodevelopmental Sciences, Institute of Psychiatry, King's College London, London, England

Jane Bunclark
Consultant Nurse for Self-Harm; Head of Nursing Mood, Affective and Personality Clinical Academic Group, South London & Maudsley NHS Foundation Trust, London, England

Lisa Conlan
Consultant Psychiatrist, South London and Maudsley NHS Foundation Trust, London, England

Rory Conn
ST5 in Child & Adolescent Psychiatry, Tavistock and Portman NHS Foundation Trust, London, England
Darzi Fellow in Patient Safety and Quality Improvement, Great Ormond Street Hospital, London, England

Sean Cross
Consultant Liaison Psychiatrist St Thomas' Hospital & King's College Hospital, London, England
Clinical Lead for Liaison Psychiatry & Director of Centre for Mental Health Simulation, South London and Maudsley NHS Foundation Trust, London, England
Visiting Lecturer, Institute of Psychiatry, Psychology & Neuroscience, King's College London, London, England

Abigail G Crutchlow
Higher Trainee in General Adult Psychiatry, South London & Maudsley NHS Foundation Trust, London, England

Matthew Fernando
ST5 Child & Adolescent Mental Health Services, South London & Maudsley NHS Foundation Trust, London, England

Laurine Hanna
Higher Trainee, General Adult Psychiatry, South London & Maudsley NHS Foundation Trust, London, England

Peter Hindley
Consultant Child & Adolescent Psychiatrist, Children's Psychological Medicine, St Thomas' Hospital, London, England
South London & Maudsley NHS Foundation Trust, London, England
Honorary Teacher, King's College London, London, England

Mujtaba Husain
ST6, General Adult Psychiatry, South London and Maudsley NHS Foundation Trust, London, England
Chair, Academy of Medical Royal Colleges' Trainee Doctors' Group (ATDG), London, England

Noreen Jakeman
Principle Pharmacist for Mental Health Services, Lewisham & Greenwich NHS Trust, London, England

Cheryl Kipping
Consultant Nurse – Dual Diagnosis, South London & Maudsley NHS Foundation Trust, London, England

Natasha Liu-Thwaites
ST6 in Psychotherapy (CBT), South London & Maudsley NHS Foundation Trust, London, England

Sean Lubbe
Staff Specialist – Aged Care Psychiatry
Conjoint Lecturer – University of New South Wales (UNSW), New South Wales, Australia
School of Psychiatry – UNSW Black Dog Institute, New South Wales, Australia

Vivienne Mak
Consultant in Liaison Psychiatry of Older Adults, South London & Maudsley NHS Foundation Trust, New South Wales, Australia

Isabel McMullen
Consultant Psychiatrist, South London and Maudsley NHS Foundation Trust, New South Wales, Australia

John Moriarty
Consultant Psychiatrist & Director of Postgraduate Psychiatric Training, South London & Maudsley NHS Foundation Trust, New South Wales, Australia
Honorary Senior Lecturer, Kings College London, New South Wales, Australia

Rory Sheehan
Specialist Registrar in Psychiatry of Intellectual Disability, North London Training Scheme for Psychiatry of Intellectual Disability, London, England
Academic Clinical Fellow, University College London, London, England

Abigail Steenstra
Psychiatry Core Trainee 3, South London & Maudsley NHS Foundation Trust, London, England

Rachel Thomasson
ST5 Liaison Psychiatry, Manchester Royal Infirmary, Manchester, Lancashire, England

Stephanie Young
Consultant in Rehabilitation Psychiatry, South London & Maudsley NHS Foundation Trust, London, England

Patient Focus Groups

Elinor Hynes
CT3 Psychiatry, South London & Maudsley NHS Foundation Trust, London, England
Focus group team lead; liaising/interviewing; transcribing and collating quotes

Zachary J Ferguson
Foundation Year 1 doctor, South Thames Foundation School, London, England
Interviewing and transcribing

Louise Bundock
CT3 Psychiatrist South London & Maudsley NHS Foundation Trust, London, England
Interviewing

Patient & Carer Views (individual quotes have been anonymised)
Alcoholics Anonymous
The Dragon Cafe service users
Family Health Isis
Marjorie Alleyne
Amelia Amarelle
Wendy Blake
Marian McEvoy
Barbara Riddell
Sarah Wheeler
Marjorie Wright

Online Video Resources

Zachary J Ferguson
Foundation Trainee, South Thames Foundation School, London, England
Camera, editing, post-production; interviewer

Matthew Fernando
Writer, clinical advisor
ST5, Child & Adolescent Psychiatry, South London & Maudsley NHS Foundation Trust, London, England

Roxanne Keynejad
CT1 Psychiatry, South London & Maudsley NHS Foundation Trust, London, England
Film team coordinator; interviewer

David McLaughlan
Research Fellow, South London & Maudsley NHS Foundation Trust, London, England
Clinical advisor, assistant coordinator; interviewer

Actors:
Sam Adamson – Alex Walker (Video 1–6)
Pat Imamura – Nurse Tracy (1,2)
Raj Shah – Dr Tom (1,2)

Megan Fisher – Dr Helen (3,4)
Roxanne Keynejad – Nurse Alana (3,4)
Tijan Chee – Dr Li (5,6)
Matt Fernando – Rob, nurse (5)
Katy Lowe – Nurse Gabrielle (5)
Emma Louise Johnston – Nurse Wilma (5)
Emily Hackett – Nurse Xena (5)
Josef Prochaska – Nurse Fernando (5,6)
Ronald Oguntoyinbo – Care coordinator & social worker, Richard (6)
Jennifer Seal – Pharmacist Holly (6)
David O'Flynn – Dr Ralph (6)
Ruth Ann Harpur-Lewis – Claire, psychologist (6)
Sarah Stringer – Catherine, Alex's sister (6)
Hannah Nice – Emily, occupational therapist (6)

Multidisciplinary Team Interviews

Barbara Wood, Consultant Psychotherapist
Dele Olajide, Consultant Psychiatrist
Irene Sclare, Consultant Psychologist and researcher
Cheryl Walder, Child and Adolescent Mental Health Service Team Manager, Registered
Mental Health Nurse
Orla Jordan, Social Worker
Nicky Smith, Approved Mental Health Professional
Emmanuel Lahai-Taylor, Psychiatric Liaison Nurse
Jane McGrath, Service user Representative, West London Mental Health Trust, NHS Dignity Inspector and
Patient and Public Involvement Member of NHS Alliance

Also thanks to Paul Wilkinson, Dr Martin Baggaley and staff at the Ortus Centre for their throughout the filming process.

Foreword

When I was doing my house jobs (as we called them in those days before the start of the First World War) and during years as a medical SHO, every doctor I knew carried a copy of Robinson and Stott's *Medical Emergencies* in the pocket of their white coat. Unlike every other textbook that we owned, this one told you what to do when in trouble. It also had a brilliant index, including my favourite entry, "Blue, patient turning: 22–24".

And now Sarah Stringer ("Strings") and her colleagues have produced the same for clinical psychiatry. It is not difficult to describe the main mental disorders, list the various available treatments, or even give a guide to the current status of mental health law. What is difficult is learning how to actually do the job. Many people who are not in the trade think they know a lot about psychiatry – it seems to be a perennial source of discussion, argument and debate – much of which is readily understood by the general public. This is in stark contrast to ophthalmology, clinical oncology or cardiac anaesthesia: although these subjects are of great interest to people, you have to be a member of the club before you can take part in the debates, and that takes years.

But if psychiatry is a matter of public interest, debate and discourse, very few people really know what a psychiatrist actually does. And I am afraid that the ever diminishing time given over to psychiatry in medical schools rarely provides answers, any more than a medical student's exposure to surgery is much help if they actually decide to become a surgeon.

This is the book that tells you how it is. What psychiatrists do, and how you can become one. It describes who is who in the multi disciplinary team, how to handle your first night on-call, how to deal with someone who is angry (whether a patient or colleague), how mental health services function in real life, what to do when landed with your first follow-up clinic, and why it is essential to make friends with your administrator. It is also replete with sensible advice – not from people like me, whose advice is about as helpful to a doctor starting their first psychiatry post as the advice of a General to a young officer fresh out of Sandhurst. No, you want to hear from people who have just found their own feet, and who know how it *is*, not how it *was*. And you also want to hear it from the other side – what it is like to be a patient, and what they and their families value in their psychiatrist. This book does all that.

But having said that, there is much in this book that does remind me of my first faltering steps on the road to becoming a proper psychiatrist. The health service may have changed, the jargon shifted, the forms are different – but this book also conveys some of the essential truths about what makes a good psychiatrist, and how you can achieve that. Learning how to talk to patients in distress, how to make a good differential diagnosis, how to deal with the strains, but most of all, why it is a privilege to be a psychiatrist.

Professor Sir Simon Wessely
Chair, Psychological Medicine, Institute of Psychiatry, King's College London
President, Royal College of Psychiatrists

Acknowledgements

Mujtaba Husain

- Initial planning and idea development – thank you!

Expert Advisors

- Daniel M Bennett
- Ann Bessell
- Emmeline Brew-Graves
- Annis Cohen
- Penny Collins
- Frances Connan
- Jo Cresswell
- Duncan Doyle
- Robert Flanagan
- Robert Flynn
- Amanda Foakes
- Sarah Grice
- Brian Hana
- Simon Harrison
- Claire Henderson
- Penny Henderson
- Andrew Hodgkiss
- Stania Kamara
- David McLaughlan
- Jack Nathan
- Edward Noble
- Victoria Oldfield
- Elizabeth Parker
- Dimitrios Paschos
- William Pitcher
- Barry Purdell
- Alison Roberts
- Dene Robertson
- Cameron Russell
- Alice Roberts
- Trudi Seneviratne
- Ruth Sugden
- Tracey Taylor
- Chris Tris
- Zoe Wake
- Lucy Wilford
- Charlotte Wilson-Jones
- Felicity Wood
- Deborah Woodman
- Adam Winstock

Breaking the ICE Test Pilots

- Roxanne Keynejad
- Julia Temitope Ogunmuyiwa
- Michael Utterson

SS: Many thanks to all who've taught me how to be a psychiatrist over the last eleven years: patients, students and colleagues. Thank you to those who supported me to walk cheerfully, live adventurously, and to edit this book without taking a hammer to my laptop: Martin, Pat, Caroline, and my much-loved Stringer Clan. Finally, great gratitude to Beth (the secret fourth editor) – your tolerance, proof-reading and ability to provide tea via some sort of invisible conveyor belt have been an essential part of the process. (And yes, I promise not to write another book for at least a while ...)

JH: To my dear family and friends – thank you very much for your support and patience. See – the book did get finished! Thank you also to the many patients, colleagues, and students who have offered inspiration for the book; you continue to make working in psychiatry stimulating, surprising, and rewarding.

AB: I would like to thank Bernadette Burnside, who gave me my middle initial in the hope it would read well on the cover of a book. I believe she was hoping for something more like 'War and Peace', but in the meantime, I hope this will suffice. For someone who has been supportive of my publishing career for more than 30 years with scant return, she certainly deserves all the thanks I can give. Thanks are also due to the surprising, challenging and inspirational patients and colleagues that I have been lucky enough to work with daily, never forgetting my acute Trust colleagues.

Abbreviations

ADLs	activities of daily living
AMHP	Approved Mental Health Professional
bd	*bis die* (twice daily)
BMI	body mass index
BNF	British National Formulary
BP	blood pressure
BPAD	bipolar affective disorder
CAMHS	child & adolescent mental health services
CASC	Clinical Assessment of Skills & Competencies (exam)
CBT	cognitive behaviour therapy
CC	care coordinator
CG	Clinical Guideline (NICE references)
CIWA-Ar	Clinical Institute Withdrawal Assessment of Alcohol Scale, Revised
CMHT	community mental health team
CPA	Care Programme Approach
CPN	community psychiatric nurse
CRP	C reactive protein
CT	computed tomography
CT1-3	Core Trainee years 1–3
CTO	Community Treatment Order
CXR	chest X-ray
DHx	drug history
DLB	dementia with Lewy bodies
DoLS	Deprivation of Liberty Safeguards
ECG	electrocardiogram
ECT	electroconvulsive therapy
ED	emergency department ('casualty' / 'accident & emergency')
eGFR	estimated glomerular filtration rate
EPSE	extrapyramidal side effects
ERT	emergency response team
ESR	erythrocyte sedimentation rate
EUPD	emotionally unstable personality disorder ('borderline personality')
EWS	early warning scoring
FBC	full blood count
FHx	family history
FGA	first generation antipsychotic
GAD	generalised anxiety disorder
GHB	gamma-hydroxybutyric acid
GBL	gamma-butyrolactone
GMC	General Medical Council
GP	general practitioner
GUM	genitourinary medicine
HCR-20	Historical, Clinical, Risk Management–20 scale (forensic risk assessment)
HIV	human immunodeficiency virus
HONOS	Health of the Nation Outcome Scales
HPC	history of presenting complaint
HR	heart rate
HTT	home treatment team (crisis team)
IAPT	Improving Access to Psychological Therapies

IM	intramuscular
IMCA	Independent Mental Capacity Advocate
IMHA	Independent Mental Health Advocate
IQ	intelligence quotient
IV	intravenous
LD	learning disability (also known as intellectual disability)
LFT	liver function tests
M-ACE	Mini-Addenbrooke's Cognitive Examination
MAPPA	Multi-Agency Public Protection Arrangements
MCA	Mental Capacity Act
MC&S	microscopy, culture & sensitivity
MHA	Mental Health Act
MHOA	mental health of older adults
MMSE	mini mental state examination
MOCA	Montreal Cognitive Assessment
MRCPsych	Member of the Royal College of Psychiatrists
MRI	magnetic resonance imaging
MSE	mental state examination
MSU	mid-stream urine
NHS	National Health Service
NICE	National Institute for Health & Care Excellence
NMS	neuroleptic malignant syndrome
OCD	obsessive compulsive disorder
od	*omni die* (daily)
OT	occupational therapist
OTC	over-the-counter
PICU	psychiatric intensive care unit
PLN	psychiatric liaison nurse
PMHx	past medical history
PO	*per os* (by mouth)
PPHx	past psychiatric history
PRN	*pro re nata* (as required)
PTSD	post-traumatic stress disorder
qds	*quater die sumendum* (take four times a day)
RC	Responsible Clinician
RCPsych	Royal College of Psychiatrists
RMN	registered mental health nurse
RR	respiratory rate
RT	rapid tranquilisation
SGA	second generation antipsychotic
SHO	senior house officer (older term for Core Trainee)
SHx	social history
SI	serious incident
SMART Goals	Specific, Measurable, Achievable, Realistic, Time-Limited
SMI	severe mental illness
SS	serotonin syndrome
SSRIs	selective serotonin reuptake inhibitors
TCAs	tricyclic antidepressant
tds	*ter die sumendum* (take three times a day)
TFT	thyroid function tests
TTA/Os	to take away/out (discharge medication)
UDS	urine drug screen
U&E	urea and electrolytes
WCC	white cell count
WPBA	workplace-based assessment

About the companion website

This book is accompanied by a companion website:

www.psychiatryice.com

The website includes:

- PowerPoint of all figures from the book for downloading
- PDFs of all tables from the book for downloading
- Videos following the progress of Alex Walker, a young man with psychosis
- Interviews with different MDT members
- Service user interviews
- Interactive patient management problems

PART I
Introduction

CHAPTER 1

Welcome

Sarah Stringer

King's College London, London, England

> Standing on the edge with my patients – abiding with them – means that I must harbour a true awareness that I, too, could lose my child through the play of circumstance over which I have no control. I could lose my home, my financial security, my safety. I could lose my mind. Any of us could.
>
> **Christine Montross**

When you say you're a psychiatrist, people either run towards you or away from you. Some tell their life stories, hoping for wise insights or solutions; others ask if you're about to read their mind, analyse or section them. Medical colleagues may be equally fascinated or unnerved by your new 'powers'. This says lots about the stigma and ignorance in mental health, but doesn't tell you what your new job actually involves. That's where this book comes in.

Breaking the ICE isn't a textbook, but a handbook: rather than focusing on facts and figures, it explains *how* to be a psychiatrist. There are three sections:
- *Introduction:* overview of your role; psychiatry refresher
- *Common Tasks:* day-to-day work, whether based:
  - In a Community Mental Health Team (CMHT)
  - On a psychiatric ward
  - On-call in the general hospital and Emergency Department (ED)
- *Emergencies:* rarer, urgent situations – in the CMHT, Ward, or while on-call.

We recommend you read the Introduction before starting. Then, dip into the relevant *Common Tasks* once you've worked out what your job involves (first 1–2 weeks). It's probably worth skim-reading the *Emergencies* before your first on-call shift, and within your first month.

To prevent repetition:
- The Introduction covers key assessment and management principles – we'll relate back to these throughout the book
- Topics are placed in the setting where you're most likely to manage them *yourself*. With psychosis, for example:
  - *On-call* – assessing someone with a first episode of psychosis (Ch.53)
  - *CMHT* – psychosis management – initial (Ch.23) and longer-term (Ch.24)
  - *Ward* – most psychosis management decisions are made in team ward rounds, but you'll often be alone if and when neuroleptic malignant syndrome strikes (Ch.67)
- Each chapter starts by highlighting related topics
- At the end of chapters, we've addressed *What ifs … ?*
  - Situations where real life doesn't run smoothly
  - Important points if seeing this person elsewhere, e.g. CMHT instead of ED.

Psychiatry: Breaking the ICE – Introductions, Common Tasks and Emergencies for Trainees, First Edition.
Edited by Sarah Stringer, Juliet Hurn and Anna M Burnside.
© 2016 John Wiley & Sons, Ltd. Published 2016 by John Wiley & Sons, Ltd.
Companion Website: www.psychiatryice.com

Nonetheless, you will find areas of repetition, especially if you read the book cover-to-cover. This is because we expect you to dip in and out of chapters, as needed, and we don't know which chapters you'll meet first. Our apologies if this is slightly annoying as you grow more familiar with the structure of assessments, but we'd rather state the obvious than leave you with major gaps. Additionally, since *Breaking the ICE* is aimed at all trainees (including doctors who may have never worked in the UK before), you might find you already know some of the basics – feel free to skip over them (we won't be offended).

Finally, we've gathered the views of patients and colleagues from focus groups and online responses – and peppered the book with them. They include tips, personal experiences of mental illness, and warnings to help you avoid common mistakes. Some are uncomfortable to read – but if you can take them on board, we think they'll change your practice for the better.

Whether you're planning a career in psychiatry or just passing through, we hope you enjoy your placement. And in case you're wondering, you can only read minds after passing the MRCPsych exam.

Reference

Montross, C. (2014) *Falling into the Fire: A Psychiatrist's Encounters with the Mind in Crisis*. Oneworld Publications, London.

CHAPTER 2

Mental health services overview

Christina Barras[1], Rory Conn[2], Laurine Hanna[3], Abigail G Crutchlow[3], and Juliet Hurn[3]

[1] South West London & St George's Mental Health NHS Trust, London, England
[2] Tavistock and Portman NHS Foundation Trust, London, England
[3] South London & Maudsley NHS Foundation Trust, London, England

Ninety per cent of people with mental health problems are treated in primary care; <5% see a psychiatrist and fewer still require admission (Mental Health Foundation, 2007). You'll meet people who've been under psychiatric services for years, but try to remember you *won't* see the many more who've recovered and lead lives without any psychiatric input.

Psychiatric services are provided by mental health Trusts, not the 'acute' Trusts covering physical health. Each Trust organises sub-specialties according to service-lines/directorates, e.g. general adult, older adult. Within these, individual teams or wards provide services across defined geographical areas (Figure 2.1, Table 2.1, Box 2.1).

CMHTs are the bedrock of specialist psychiatric care. Admission is needed when people:

- Can't be properly assessed or treated in the community
- Pose high risks to themselves or others.

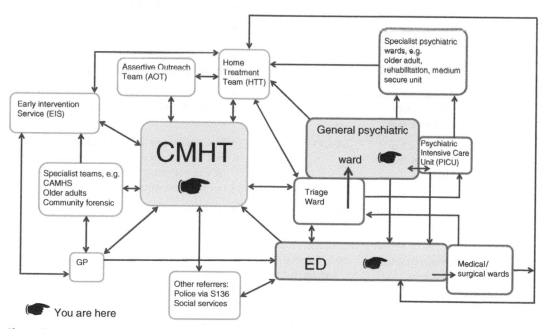

Figure 2.1 Mental health services and flows between them. (*Source*: Image created by Juliet Hurn and Beth Bridewell Mason.)

Psychiatry: Breaking the ICE – Introductions, Common Tasks and Emergencies for Trainees, First Edition.
Edited by Sarah Stringer, Juliet Hurn and Anna M Burnside.
© 2016 John Wiley & Sons, Ltd. Published 2016 by John Wiley & Sons, Ltd.
Companion Website: www.psychiatryice.com

Table 2.1 Common psychiatric services.

Site	Service	Usual criteria	Purpose and features
Community	General adult CMHT	18–65s	• The standard CMHT: works with a range of mental health problems, over a catchment area • Some Trusts subdivide into teams providing: ○ Initial assessment and shorter periods of treatment, e.g. Assessment and Brief Treatment (ABT) ○ Complex/longer-term care, e.g. Continuing Care/Support and Recovery • Other Trusts have diagnosis-based CMHTs
	Home Treatment Team (HTT; crisis team)	Over 18s, on the cusp of admission or discharge	• Alternative to admission (±*gate-keep* by assessing all patients before admission) • Can support early hospital discharge • Home visits – sometimes several times a day – for assessment, support, and medication supervision • Input from days to weeks
	Early Intervention Service (EIS)	Young (e.g. 16/18–35s) with prodrome/first or second episode of psychosis	• Optimises psychosis diagnosis and treatment • Aims to improve prognosis by keeping duration of untreated psychosis (DUP) <3months • Small caseloads (higher levels of support) • Input varies, e.g. 2–5 years • Discharges to GP or longer-term community team
	Assertive Outreach Team (AOT)	18–65s who are hard to engage	• Intensive, long-term support for patients who are chaotic, risky, or prone to frequent/long admissions • Small caseloads • Usually only accepts referrals from CMHTs
	Child and Adolescent Mental Health Service (CAMHS)	<18s	• Close links with paediatrics, schools and GPs • Emphasises family working and psychological interventions
	Mental Health of Older Adults team (MHOA)	>65s/75s	• New onset mental illness in older adults, *or* 'graduates' from general adult services who have become old *and* frail/cognitively impaired • Dementia specialists
	Forensic Community Team	Significant offending *and* mental illness	• Strong links with police, probation, Multi-Agency Public Protection Arrangements (MAPPA), etc • Small caseloads
	Learning Disability (LD) team	LD *and* mental illness/complex needs	• Moderate/severe LD (mild LD usually treated by generic CMHTs) • Strong links with LD Social Services and third sector, e.g. Mencap
	Substance Misuse Service (Addictions/Dual Diagnosis)	Alcohol/drug use	• Assessment and treatment of substance misuse problems, including motivational interviewing (p74), detoxification and substitute prescribing • Increasingly run by third sector/private companies • Comorbid mental illness is often treated by CMHTs

Table 2.1 (*continued*)

Site	Service	Usual criteria	Purpose and features
Inpatient	General adult wards (Acute/Locality)	18–65s	• Inpatient assessment and management • Any diagnosis • Informal (voluntary) or detained • Staff manage the door (but not 'locked') • No time limit on stay
	Triage ('*tree-arj*')	New general adult admissions	• Rapid assessment, identify patients needing: ∘ Prompt treatment ∘ Swift discharge ∘ Transfer to acute ward for longer admission • Daily consultant ward rounds • Higher levels of nursing staff • <1 week stay
	Psychiatric Intensive Care Unit (PICU; '*pee-queue*')	Higher risk, detained patients	• Manages risky behaviours, e.g. aggression, absconding • Locked ward • Higher levels of nursing staff and senior medical cover • May contain s136 suite and seclusion room
	Rehabilitation ('*rehab*')	Complex, severe and enduring mental illness (usually psychosis)	• Long stay, e.g. one to two years • Occupational therapy focus • Thorough preparation and treatment before discharge, often to supported accommodation
	Old Age Wards	See MHOA Team	• Intensive nursing support for physical care and activities of daily living • Specialist dementia care
	Child and Adolescent Wards	All <18s	• Specialist care of children and young people • Usually have a teacher/'school' on site • Some Trusts separate children from adolescents
	Specialist wards	Regional / national catchment area	• Care of particular problems, e.g. personality disorders, challenging behaviour, eating disorders, LD, substance misuse, neuropsychiatry • Patients must usually meet strict admission criteria and have funding agreed beforehand
Acute hospital	Liaison psychiatry/ Psychological Medicine	Patients presenting to ED/medical or surgical wards	• Work closely with physicians to assess and treat people with psychiatric problems in the general hospital • May offer specialist clinics, e.g. self-harm follow-up, medically unexplained symptoms • May have an extended remit under the new Rapid Assessment Interface and Discharge (RAID) model, with a focus on avoiding admissions and reducing length of stay or frequent attendances.

The hospital ($\pm$ ward) is determined by the patient's address, General Practice (GP) or CMHT. Remember this when on-call, as bed managers need these details to check whether someone 'belongs' to your unit, or needs admission elsewhere in the country.

Box 2.1 Recent service provision trends

Community services were traditionally provided by a single, catchment-based CMHT.
- In the 1980s, many CMHTs divided into teams providing shorter and longer-term care, e.g. ABT versus Continuing Care
- *Modernisation teams* were developed in the 1990s (AOT, HTT, EIS)
  - These were disbanded in some areas, due to cost or an inconclusive evidence-base
- Some Trusts now provide diagnosis-led services, often posing tricky boundary problems, e.g. personality disorders, psychosis
- Great variety across the country, especially:
  - Specialist service provision
  - Inpatient service configuration, e.g. triage wards; unisex/mixed wards.

Whatever your set-up, try to understand the flow between services and teams, and remember that good communication across these boundaries is essential. Service interfaces are hot-spots for problems and negative patient experiences, e.g. meeting new staff, re-telling stories. The separation of mental health and acute Trusts widens the gap between physical and mental health, causing difficulties – as you'll see if trying to access medical notes on 'mental health' patients when on-call.

Further reading

Mental Health Foundation (2007) *The Fundamental Facts: The Latest Facts and Figures on Mental Health*. Sainsbury Centre for Mental Health, pp. 45–46.
Department of Health (2011) *No Health Without Mental Health – a cross-government mental health outcomes strategy for people of all ages*. HM Government, London.

CHAPTER 3

Your team

Christina Barras[1], Rory Conn[2], Laurine Hanna[3], and Abigail G Crutchlow[3]

[1] South West London & St George's, Mental Health NHS Trust, London, England
[2] Tavistock and Portman NHS Foundation Trust, London, England
[3] South London & Maudsley NHS Foundation Trust, London, England

> **TIP:** Become a part of your team. Too many trainees are distant figures who don't involve themselves closely with their nursing and other colleagues. I'm always worried when I phone a ward and they don't know their junior doctor's name.
>
> **Greg Shields, CT3**

Teams are generally less hierarchical than in other areas of medicine, taking a truly multidisciplinary approach, and rarely worshipping doctors. Many colleagues are extremely experienced – so discuss management with them, particularly when they know patients well.

In any team, there may be multiple consultants responsible for patient care; they're usually keen to be contacted with questions or concerns. One named consultant will provide your weekly clinical supervision. You may also have:

- Middle grade doctors, e.g. specialty/higher trainees ('registrars'), staff grades or associate specialists. They lead in the consultant's absence and are usually section 12 approved, so can undertake Mental Health Act (MHA) assessments (but *can't* approve s17 leave or discharge detained patients).
- Junior doctors, e.g. foundation trainees, core trainees (CTs), GP trainees.

Ask what your colleagues do, how they can help, and what they expect from you. Friendly professional relationships improve patient care, so proactively offer support, joint assessments and face-to-face handovers whenever possible. Courtesy is essential: medicine is a small world, and psychiatry even smaller. Respectful practice will do more for your reputation than playing the "Doctor card":

- It should be obvious, but please, sorry and thank you are expected basics
- Thanking colleagues is positively reinforcing (p76)
- When grabbing yourself a cup of tea/coffee, ask if anyone else wants one.

> **TIP:** The best trainees talk to the cleaners, porters and healthcare assistants, not just the 'important' people like consultants. We all notice that.
>
> **Martin Baggaley, Medical Director**

Psychiatry: Breaking the ICE – Introductions, Common Tasks and Emergencies for Trainees, First Edition.
Edited by Sarah Stringer, Juliet Hurn and Anna M Burnside.
© 2016 John Wiley & Sons, Ltd. Published 2016 by John Wiley & Sons, Ltd.
Companion Website: www.psychiatryice.com

Table 3.1 Team members (C = CMHT; W = ward).

Title	C	W	Role/responsibilities
Team manager	✓		• Usually nurse/social worker • Overall service responsibility • Line manages and supervises all care co-ordinators • Service practicalities e.g. referrals, complaints, developing care pathways, implementing and reviewing service targets • Very experienced
Ward manager		✓	• Inpatient team manager, but usually a nurse and only supervises nurses
Care coordinator (CC)	✓		• Usually nurses/social workers; sometimes OTs, psychologists • Coordinate care for their caseload (20–30+ patients), including home/hospital visits • Manage Care Programme Approach (CPA) process (Ch 19) • ±Assess new patients • ±Specialist training, e.g. psychotherapies, substance misuse
Registered Mental Health Nurse (RMN)	✓		• *Community Psychiatric Nurses* (CPNs) • Care-coordinate • Administer medication/depots
		✓	• Administer medication, spend therapeutic time with patients, monitor mental states and risk • Highly experienced in managing psychiatric emergencies • *Emergency Response Team* (ERT) = nurses who attend psychiatric or medical emergencies across the unit
Social worker	✓	✓	• May care-coordinate (CMHTs) • Specialist assessment and management of social needs • Make up the majority of *Approved Mental Health Professionals (AMHPs):* experts on mental health law who undertake MHA assessments
Occupational Therapist (OT)	✓	✓	• Assess level of function: activities of daily living (ADLs), cognitive and social abilities • Support functional and occupational skills development
		✓	• Ward OTs run activity groups and outings to help with recovery • *Activity coordinators* may or may not be trained OTs (if not, they'll focus on activities and outings)
Clinical psychologist	✓	✓	• Provide psychotherapy (group/1:1) e.g. cognitive behavioural therapy (CBT), family therapy, cognitive analytic therapy • Run groups, e.g. mindfulness, self-esteem, recovery • Specialist assessments ± management, e.g. challenging behaviour, neuropsychiatric testing • Facilitate team reflection and support with difficult dynamics
Pharmacist	✓	✓	• Review drug charts • Pharmacological advice • May offer clinics or appointments for patients to discuss medication

Table 3.1 (*continued*)

Title	C	W	Role/responsibilities
Support worker/ healthcare assistant (HCAs)	✓	✓	• Support patient care, e.g. facilitate attendance at appointments; escort patients on leave, complete observations on wards • Not qualified nurses, but often have useful insights and sometimes years of experience.
Vocational worker	✓	✓	• Advice and support on education and employment, e.g. help getting into training; support at work/college
Benefits advisor	✓	✓	• Financial advice, e.g. debt management, benefits
Advocates	✓	✓	• Advocate for patients' needs/rights (p84) • Varied focus, e.g. Black and Minority Ethnic patients, learning disabilities • *Independent Mental Health Advocate (IMHA)*: explain and help people exercise their rights under the MHA; support patients' involvement in care planning • *Independent Mental Capacity Advocate (IMCA)*: advocate for patients who lack capacity and don't have carers to advocate around best interest decisions
Administrative staff	✓	✓	• *Administrators* facilitate correspondence, diary/appointment management, meeting minutes • May support wider team functions e.g. CPA management, data entry
	✓		• *Receptionists* manage visitors to team base • Vital supportive role to waiting patients/carers
		✓	• *Ward clerks* keep the ward running; help you wrestle dodgy printers and fax machines • More informal relationship with patients – can provide helpful insights
Other staff	✓	✓	• Remember you still have access to all the MDT staff you had as a medic, e.g. physios, chiropodists, Speech and Language Therapists (SALT)

TIP: When a colleague asks for advice/support, ask, "What do *you* want to do?" Most of the time, it's the same thing you'd have done. Sometimes they've a much better idea than you. *Occasionally* you'll change their plans ... but this won't make you appear controlling.

TIP: We're privileged to have the best job: of listening to people tell us stories. It can be as joyful and fulfilling as it can be frustrating, stressful and tiring. Many of your colleagues will be devoted, skilled and funny. You can have fun. This is extremely important, and easy to forget.

Elizabeth Venables, Consultant Psychiatrist

TIP: Mental health difficulties can cause or exacerbate underlying communication difficulties. SALT can assess and provide advice, exercises, tools, strategies to improve communication. Remember to refer to us!

Anna Volkmer, SALT

TIP: Socialising with colleagues can help understand them, particularly when you're confused by their decisions. I've always found my sense of integration and wellbeing in a team is enhanced when there's some sort of social occasion early in the placement. Developing a sense of bonding seems a more rapid and healthy process outside the formal structures of hierarchy.

Bradley Hillier, Forensic ST6

CHAPTER 4

Your role

Christina Barras[1], Rory Conn[2], Laurine Hanna[3], and Abigail G Crutchlow[3]

[1] South West London & St George's Mental Health NHS Trust, London, England
[2] Tavistock and Portman NHS Foundation Trust, London, England
[3] South London & Maudsley NHS Foundation Trust, London, England

---

PATIENT VIEW:

So what you want is a good listener, someone who understands the problems, the wider implications for the patient and their family in society. But somebody who's also able to pick up physical problems. I'd want to see someone who'd know if my symptoms were due to a brain tumour. I'd want to see someone who could prevent a suicide by being able to prescribe. What you're looking for is someone who's a good diagnostician, who is human.

'Jennifer'

General

Coming from medicine or surgery, psychiatry can be something of a culture shock. In CMHTs or psychiatric units, you'll often be hailed as the most senior medic in the building: even consultants may defer to your (more recent) expertise! The situation reverses when on-call in ED, with medics viewing you as the most senior *psychiatric* opinion in the hospital. Both situations can feel daunting and somewhat absurd. Stay grounded. You're a newbie with contacts: you *won't* have all the answers, but you can find them using your 'membership' of both medical and psychiatric teams.

As you've seen, you're working with many highly specialist non-medics, whose skills overlap or overshadow yours. It helps to consider how you fit in.

Firstly, you're a medically trained doctor, so well placed to bridge the perceived gap between medical and psychological issues. Good mental health is a complex blend of biological, psychological and social factors, and management plans should reflect *all* these issues. Your medical training will save lives, improve the quality of lives, prevent iatrogenic harm, and decrease team anxiety that 'something organic is being missed'. So don't forget or disown your medical training; it's an essential part of your identity *and* holistic patient care.

In recognising the importance of your medical background, you must also recognise its limitations. Although you've learned *some* social and psychological principles and skills, you're still a beginner, compared with colleagues. The best psychiatrists don't hide behind medications and biology, but use their training to develop a varied repertoire of psychosocial approaches and tools. If you do this:
- Colleagues and patients will see you as *useful* – not 'just' a prescription service
- Medics will be a little in awe of you, as you step in to manage hairy situations with skills, not pills (it looks a bit like magic).

Psychiatry: Breaking the ICE – Introductions, Common Tasks and Emergencies for Trainees, First Edition.
Edited by Sarah Stringer, Juliet Hurn and Anna M Burnside.
© 2016 John Wiley & Sons, Ltd. Published 2016 by John Wiley & Sons, Ltd.
Companion Website: www.psychiatryice.com

Finally, psychiatrists are also leaders. Consultants are ultimately responsible for managing risk and drawing together the team's skills as safe, individualised, holistic care. In your consultant's absence, colleagues may seek your advice, especially when things become risky or complicated. Learn from your consultant and assume more leadership responsibilities as you progress. Part of your leadership role is through role modelling – particularly when on-call in the general hospital. By demonstrating patience, compassion and expert communication skills, you can fight stigma and improve the way people with mental health problems are treated in general hospitals. If medical staff like and respect you, they'll follow your example.

> **TIP:** When with a patient, you're in different roles, but try to keep this to the minimum difference needed *to do the job well*. You're essentially engaged in a human conversation, and need to preserve humanity.
>
> Duncan Doyle, AMHP

Specifics

Your first placement is normally a general adult ward or CMHT. If you don't have on-call duties, try to shadow on-call psychiatrists, to understand what's expected out-of-hours. Wherever you are, your role involves:
- Assessing
  - New referrals (ward: clerking admissions)
  - Mental states
  - Physical health
  - Risk
- Attending and documenting team meetings (ward: ward rounds)
- Presenting findings to your team
- Liaising with CCs, referrers, carers, medics, housing officers, etc
- Prescribing and reviewing medications
- Developing/facilitating management plans
- Admin:
  - Writing prescriptions/drug charts
  - Letters to GPs (CMHT review letters; ward discharge summaries)
  - Referrals to medical specialists, other teams, e.g. HTT
  - Reports, e.g. for solicitors, tribunals, benefits agencies.

> **TIP:** A good relationship with the administrator is key to a smooth-running post. Check the administrative tasks you must complete for all patients and don't make administrators chase you for paperwork.

There are some tasks specific to your job:
- CMHT:
  - Outpatient clinics (Ch.18)
  - Home visits (Ch.20)
- Ward:
  - Assessing suitability for leave or discharge (p216–217)
  - Seclusion reviews (Ch.39)

- ○ Co-facilitating ward groups, e.g. OT, mindfulness
- ○ Providing duty doctor cover
- On-call:
  - ○ Assessment and initial management in the time-pressured ED environment
  - ○ Advising medical staff on psychiatric management
  - ○ Overseeing transfers between the general hospital and psychiatric unit.

Your other key role is to learn – through work itself, clinical supervision, and regular, structured teaching. Lectures, case presentations, journal clubs and clinical skills training will inform your day-to-day practice and help with exam preparation.

PATIENT VIEW:

I know doctors must be detached, but some are so very *cold*. They seem to not care and have no regard for my privacy when openly and loudly discussing my problems with others. I've also seen some doctors who are fantastic: warm and friendly in their words and body language; who seem to genuinely care and want to help however possible. I have also found nurses in hospitals to be outstanding. They are friendly, non-judgmental and are okay to sit with you and hold your hand and listen if you get upset.

'Rose'

CHAPTER 5

Getting started

Mujtaba Husain[1], Christina Barras[2], Rory Conn[3], and Laurine Hanna[1]

[1] South London & Maudsley NHS Foundation Trust, London, England
[2] South West London & St George's Mental Health NHS Trust, London, England
[3] Tavistock and Portman NHS Foundation Trust, London, England

Speak to your predecessor before starting, for basic information about the job, including your day-to-day work and any tips. Organise a clinical handover (face-to-face/telephone/list of outstanding jobs) and agree where they'll leave any keys or swipe-cards.

Your first day or two will probably be an induction whirlwind, covering everything from pharmacy procedures and psychiatry refreshers to IT access. Make sure you know how to:

- Access
  - Patient records
  - Trust protocols
  - Patient information leaflets (PILs)
- Order and check medical investigations
- Get help in an emergency:
  - Psychiatric e.g. Emergency Response Team (ERT)
  - Medical, e.g. call 999; 2222 for crash team/ERT
- Contact your clinical and educational supervisors.

TIP: Swap contact details with other trainees at induction. It's easy to feel isolated if only crossing paths at teaching and handovers – especially when working in CMHTs. Regular lunches solve more than hunger.

TIP: Make sure you do all the mandatory training in the first week to avoid disruptions.

Anoop Saraf, Consultant Psychiatrist

After induction you'll have your first day in the CMHT or ward. A senior colleague should give you a tour, covering:

- Staff names (take notes)
- Door codes, keys, swipe-cards
- Location and use of alarms
- Your computer/room
- Timings: team handovers, team meetings/ward rounds
- Where to get lunch and take breaks.

Psychiatry: Breaking the ICE – Introductions, Common Tasks and Emergencies for Trainees, First Edition.
Edited by Sarah Stringer, Juliet Hurn and Anna M Burnside.
© 2016 John Wiley & Sons, Ltd. Published 2016 by John Wiley & Sons, Ltd.
Companion Website: www.psychiatryice.com

Build and carry a contact list of useful phone numbers and e-mail addresses (Appendix F). Never share or document colleagues' mobile numbers without checking – they may be personal rather than work numbers. Meet with teammates early on, to discuss their role and caseload (CMHT) or named patients (ward).

Meet your consultant in the first week to discuss:
- How to contact them (exchange phone numbers)
  - Who to contact if they're unavailable
- Your timetable
- Your day-to-day duties in the team
- Supervision arrangements
- An overview of your Trust's organisation and how your team fits in

TIP: At first meeting, ask your consultant: "What are your expectations of an SHO? What is/isn't acceptable? What do/don't you like trainees saying or doing?"

Piers Newman, Psychotherapist

Pin a copy of your weekly timetable and bleep/telephone number in the team or nursing office so colleagues know when you're around and how to contact you. Warn them of protected teaching and leave, so they can arrange cover or work around these.

TIP: The RCPsych PILs can be used as a free Smartphone application

CMHT extras

In the absence of daily handovers, you risk becoming the Invisible Doctor, especially if you have your own office.
- Start the habit of a morning cup of tea and informal catch-up with teammates to check any concerns, write prescriptions or book appointments
- If you have an office, leave your door open, unless needing privacy/silence
- If using an electronic diary, consider giving the administrator, team leader and consultant 'read access'. This ensures they know what you're up to, and can cancel appointments if you're off sick.

Clinics (Ch.18) and home visits (Ch.20) may be new experiences. Check how teammates will book you for these, and remember to factor journey times into your diary.

Find out when the CMHT closes (usually 5pm) and how/when to set alarms or lock up if last out. If you *have* to leave by 5 pm, all the better for your time management skills!

Ward extras

Each morning, take a handover from the nurse in charge. Check specifically for:
- New or planned admissions
- Morning blood tests
- People needing psychiatric, physical or medication reviews.

You can then plan your work around any fixed commitments. Consider offering a slot each week for patients to book *themselves* in to discuss any worries.

You'll usually share your ward with another trainee, and life's much easier when you look after each other, e.g. with cross-cover.

TIP: Hiding in the office may be an effective way to keep on top of paperwork, but making time regularly in your day to engage with patients and ward staff will pay greater dividends. It helps you build alliances with hard-to-reach patients; work more coherently within the multidisciplinary team; more accurately monitor people's responses to treatments; and reduce anxiety in staff and patients.

Marcella Fok, ST5

On-call extras

See Ch.50 to plan your first on-call shift.

CHAPTER 6

Safety and verbal de-escalation

Sarah Stringer

King's College London, London, England

TIP: Always trust the little voice in your head.

Gemma Hopkins, ST5

Safety

People with mental health problems are more often *victims* than perpetrators of violence. Nonetheless, sensible precautions reduce your risk of harm.
- Avoid anything around your neck that could be grabbed, e.g. ties, stethoscopes
- Check where alarms are and how they work ± carry a personal alarm
- Before assessing anyone:
  - Check history of aggression (staff and notes)
  - Consider taking a teammate – never be embarrassed to ask
  - Avoid remote meeting rooms/meeting out-of-hours
  - Ensure colleagues know where you are and can easily observe you, e.g. via a viewing window
  - Ask a *specific* person to check on you
  - Sit nearest the door and within reach of an alarm
- End the interview if:
  - You *feel* unsafe for any reason. Listen to your 'gut' feeling; don't be a hero.
  - There are signs of arousal which may precede aggression (Figure 6.1)
    - Restlessness, standing, pacing, erratic movements
    - Entering personal space/blocking exits
    - Standing over/'squaring up' to staff
    - Tense/twitching muscles, clenched fists
    - Fast breathing, dilated pupils, sweating
    - Staring *or* avoidant eye contact
    - Face: angry, reddening or blanching
    - Anger, irritability *or* fear
    - Louder speech, shouting, swearing, insults, sarcasm *or* going silent
    - Verbal threats, e.g. *I'm going to hit you!/You'll wish you hadn't done that!*
    - Shows of strength or violence, e.g. punching walls, banging fist on table
    - Behaviours known to precede *previous* violent outbursts.

Psychiatry: Breaking the ICE – Introductions, Common Tasks and Emergencies for Trainees, First Edition.
Edited by Sarah Stringer, Juliet Hurn and Anna M Burnside.
© 2016 John Wiley & Sons, Ltd. Published 2016 by John Wiley & Sons, Ltd.
Companion Website: www.psychiatryice.com

Community posts are more 'normalised' environments, so it's easy to overlook risks. Read the lone working protocol, always sign in and out, and don't book appointments after the CMHT closes. Activated alarms may sound throughout the building – check who attends (usually everyone) and how to identify the source.

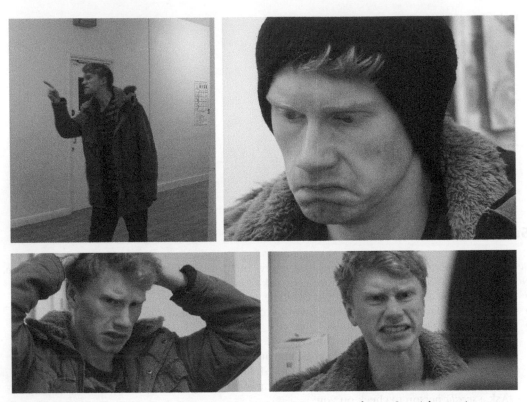

Figure 6.1 Signs of arousal. (*Source*: Photographs by Zachary J Ferguson and actor Sam Adamson.)

Verbal De-escalation

TIP: At a psychiatric emergency, the first procedure is to check your own mental status.

Samuel Shem, *Mount Misery*

Verbal de-escalation is the skill of talking someone down. You'll learn it in mandatory 'breakaway' training, but before using it, try to observe experienced colleagues in action (and watch Video 4). Never deal with aggression alone – get out or get help. If the staff present can't handle the situation, delegate someone to call the ERT or police.

In fraught situations, only one person should talk – preferably someone who already has a good relationship with the patient. If there isn't an obvious leader, people may look to you. Ensure colleagues remain attentive and concerned throughout: their behaviour or conversation can distract and dangerously undermine a de-escalation attempt.

The aims of de-escalation are to:
- Keep everyone safe, e.g.
  - Stall for time while awaiting back-up
  - Distract from violent behaviour
- Help the person:
  - Manage their emotions and regain control
  - Problem-solve
- Avoid restraint or rapid tranquilisation. These only reinforce the idea that action – not discussion – solves problems
- Assess mental state and gain further history.

Approach

PATIENT VIEW:

If you've got an animal who's frightened, and you want to get them to feel relaxed around you and you go in with a club and say, "Come here!" you're going to scare it and make it react to your aggression. You need to be sensitive and gentle to get a sensitive response.

'Shiloh'

Match body language to your stated wish to help, otherwise the person won't trust you.
- Hand someone your bleep/mobile to prevent distractions
- No sudden moves
- Increase personal space
  - >2 arm-lengths; out of punching/kicking range
  - If the patient warns you to back off, obey
- Stand at an angle: less threatening and decreases your size as a target
- Legs: slightly bent, one foot behind you – easier to step back if they lunge
- Hands:
  - Visible, palms out – showing you're not hiding a weapon
  - Below waist height – less threatening ± can block kicks
  - Don't point at the person
- Eye contact: available, but not constant staring
- Face: concerned and calm
- Voice: soft, clear, interested and gentle (but *not* patronizing)
- Stay polite and respectful, even when firmly setting boundaries
- Don't provoke, challenge or insult the patient. Humour is risky.
- Don't be defensive: this isn't about you or your department, even if it seems to be.
- *If* you can both sit down, try to – it's a less confrontational position

Follow the steps in Table 6.1 and aim to create the loop in Figure 6.3.

If verbal de-escalation doesn't work, get out and get help (Ch.74)

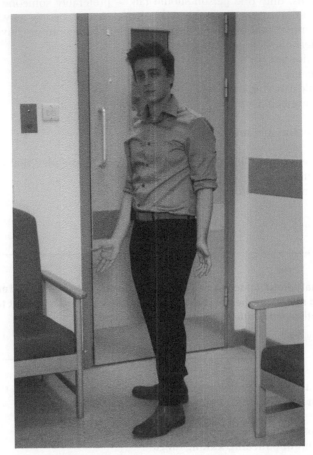

Figure 6.2 Non-confrontational engagement. (*Source*: Photograph and modelling by Zachary J Ferguson.)

Table 6.1 De-escalation steps.

Step	Details/*examples*
1. Introduction	*Hello Harry, I'm Dr X. I want to keep everyone here safe. The staff are worried about you. Can you tell me what's wrong?*
2. Allow time to vent	Let them get things off their chest
3. Be concise and repetitive	Repeat simple, short messages Give time to process and respond to messages
4. Identify needs	*What do you need at the moment? I want to help you, if possible* ± *If we can't sort it out today, at least we can work out the next steps*
5. Identify feelings	If they don't know or aren't clear about their needs, suggest things based on what you know or can read from their body language, e.g. *Are you angry about something?*
6. Listen carefully	Show active listening Empathise Summarise key points, e.g. • *Can I check I've got it right? You're hungry and tired and need help with housing.*

Table 6.1 (*continued*)

Step	Details/*examples*
7. Agree whenever possible	This lessens confrontation. You can agree with different things, e.g.
	• *You* have *waited a long time* (facts)
	• *Waiting's very frustrating, especially when you're in pain* (feelings)
	• *I believe everyone should be seen as quickly as possible* (principles)
	• *I bet most people would be upset if they'd waited that long* (the odds)
	If it's impossible to agree, agree to disagree and move on
8. Set clear boundaries	Do this calmly but assertively, without threats, e.g.
	• *It's hard for me to concentrate when you're shouting* ($\pm$ *because you're scaring me*).
	• *I need you to stop shouting, so I can help you out*
9. Offer choices	The patient may see their only choices as fight or flight
	Offer realistic alternatives which you can provide quickly, e.g. somewhere quiet to talk, refreshments, medication to relax them
	Even when medication's necessary, always offer tablets before injections.
10. Offer hope	Be clear that you believe things *will* get easier, and that your plan will help

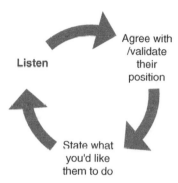

Figure 6.3 Verbal de-escalation 'loop' of conversation.

Debrief

Afterwards, meet with staff:
• Is everyone OK?
• What went well?
• What could have been done better?
• What can be learned, e.g. early warning signs, triggers?
• Plan to prevent/manage future outbursts.

Debrief with the patient, once calmer:
• Let them explain how they were and *are* feeling
• Explain why you needed to do what you did
• Suggest ways to prevent future outbursts, e.g. asking staff for help, requesting a time out/PRN sedative medication
• Ask how they'd like to be managed if this situation happened again.

PATIENT VIEW:

There were times I was attacking people. It wasn't because I am some nasty person, but I genuinely thought everyone was about to attack me. I heard them talking about me: how bad I was, how I should be in prison ... I was picking up danger from everywhere. I had fear from every single person, like they were snipers. Plus, I couldn't escape from the wards. Fight or flight.

'Marcus'

TIP: When patients come across as angry or aggressive, it's often because they're afraid or anxious. The same is also true of hostile colleagues – they may feel they're not coping or out of their depth. Empathy and a willingness to listen are often effective remedies.

David McLaughlan, CT3

Further reading

Richmond, J.S., Berlin, J.S., Fishkind, A.B. *et al.* (2012) Verbal de-escalation of the agitated patient: Consensus Statement of the American Association for Emergency Psychiatry Project BETA De-escalation Workgroup. *The Western Journal of Emergency Medicine*, **13** (1), 17–25.

CHAPTER 7

Boundaries, time management and burnout

Sarah Stringer[1], Christina Barras[2], Rory Conn[3], and Laurine Hanna[4]

[1] *King's College London, London, England*
[2] *South West London & St George's Mental Health NHS Trust, London, England*
[3] *Tavistock and Portman NHS Foundation Trust, London, England*
[4] *South London & Maudsley NHS Foundation Trust, London, England*

> **TIP:** You can say *no* to interactions you think are unacceptable. You need a firm but kind manner, and a calm sense of your own authority. You'll also need the support of colleagues and supervision to help arrive at this sense of authority and ability to exercise this kindly. Reflect on 'where you're at' in the process of establishing your own authority in general relationships: are you always being walked over? Can you be firm without being aggressive? This is a journey for the self, which is linked to – but not the same as – authority as a psychiatrist.
>
> Duncan Mclean, Consultant Psychotherapist

Boundaries

Boundaries separate your professional and personal identity, protecting you and your patient. They say lots about the kind of doctor you are, and will be interpreted in different ways by patients. It's hard to get the balance between being cold and aloof *or* overfamiliar and inappropriate. The trick is being:

- Human, but professional
- Hard-working, but realistic
- Helpful, but not paternalistic
- Open, honest and genuine, whilst protecting things which are personal to you
- Friendly, but not taking over the role of 'friend' from a patient's own social network.

Remember:

- Patients *will* be curious about you
- All your resources are finite, e.g. energy, time, compassion
- Your first year in psychiatry creates patterns which are hard to reverse later.

Negotiating relationships with your patients can be difficult and one size doesn't fit all. Some patients may want to be your friend or even your partner, but to help them, you must ensure they can see you as their doctor. You'll need to work out the subtleties around your own style, but the tips in Table 7.1 may help.

Table 7.1 Guidance on boundaries.

Issue	Advice
Boundaries	• Discuss boundaries in supervision • Make boundaries explicit as needed, e.g. how or when people can contact you; appropriate/ inappropriate behaviour • Address the subtle erosion of boundaries, e.g. appointments over-running; frequent, lengthy telephone calls between appointments • When asking someone to stop doing something, explain *what* they're doing, *why* they must stop, and *what* will happen if they continue • Don't make your personal number available to patients; think carefully before passing your work number/e-mail to patients • It's never OK to date or have sex with a patient/carer, no matter how minor or distant your clinical role
Attitude	• Respect your patients *and* yourself: no-one should be walking over anyone • Treat people equally. It's not fair to spend hours with a 'favourite' while avoiding patients you dislike. • Find a role model or mentor, preferably someone who isn't burned-out or being investigated by the GMC! Seek advice and follow their example.
Secrecy	• Never ask patients to keep secrets. If *asked* to keep a secret, explain confidentiality limitations • Never do anything with a patient that you'd hide from your team

Touch	• Can be comforting *or* misunderstood/inappropriate
	• Don't do it if:
	  ◦ It makes either of you uncomfortable or excited
	  ◦ You'd stop – or have to explain yourself – if someone walked in

Reliability and expectations	• Do what you say you'll do • Don't offer anything if you doubt you can do it • Remember that your behaviour sets up expectations ◦ When you leave, it's hard for staff and patients if you've spent months being a 'super-human' doctor • Don't play into idealisation, e.g. being a 'perfect' doctor. Be wary whenever anyone says you're the *only* person who's ever listened, understood, cared or helped them – it's only a matter of time before you'll fall from this pedestal to join the 'denigrated' majority. • Be honest about your mistakes, doubts and failings

Patients may ask you personal questions, but what you share is up to you: you've a right to privacy. Before disclosing personal information, ask yourself:

• *Why do they want to know?*
• *Do I want to tell? Why?*
• *Will it help them?*
• *Could this harm them or me?*
• *Am I happy for* every *patient/colleague to know this about me?* (Patients owe you no duty of confidentiality).

Remember that defensiveness only makes you more tantalising! So, if a patient asks whether you're married, you can:

• Answer *yes/no* (but expect further questions)

- Deflect with a smile or an earnest return to topic
  - *We're here to talk about you*
- Explore their reasons, e.g.
  - *I can answer that, but I wonder why you wanted to know*
  - *It sounds important for you to know. I wonder what you were thinking about when you asked that question?*
- Firmly state boundaries, e.g.
  - *I'm not going to talk about my personal life.*

> **TIP:** Think about what you want to reveal to patients *and* staff... If *nothing*, that reveals an awful lot about you.
>
> Piers Newman, RMN and Psychotherapist

> **TIP:** Patients can have a way of making you feel angry, sad, excessively worried about them, or even have sexual feelings towards them. To experience these feelings is normal; to act on them is highly dangerous. If you have strong feelings of any sort towards your patients talk to your supervisor and get the necessary support, through psychotherapeutic supervision, Balint groups, etc. Make sure you're safe, e.g. consider transferring their care to someone else, or taking a chaperone.
>
> Daniel Harwood, Old Age Consultant

Time management

Without good time management, you'll feel constantly pressurised and rushed, risking rash decisions. Manage expectations by clarifying your timetable, e.g. Table 7.2. Though wonderful to review patients, 9am–5pm, every day, it's not possible – you must make space to:
- Breathe and reflect
- Eat, drink, use the toilet
- Complete admin (two sessions/week): if you don't write up the patients you've seen, legally you *haven't* seen them
- Be on-call, e.g. stop seeing patients by 4pm if you need to take the bleep at a different site for 5pm
- Take leave.

Once colleagues understand your timetable, they'll work within it, and you'll have fewer issues with patients being 'dropped' into your lunch break. Also, once you've gained a sense of control, it's easier to be flexible. Flexibly responding to crises does wonders for your reputation, and the team will *appreciate* you making exceptions, rather than taking you for granted.

Table 7.2 Sample CMHT timetable.

	Monday	Tuesday	Wednesday	Thursday	Friday
AM	Outpatient clinic	Team meeting	Protected teaching	Clinical supervision New patient assessment	Outpatient clinic
NOON	Lunch	Lunch	Lunch	Lunch	Lunch
PM	Home visits	Emergency reviews / Admin	Protected teaching	Home visits	Admin

> **TIP:** Keep a *Not To Do Folder* of everything you say *no* to. Be proud of it, and when feeling stressed, look inside and notice how much worse things would be if you'd said *yes*...

Prioritize tasks to use your time most effectively. When *fraught*, ask yourself:

- *Is this urgent?* (If so, do it now)
- *Is this a rate-limiting step?* (If so, do it soon)
- *Must this be done perfectly?* (If not, aim for 80%)
- *Am I the only one who can do this?* (If not, consider delegating/sharing)
- *Will this cause problems if left until tomorrow?* (If not, it can wait).

However, remember you'll save time by completing letters or notes the same day you see patients. They take ages if they build up, as you'll struggle to remember what was said.

Finally, take a look at Figure 7.1:

- What do you notice about the innermost circle, compared with the outermost circle?
- Which circle do you think people worry about most?

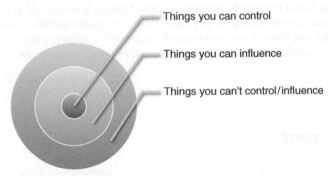

Figure 7.1 Circles of concern/influence. (*Source*: Adapted from Covey 2004.)

There are few things you can *control*: your own thoughts, behaviours and immediate environment. However, they're worth focusing on, as you *can* change them, e.g. revising for your MRCPsych.

Put *some* time into the things you can *influence* (e.g. people, policies) whilst recognising your limitations, e.g. you can only *advise* your stressed colleague to knuckle down for the exam.

Finally, there are things you *can't control or influence*. When stressed, it's tempting to focus on these, wasting time and energy without changing anything. Recognising they're beyond your control gives you permission to stop worrying about them, e.g. brand new questions in the exam which redefine 'clinical relevance'.

Focus on the things you can change. If you find this approach helpful, share it with patients.

Burnout

> **TIP:** Mental illness is disturbing, and it's normal and healthy for a psychiatrist to feel disturbed by their patients. The point is not to become immune to this disturbance, but rather to remain disturbed yet endeavour to do your job properly at the same time.
>
> Marcella Fok, ST5

We *all* risk burnout if we don't look after ourselves. Signs include:

- Feeling drained, unmotivated, irritable, tearful, pessimistic or disinterested
- Struggling to connect with people

- Losing compassion or patience
- A sense of dread at the thought of work
- Physical health problems.

There's obvious crossover with depression, but burnout isn't easily treated – it's a sign that you've drained yourself dry, and can be irreversible. Fortunately, you can spot and prevent patterns which lead to burnout:

- Work invades your home, e.g. taking work home, being contacted when off-duty by staff or patients
- You start early, stay late, or never have a lunch break. This *isn't* evidence of your dedication, but poor time management/excessive workloads.
- You must do everything 'perfectly' (be *good enough*; 100% isn't realistic 100% of the time)
- You say *yes* to everything.

Take holidays and when you're off work, be *off* work: turn off your work mobile; set an out-of-office message and don't check work e-mails. Learn to say *no*. If your workload's unmanageable, discuss it in supervision, finding ways to delegate, share tasks and manage time more effectively. If your consultant can't help, talk to your Training Programme Director about the post. See Resources for professional support.

> **TIP:** You're the worst people for looking after yourselves! You can best support me by going home when you're unwell, so I don't have to worry about you. You're needed for your capacity to work, not simply your presence.
>
> **Piers Newman, Family Therapist**

> **TIP:** An antidote to most things, for most people, is to get outside and dig a hole, or plant a tree, or ride a horse, or walk your dog, or stir your compost bin, etc.
>
> **Elizabeth Venables, Consultant**

> **PATIENT VIEW:**
>
> We bring a lot of bad stuff, and not being rude to anyone, we dump it on you. You have to carry this around, so for your own mental health, go and talk to someone. Simply to be told, it's not you, it's your patient, your patient is transferring stuff onto you. If you can't see a more senior psychiatrist or psychologist, use each other. You're at the same level, you have similar problems, go and talk to each other. Treat each other as patients.
>
> **'Tolu'**

> **TIP:** Doctors have one of the highest rates of mental health and substance misuse problems of any professional group, particularly psychiatrists, anaesthetists and GPs. Although it can seem like the potential end of a career, doctors should know that this is increasingly being viewed as a health issue and addressed compassionately and supportively by the Royal College, BMA and GMC. Lots of Trusts have pastoral care services and run staff health and wellbeing groups. I'd encourage people to see what's available locally, and not be deterred if this is presented as 'spiritual'.
>
> **Bradley Hillier, Forensic ST5**

TIP: Psychiatry carries a different *quality* of stress to the rest of medicine. Expect debate, eclecticism and awkward reconciliation. There can be a feeling of *more questions than answers*, which can be slightly overwhelming at times. So it's important to try and develop some comfort in dealing with often profound uncertainty.

Liam Gilgar, CT2

Further reading

Royal College of Psychiatrists (2013) CR180 Vulnerable patients, safe doctors: good practice in our clinical relationships, 2nd edn, Royal College of Psychiatrists, London.

Covey, S.R. (2004) *The 7 Habits of Highly Effective People*, Simon and Schuster, London.

Useful resources, including mindfulness and compassion focused therapy:
  ○ www.psychology.tools/

Balint group information:
  ○ www.balint.co.uk

The British Medical Association's confidential burnout questionnaire:
  ○ https://web2.bma.org.uk/drs4drsburn.nsf/quest?OpenForm

Doctor support services:

BMA Doctors for Doctors 08459 200 169

British Doctors and Dentists Group (dependency problems) 07792 819966

Family Support Group 07818 475825

Doctors Support line 0844 395 3010 (evening telephone service)

MEDNET (covers London and KSS Deaneries) 0208 938 2411

Practitioner Health Programme (doctors in London, Brighton, Hove and KSS): www.php.nhs.uk

Sick Doctors Trust (dependency problems) 03704 445163

CHAPTER 8

Psychiatric assessment

Sarah Stringer[1], Mujtaba Husain[2], Penelope Brown[2], and Sean Cross[2]

[1] King's College London, London, England
[2] South London & Maudsley NHS Foundation Trust, London, England

We're assuming you have a basic knowledge of psychiatry, even if it's a little rusty. This section summarises key points, but for comprehensive coverage, see Further Reading.

Preparation

Gather information
Whether it's a swift verbal handover or a thorough read of the notes, try to establish:
- Reason(s) for presentation today
- Key problems and symptoms
- Past diagnoses
- ± Relapse signature, i.e. *this* person's typical signs when *they're* getting unwell
- Risks.

You don't need to read *everything* – focus on key documents.
- Referral letter/paramedic notes/MHA section papers
- Last discharge summary/outpatient letter
- Care Programme Approach (CPA) plan/crisis plan
- Risk assessment
- Recent contacts (past week for inpatients; past 1–2 months for outpatients).

If they're known to another Trust, contact their team and speak to the Duty Worker, CC or consultant. Once discharged, the GP usually has copies of letters, whilst Medical Records holds comprehensive notes.

> **TIP:** Especially in the community, don't assume everyone knows the patient, just because they've been under services for years. Whenever possible, reassess the history and draw a *timeline*, illustrating the person's changes in function/health, related to social circumstances, medication, psychological input, etc. This can bring a fresh view, especially to chronic problems.
>
> **Juliet Hurn, Editor**

Plan the assessment
Balance privacy with safety, remembering that mental health and personal problems may fascinate other patients and uninvolved staff; try to prevent your patients becoming a source of entertainment, especially if loud or disinhibited.

Psychiatry: Breaking the ICE – Introductions, Common Tasks and Emergencies for Trainees, First Edition.
Edited by Sarah Stringer, Juliet Hurn and Anna M Burnside.
© 2016 John Wiley & Sons, Ltd. Published 2016 by John Wiley & Sons, Ltd.
Companion Website: www.psychiatryice.com

Meet patients with other people when helpful for context or reassurance, e.g. relative, CC. Explain that they can ask carers to leave at any point, to discuss sensitive matters, and let carers speak to you privately as needed. Assessments aren't always suitable for patients' children, so consider asking a relative or colleague to look after them when appropriate.

Psychiatric history

> **PATIENT VIEW:**
>
> There's immense power in the role of the psychiatrist. If you're sitting with someone who's unwell, every single moment you have with that person, you can either nudge them towards getting better or you can shut them off and send them further into their illness. It's critical that every moment with them, you think, *How do I enhance a sense of connection?*
>
> **'Molly'**

1. Approach

The first step is engagement – without it, your knowledge is useless. Whether this is someone's first experience of psychiatric services, or the continuation of many years' contact, they may be frightened, wary or angry about seeing you. Meet them with compassion, gentleness and curiosity, aiming to connect, help them tell their story and make sense of their experiences. Get this right, and symptom coverage will then come naturally, and often more quickly. Remember, running through a rapid 'check-list' of questions is helpful in medical emergencies, but makes psychiatric interviews almost impossible.

Empathise

To empathise, you must (metaphorically) spin yourself round to sit in your patient's seat, and see the situation through their eyes. What does their world feel like? Why are their problems so difficult for them? You must then *communicate* your empathy, through your facial expression, tone of voice, body language, use of silence and empathic statements. Try to avoid dry, stock phrases (e.g. *That must be very distressing*); say things which fit you and this patient in this moment. Being genuine is essential, and it's ultimately less important to say the right thing than to say it the right *way*.

> **PATIENT VIEW:**
>
> We're all people, you're all people, and when you're broken, in whatever way you want to take that … Being harsh, being judgmental, being negative, doesn't really harm the person you're talking to, it harms *you*. It makes you cold, it makes you less a doctor.
>
> **'Liz'**

TIP: Patients tell us awful things – try to remember to be at least a little shocked. Not so shocked they feel they can't say more, but shocked enough to validate their disclosure and justifiable distress. You can rapidly become 'unshockable' in psychiatry, leaving patients cold.

Sharon Brown, Consultant

Find a shared agenda

Part of empathy is recognizing that your patient is (probably) not a psychiatrist with a medical perspective; they have their own understanding of why they're talking to you, and their own agenda for the interview. Without a joint reason to talk, or *shared agenda*, the interview will break down.

You may feel you're going round in circles or that there are two separate conversations going on, e.g. you keep asking about first rank symptoms, while your patient keeps talking about a rat infestation. This 'stuck record' suggests you lack a shared agenda.

Empathy bridges this gap. Someone whose flat is infested with rats (real or imagined) is not interested in ploughing through a list of first rank symptoms. Concentrate on your patient's agenda first, and let your medical agenda sit in the background, simply *noticing* the possible medical relevance.

Once your patient knows you've understood their problem, you can start to develop a shared agenda. People are more likely to work with you if they can see a logical reason to do so. Try connecting your two agendas, e.g.

- *I want to try and help you with [X], but I'll need to ask you a few questions. Is that OK?*
- *People coping with this level of stress can experience lots of things. Can I check if any of these have happened to you?*

You can then continue your assessment *with* your patient, rather than dragging them along behind you.

PATIENT VIEW:

I think assessments are humiliating: they make you go over everything again despite having all your notes. You're left feeling empty, and having to wait for some sort of diagnosis to come. You're not treated like somebody who matters, who needs help and support. It's as if you're treated not as a person, and not with warmth and humanity. You're treated as a case.

'Mags'

---

2. Content

There are many headings in psychiatry, and it can help to note them on a few sheets of paper, stapled together before the interview. Rather than rigidly going through each section, you can fill in areas as they pop up, and cover gaps towards the end. Example questions are written in italics.

TIP: Curiosity skilled the CT.

Background information

Summarise briefly, e.g. Mei Ying is a 21-year-old Chinese woman, admitted informally on 31st December. She is known to the South CMHT with a history of psychosis, but disengaged and became homeless a month ago.

Presenting complaint (PC)

- *What's the main problem at the moment?*

Write verbatim, e.g. "I'm frightened."

History of presenting complaint (HPC)

This is the most important part of the history: the story of their problems/symptoms. It helps you understand their needs and form differential diagnoses.

- Start with open questions
- Follow the story with logical curiosity, e.g. *Why? How? What happened next?*
- Then check specific symptoms, duration and any triggers, e.g. stress, drugs, life events.

Past Psychiatric History (PPHx)

Don't ask if they have a 'psychiatric history'. Try to ask more normal questions.

- *Has anything like this ever happened before?*
- *Have you ever needed help for stress or mental health problems?*

- *Were you given a diagnosis?*
- *Were you given any treatment (e.g. talking therapies or medication)?*
- *What helped?*
- *Were you ever admitted to a mental health hospital?*
  - *Was that voluntary or under a section?*
  - *How long was the admission?*
  - *What happened in hospital?*

Past Medical History (PMHx)

Look for:
- Triggers for mental illness, especially chronic $\pm$ painful medical problems
- Organic causes of psychiatric symptoms, e.g. head injury, epilepsy, systemic illnesses like hyper/hypothyroidism
- Comorbid medical risks, especially cardiovascular (p49)
- *Have you had any physical problems?*
- *Do you see your GP for anything?*

Drug History (DHx)

Check all medications, including over-the-counter (OTC) and herbal remedies. Save time by asking if they're carrying their medications/a list/recent prescription.
- *Which medicines do you take?*
- *Have there been any recent changes?*
- *It's hard to always take tablets. Do you have any difficulties taking all your medicines every day?*
- *Are you allergic to any medications? Have you had any bad side effects?*

Family History (FHx)

Drawing a genogram can help.
- *Who's in your family? Do you have children?*
- *Does anyone have physical health problems?*
- *Has anyone suffered with stress or mental health problems?*

Personal history

The amount of information you can or should cover depends on time pressures and rapport. Do what feels helpful to understand the person. The basic areas are:
- *As far as you know, were there any complications with your birth?*
- *Do you know when you started walking and talking?*
- *How was your childhood?*
- *How was school?*
- *How did you do in school?*
- *What kind of work have you done?*
- *Have you had relationships? What were they like?*

Substance misuse

Check drugs, alcohol, smoking and (if sleepless or anxious) caffeine. Legal highs, OTC medications and cannabis may not be viewed as 'drugs' unless you ask specifically.
- *Do you drink alcohol?*
- *Do you use any drugs?*
- *Have you used anything in the past?*

If they do, check for contact with substance misuse services, and take a more detailed history, covering the last *five days'* use. For each substance, check *TRAPPED* (TAPPED for alcohol):
- **T ype**
- **R oute** – PO/IV/IM/SC/snort. If injecting, do they share needles?

- **A mount** – weight (grams or fractions of an ounce); alcohol in units
- **P attern** – frequency of use and duration at this level
- **P ast abstinence** – formal/self detox? Duration? Reasons for relapse?
- **E ffect on life** – compare periods of use and abstinence if possible
- **D ependency** – three or more in the past year of:
  - ○ Tolerance
  - ○ Withdrawal/use to prevent withdrawal
  - ○ Craving (compulsion to use)
  - ○ Salience (primacy; the drug takes priority over everything else)
  - ○ Loss of control
  - ○ Use despite harm.

TIP: Many people minimise substance misuse, especially when speaking to doctors. Try: *"Has it ever been more than that?"* and *"What's the most you've ever used/drunk?"*

Forensic History

- *Have you ever been in trouble with the law?*
- *Do you have any convictions?*
- *Have you ever been to prison?*

Pre-morbid personality

- *What were you like before all this started?*
- *How would other people describe you?*

Social History (SHx)

- *Where do you live?* (owner, lodger, council tenant etc.)
- *Who lives with you?*
- *Who are you close to? How often do you see them?*
- *Are any of your relationships strained at the moment?*
- *Are you working?*
- *Do you receive benefits?*
- *Have there been any financial/housing problems?*
- *Take me through a typical day.* (Particularly important for exploring routines and ADLs, e.g. where there is substance misuse or cognitive impairment).

TIP: People are usually comfortable answering all kinds of questions if you're comfortable asking them. If you're feeling awkward, try:
- *This is something I ask everyone …*
- *When people feel* [stressed, low etc. – use their words] *they might* [drink more/feel suicidal, etc.]. *Has that happened to you?*
- *We've covered a lot, but have I missed anything important?*
  Don't rush past difficult topics – an attentive silence may help someone summon the courage to talk.

PATIENT VIEW:

Ask, "What happened to you?" rather than, "What's wrong with you?"

'Shawki'

Mental state examination (MSE)

TIP: Never write off someone's 'symptoms' as meaningless nonsense: everything has a meaning, either from the patient's past, or in their current lived experience.

Alex Langford, CT3

The MSE is a snapshot, describing your patient exactly as they present at interview. A good MSE helps colleagues spot your patient, *and* compare their presentation at a future date. Most of the information will be clear from your interview so far, but the MSE reminds you to screen for things you may have forgotten.

Appearance and behaviour (A & B)
- Age, ethnicity, build; distinguishing features, e.g. tattoos, scars
- Clothing – well-kempt/dishevelled; unusual e.g. pirate hat
- Body language, including eye contact, facial expression, posture, psychomotor agitation/retardation
- Unusual movements or medication side effects
- Behaviour, e.g. dancing, eating, crying, visibly distracted by hallucinations
- Rapport and interaction, e.g. cooperative, guarded
- Intoxicated or withdrawing from alcohol or drugs
- Odours.

Speech (S)
- Rate – slow, normal or fast
- Tone – emotional quality of the speech, e.g. annoyed, sarcastic, gloomy
- Volume – soft, normal, loud
- Flow – spontaneous, hesitant, garrulous
- Formal thought disorder, e.g. poverty of thought, flight of ideas, loosening of associations/derailment, circumstantiality, tangentiality.

Mood (M)
- Subjective – *How do you feel at the moment?* (E.g. "Awful!")
- Objective – your view of their mood, e.g. angry, depressed, elated
  - Affect – flattened, normally reactive, labile.

Thought (T)
- Worries, preoccupations, obsessions
- Delusions
  - Type, e.g. grandiose, persecutory, nihilistic; thought interference, passivity
  - Give examples, e.g. Believes the Triads released rats into her hostel
- Over-valued ideas
- Thoughts of harm to self or others.

Perception (P)
- No illusions or hallucinations in any modality *or* …
- Hallucinations/illusions
  - Check auditory, visual, olfactory, gustatory and tactile/deep somatic
  - Describe, e.g. Triads' voices (second person), plotting to kill her
- Depersonalisation/derealisation.

Cognition (C)

- Grossly oriented to time, place and person; good concentration and memory *or…*
- Score formally if any concerns, using your Trust's preferred scale, e.g.
  - *Mini Mental State Examination* (MMSE) – recent copyright fees have decreased usage; check if your Trust has paid to use it!
  - *The Montreal Cognitive Assessment* (MOCA) – free and increasingly used (Appendix D1)
  - *The Mini-Addenbrooke's Cognitive Examination* (M-ACE) – free (Appendix D2).

Insight (I):

- *What do you think is causing this problem?*
- *Is it possible this could be a mental health problem?*
- *What would help?*
- *Would you be willing to try* [medication, psychology, etc]*?*

Say what you see – it's better to describe things than use clever (sometimes wrong) psychopathological labels. Descriptions build a better picture of your patient, and let colleagues draw their own conclusions about the psychopathology. Even when using terminology, description is key.

Physical assessment

New patients or those with a changed presentation should be offered a full physical examination and appropriate investigations. This is always your job in psychiatric units, but in some CMHTs you might ask their GP to facilitate. Look for:
- Physical problems *causing* psychiatric symptoms, e.g. delirium, hypothyroidism, substance misuse
- Comorbid illness requiring attention
- Medication-related issues:
  - Medical contraindications
  - Baseline checks for later comparison
  - Side effects, e.g. EPSEs, metabolic syndrome.
  - See Ch.11 for further details.
Investigations depend on the presentation, but routinely include:
- Physical observations – HR, BP, temperature, SaO_2
- Blood sugar
- Urine dip ± urine drug screen (UDS)
- Blood tests, e.g. FBC, U & Es, LFTs ± TFTs, glucose, lipids, drug levels
- ECG.
- Other investigations can be organised as indicated (Appendix A).
Document recent investigation results in your summary, since these may be hard to access later, e.g. if transferring the patient from ED to a psychiatric ward.

Collateral history

Friends, family, GPs and CCs may shed new light on the nature and extent of problems, or highlight concerns you've overlooked. Carers can describe the realistic level of support available at home, sometimes making the difference between admission and discharge.

Openly seek the patient's permission to contact non-health professionals *before* doing so. You can only contact people against the patient's will in order to prevent harm, and should only share the information necessary to manage this risk. For example, you might warn a patient's housing officer that he's at risk of assault, but shouldn't fax him a full psychiatric history.

You don't need consent to *listen* to people who approach you, though it helps to check whether you can share their concerns directly with the patient. If you *receive* sensitive collateral information (e.g. may lead to violence if the patient hears about it), you may need to record this in a separate 'third party information' section of the notes (check Trust policy).

When you can't immediately gain collateral information, include known contact details in the management plan for follow-up, e.g. name, relationship, telephone number/e-mail address.

PATIENT VIEW:

I was hypomanic and telling them so, but I felt it was only when a history was taken from my partner that it was believed. I just felt it was an insult to my integrity. So, sometimes it's about how a process is explained – and this wasn't explained to me.

'Cathy'

Risk assessment

Risk is the likelihood of harm. Risk assessment and management are key tasks, but often the most anxiety-provoking: *what if something goes wrong because of something I do or don't do?* This anxiety is both normal and useful: Trust your 'gut feeling', and seek advice when feeling uneasy.

It's hard to judge risk when you start. Relatively benign situations may terrify you, or you might develop a false sense of security from watching experienced staff make swift and seemingly intuitive decisions. Calibrate your anxiety by presenting assessments and asking senior colleagues how concerned you *should* be about each patient.

1. General principles
There are some important principles to bear in mind:
- *We can't eradicate risk*
  - As long as people live, they'll take risks
- *We can't predict the future with much certainty*
  - This is because risk events are rare, even in high-risk populations
- *Risk can be decreased by minimising risk factors and maximising protective factors*
- *Extreme responses aren't helpful*
  - You can't ignore your responsibilities to work with risk, *or* keep everyone in hospital forever to 'protect' them
- *Risk assessments aren't simply decisions made by a doctor about a patient*
  - Wherever possible, risk management should be shared with patients, carers and colleagues
- *Positive risk taking is often needed*
  - This is weighing the pros and cons of one plan over another, doing what you can to reduce risk, while recognising your patient's needs and wishes
  - Where *appropriate*, you can and should take risks, e.g. trusting some patients to seek help, rather than detaining them to hospital.

Every assessment should consider the key risks of:
- Self-harm or suicide
- Harm to others, e.g. violence, sexual assault; risks to children
- Harm *from* others, e.g. neglect, abuse; assault; sexual or financial exploitation
- Self-neglect, including physical health and self-care.

Other risks include accidents, deterioration of mental or physical health, debt or eviction.

2. How is risk assessed?
There are two main ways:
- *Actuarial risk assessment*
  - A mathematical approach, assessing risk with standardised tools
  - Used more in research than day-to-day practice.

- *Clinical risk assessment*
  - ◦ Collecting risk information and interpreting it through professional judgement
  - ◦ This is what you'll do in everyday practice, though you'll sometimes supplement it with structured tools, e.g. HCR-20 in forensic psychiatry.

Your most frequent and in-depth risk assessments are likely to be:

- New patients
- Before transfer/discharge
- After a risk event, e.g. self-harm.

Risk assessment is a conversation, not a tick-box exercise. However, most Trusts expect you to formulate risk separately in a clerking, which can help you structure assessments. The best approach starts with open questions and active listening, e.g. after hearing someone's story:

- *What do you worry will happen if this situation continues?*
- *What will you do if this goes on?*

3. Risk factors

The most important risk factor for *any* risk event is a past history: *past behaviour predicts future behaviour*. The obvious caveat is that there's always a first time for everything.

Risk factors can be thought of as:

- *Static:* unchanging
  - ◦ E.g. past behaviour, gender, socio-economic status
  - ◦ They raise or lower your concern, e.g. men are more likely to kill themselves
- *Dynamic:* can change, so are a possible focus of risk management
  - ◦ E.g. by treating depression, you'll decrease the risk of suicide.
  - ◦ Identifying dynamic risk factors lets you consider:
    - Which risk factors may get better or worse
    - What might trigger this improvement or deterioration
    - What patients, carers and staff can do to influence these risk factors.

PATIENT VIEW:

Every time you see a professional, all they see is your history – you can never get away from it. If you made a mistake twenty-five years ago, the doctors are still talking about that incident as if it happened yesterday. When you're young and ignorant you make mistakes. A mistake is something we do and we don't repeat it, so when they go back to that, it's like you're never forgiven.

'Edmund'

---

4. Protective factors

These are things which decrease the risk or help the person deal with stressors. They can also be static or dynamic, and should be weighed against risk factors, as they may completely change the level of risk. For example, a man with suicidal ideation and multiple risk factors (unemployment, HIV, financial problems) may never attempt suicide because he has a supportive partner. The *loss* of protective factors (e.g. death of a partner) can destabilise someone who's been coping with risk for a long time.

5. Suicide and self-harm (Ch.51 for full details)

Always check for thoughts of suicide or self-harm, even if it seems unlikely. Depending on the situation, you can ask directly (e.g. *Have you had thoughts of killing yourself?*) or more tentatively, e.g.

- *This sounds really stressful. Do you ever feel …*
  - ◦ *… life isn't worth living?*
  - ◦ *… you want to go to sleep and not wake up?*
- *Have you had any thoughts of harming yourself?*

- *What plans have you made? What steps have you taken?*
- *Have you decided when you'll hurt/kill yourself?*
- *What exactly will you do?*
- *Is there anything stopping you?*

Thoroughly explore any intent to self-harm, since this may help you prevent, postpone, or minimise the risk.

When someone's actually self-harmed:

- Assess and treat physical consequences
- Minimise the immediate risk of repetition, e.g. remove tablets/scissors; consider asking someone to sit with them
- Gather information from medical ± psychiatric notes
- Speak to colleagues or carers who know them well.

Now gain their full story:

- What happened before, during and after the self-harm?
- What was their view of the self-harm at the time? (Lethality and function)
- Looking back, what do they think about it now?
- What are their plans for the future? Will they self-harm again?

When assessing thoughts of self-harm *or* an actual self-harm attempt, you must think about the risk factors for completed suicide (p321–322). There's no formula to calculate whether someone will kill themselves, but the more risk factors – and fewer protective factors – the more concerned you should be.

PATIENT VIEW:

When I tried to commit suicide, I had that long chat with a psychiatrist … I had in my mind how I was going to do it. Then he asked, "Have you got any thoughts of harming yourself?" And I was thinking, "Should I tell him or not? Do I really want him to know? Because if I tell him, I'm probably not going to be able to do it." Those thoughts were going through my mind.... He'd spent time talking to me and built up rapport before he asked me about suicide. I think that made it easier, to be honest.

'Paul'

---

6. Violence (Ch.80 for details)

Asking about thoughts of violence can feel uncomfortable or offensive, but becomes easier if you empathise with the reasons *why* someone might be aggressive. Again, a stepped approach may help, e.g.

- *This situation sounds stressful/frightening. Have you thought about how you could protect yourself?*
- *Have you had to defend yourself so far? What happened?*
- *Do you ever carry weapons, just in case you need them?*
- *It sounds like you don't get on with X. What contact do you have with X?*
- *Are you planning to find X?*
- *What will you do if you meet X?*
- *Would it ever come to blows/a physical fight?* (If not: *What prevents that?*)
- *Have you had any thoughts about harming X?* (If so: *Any plans?*)
- *Would you act on those thoughts/plans?* (If not: *What stops you?*).

If there's a history of violence, explore thoroughly with the patient and any available notes:

- Planned or impulsive?
- Who was the victim?
- Why did they do it?
- Were drugs/alcohol involved?
- Were they mentally ill at the time?

- What were the consequences of the violence (if any)?
- Current view of this violence (±remorse).

Your concern should increase when *anyone* has a history of violence. Be particularly worried if their current presentation is similar to previous times when they were aggressive. For example, if someone assaulted their mother when previously psychotic and using cocaine, you'd be worried to learn they're angry with their mum, psychotic and using drugs. See p478 for violence risk factors.

7. Formulating risk

'High', 'moderate' and 'low' risk are subjective labels, and their usefulness comes down to the formulation behind them: the reasons *why* you've categorised risk this way. As a rule of thumb:

- *Low*: current evidence doesn't suggest the risk event is likely
- *Moderate*: potential for risk event, especially if circumstances change, e.g. stops medication; loses custody of children.
- *High*: risk event is likely, and could happen at any time.

It's also worth thinking about the *immediate* and *long-term* risk. The more immediate the risk, the more swiftly you must act to manage it.

- *Immediate risk* – informs short-term management
- *Longer-term risk* – informs ongoing plan.

Never simply document risk as 'low', 'moderate' or 'high' – this is meaningless. Your reasons for categorising risk level should always be included as part of a risk formulation.

8. Risk management

There's no point doing a risk assessment if your management plan ignores it. Your default position should be to work *with* patients in managing risk, though this isn't always possible. Plans should always address *immediate risk* (e.g. today/this week) while considering bio-psycho-social ways to help, longer-term.

Broadly your plan will include:

- *Steps to contain the risk*
  ○ E.g. increased support from services or family; monitoring; admission
- *Steps to modify the risk*
  ○ Minimise dynamic risk factors and enhance protective factors
  ○ E.g. remove potential weapons; support around substance misuse
- *Treating mental illness*
- *Gaining further information*
  ○ E.g. from carers, health professionals, probation, police
- *Sharing risk*
- *Discuss risks with your team/seniors*
  ○ Decisions made after discussion with other professionals are more robust, defensible and successful than those made by a lone doctor
  ○ Consider referring to MAPPA (Box 8.1).

Many teams use a *zoning* system, coding patients as red, amber, or green according to their current presentation and risk (red = high; green = low). Zoning is often noted at team meetings, and each zone has an agreed level of management. For example, red zone might indicate:

- CMHT – relapsing, needs frequent reviews ± HTT/admission
- Ward – no leave; 1:1/2:1 observations ± consider for PICU.

9. Documentation

Finally, *document* your risk assessment and management plan. This ensures colleagues understand the risks and can follow the plan. Should things go wrong – which they will, at some point – a well-documented risk assessment will show you did what you could at the time. It also helps you consider whether anything else could have been done, should a similar situation arise in the future (Box 8.2).

Box 8.1 Multi-Agency Public Protection Arrangements (MAPPA)

Many agencies share the risk assessment and management of offenders posing serious risks to the public. MAPPA consists of:
- *Responsible authority*: collaboration of police, prison, probation services. Provides a MAPPA co-ordinator.
- *Duty to co-operate (DTC) agencies*, e.g. health, social care, housing.

Categories
- 1 – Registered sex offenders
- 2 – People who've been:
  - Sentenced to ≥ 1 year for violent offences, *or*
  - Admitted under s47/49 or s37 (Appendix E3)
- 3 – Any other offender posing high risk.
  Offenders are managed at three levels, according to the number of agencies involved:
- Level 1: most mentally disordered offenders. May be managed simply through CPA, while sharing information with MAPPA agencies.
- Levels 2 and 3: progressively higher levels of multi-agency involvement; regular MAPP meetings.

Box 8.2 Christopher Clunis and Jonathan Zito

Christopher Clunis was a jazz musician, diagnosed with schizophrenia in his twenties. He had a history of violence and carrying weapons, and led a chaotic lifestyle, complicated by drug misuse, homelessness, non-adherence and disengagement. Though known to probation, the police, psychiatric and social services, his history was rarely shared and professionals relied heavily on his account of events, without seeking collateral history.

In 1992, he stabbed Jonathan Zito – a stranger – in an unprovoked attack on the London Underground. Mr Zito later died, and the case received significant media and public attention, not least because Mr Zito's widow set up the Zito Trust to shed light on the failings of Mr Clunis' psychiatric care, and raise support for mental health issues.

The Ritchie Report made recommendations for improving the care and treatment of complex patients like Christopher Clunis, highlighting the importance of:
- Information sharing – agencies *and* family
- Clear documentation, especially:
  - A care plan with identified problems, therapeutic goals and a clear statement of who is responsible for what
  - Whenever care is transferred between teams
  - For violent incidents
- A trained key worker to coordinate care and communicate with all agencies
- Risk assessment, including training in identifying risk indicators and relapse signatures.

At the end of any assessment, imagine yourself in 6 months' time. Based on your thinking and documentation, would you feel comfortable justifying your actions if something bad happened? Don't be scared or practice defensively – just reflect. If it's sensible, practical and compassionate, it's a good plan. If you're unsure, double-check it with a senior.

Formulation and diagnosis

PATIENT VIEW:

I am not my illness.

'Desron'

TIP: Try to use the medical model of *mental illness* as only one of many different ways of seeing someone. Never put someone in a diagnostic box and then ascribe everything they do to that box. The box doesn't exist – we made it up.

Alex Langford, CT3

When time is short, list your differential diagnoses, always remembering organic causes, e.g.
1 Drug induced psychosis (cannabis)
2 Relapse of psychosis, secondary to non-adherence
3 Psychotic depression
When able, *formulate:* draw together the person's story as the *bio-psycho-social 4 Ps* (Predisposing, Precipitating, Perpetuating and Protective factors). Making a mental or actual table (Table 8.1) can help organise your thoughts, present succinctly to seniors and guide management.

The formulation is a descriptive summary, explaining why *this* person presents *now* in *this* way, e.g.

Mei Ying is a 21-year-old Chinese woman, admitted informally on 31 December. She's known to the South CMHT with a history of psychosis, but disengaged and became homeless a month ago.

She presents with her typical relapse signature: persecutory delusions that Triads have released rats into her hostel and watch her with cameras; auditory hallucinations of Triads plotting to kill her. Ms Ying has core, biological and cognitive symptoms of depression. Predisposing factors include a family history of schizophrenia (father), childhood abuse, and immigration from China in 2008. Precipitating factors are non-adherence (risperidone 4 mg), cannabis use, and stress (eviction from hostel; lost her waitressing job). Problems are perpetuated by ongoing cannabis use, poor insight, and isolation, including family rejection due to stigma. Protective factors include abstinence from cocaine, Buddhist faith, her trusted friend (Lee), and current wish for help.

The differential includes a drug-induced psychosis, schizophrenia, schizoaffective disorder and psychotic depression. She is at high risk of self-neglect, further deterioration of mental health and rough sleeping. There is a moderate risk of suicide and violence.

TIP: A diagnosis only tells us what the patient has in common with others, not what makes them unique.

Chris Douglas, Consultant Psychiatrist and Psychotherapist

TIP: Diagnostic hypotheses are like affairs – you must never marry them! Have multiple ideas when thinking about a patient, don't become too enamoured with your view.

Piers Newman, Family Therapist

Table 8.1 Example formulation table for psychosis.

	Biological	Psychological	Social
Predisposing	FHx schizophrenia	Childhood abuse	Immigration
Precipitating	Cannabis use/stopped risperidone	Stress	Lost job/evicted
Perpetuating	Cannabis use	Poor insight	Isolation/family rejection
Protective	Cocaine abstinence	Help-seeking/educated/resilient	Close friend/faith

> **PATIENT VIEW:**
>
> Psychiatrists ... generally speaking, they want to label, without necessarily getting to the root of *why* you're in crisis, or what's going on or changed from your normality, what pushed you to psychosis, neurosis and back again.
>
> 'Cyrus'

References

Ministry of Justice National Offender Management Service (2012) *MAPPA Guidance*.
The Report of the Enquiry into the Care and Treatment of Christopher Clunis, 1994, London: HMSO.

Further reading

Petch, E. and Bradley, C. (1997) Learning the lessons from homicide inquiries: adding insult to injury? *Journal of Forensic Psychiatry*, **8** (1) 161–184.
Webster C.D, Douglas K.S, Eaves D and Hart S (1997) *HCR-20: Assessing Risk for Violence (version 2)*, Simon Fraser University, Vancouver.

Psychiatry overview texts

Stringer, S., Church, L., Davison, S., Lipsedge, M. (eds) (2009) *Psychiatry PRN: Principles, Reality, Next Steps*, Oxford University Press, Oxford.
Gelder, M., Andreasen, N., Lopez-Ibor, J. and Geddes, J. (eds) (2012) New Oxford Textbook of Psychiatry *(Volumes 1and2)*, Oxford University Press, Oxford.

Psychopathology textbooks

Oyebode, F. (2008) *Sims' Symptoms in the Mind: An Introduction to Descriptive Psychopathology*, 4th edn, Saunders.
Casey, P.R. and Kelly, B. (2007) *Fish's Clinical Psychopathology: Signs and Symptoms in Psychiatry*, 3rd edn, RCPsych Publications, London.

CHAPTER 9

Management: General principles

Sarah Stringer

King's College London, London, England

> **TIP:** Remember that you can't solve all problems. The default instinct of a doctor is to fix a problem. We can't always do this and sometimes just listening and acknowledging a difficulty can be as effective – and being honest with the patient about your impotence.
>
> **Vish Goel, Consultant**

Medical training often emphasises *cure* as the ultimate goal. In psychiatry, you *will* cure some people, but not everyone; many mental illnesses relapse and remit like migraines, or grumble along like diabetes. Additionally, some patients don't want to be 'cured', since they don't believe they're ill. Simply put, this isn't surgery. Psychiatry is more challenging than whipping out a gallbladder, but you're much less likely to get covered in blood.

Cure sometimes, relieve often, comfort always.

(*Edward Troudeau*)

Relief of symptoms and their impact on life are key for everyone, whether part of a cure or not. A man with Obsessive Compulsive Disorder (OCD) may want to be cured of all intrusive sexual thoughts, but this isn't possible – everyone has intrusive thoughts. However, the relief from learning that his thoughts don't mean he's a paedophile may be life changing (Ch.56).

Sometimes you can't provide cure or relief, e.g. following a suicide. Helplessness is a difficult feeling for doctors, but this is where comfort prevails. Listening and recognizing that someone's feelings are legitimate and appropriate can be more effective than everything else on your management plan. The fact that you're a doctor isn't irrelevant. Although your humanity should be equal to that of any stranger in the street, there's sometimes something profound about a doctor choosing to *be* with someone instead of *doing* something.

The recovery approach

A recovery-oriented approach recognises that people with mental health problems are each on an individual journey, with personal goals. Recovery is about what *they* feel will help them move towards a more satisfying, meaningful life, rather than focusing exclusively on a cure or even symptom reduction. Important components of recovery include preserving or developing:
- Hope
- A sense of self

Psychiatry: Breaking the ICE – Introductions, Common Tasks and Emergencies for Trainees, First Edition.
Edited by Sarah Stringer, Juliet Hurn and Anna M Burnside.
© 2016 John Wiley & Sons, Ltd. Published 2016 by John Wiley & Sons, Ltd.
Companion Website: www.psychiatryice.com

- Coping strategies
- A stable base, e.g. safe home
- Social inclusion – challenging stigma and gaining a place in society
- Empowerment – increasing the person's strength, self-management or self-efficacy
- Supportive relationships – with family/friends, not simply health professionals
- Meaning, e.g. sense of purpose.

You want to get what *you* want from life; build confidence in *your* abilities; and rely on your *own* resources and relationships. 'Patients' are the same: there's more to life than medication and outpatient appointments. Rather than taking over or expecting someone to fail without you, work hard to be only a small part of their life. Ultimately, the better you do your job, the less your patients will need you.

PATIENT VIEW:

I might not reach the level of somebody else, but I can still reach my own potential because everybody's got different levels and they should support me and encourage me to try.

'Rahim'

PATIENT VIEW:

The doctor laughed at my ambition of video game making and wanted me to find a 'serious job.' Instead, today I've earned more money on mobile games in one year than what he would earn in 20 years on salary.

'Leon'

Shared plans

A plan is more likely to work when you and the patient agree it's helpful. Since people present with problems, it's easy to overlook their strengths, ideas and coping strategies. As you did with the shared agenda, listen to their ideas for tackling any problem, with your medical agenda in the background. Once you've understood what they think may help, you can then try to find a shared management plan by bringing in your medical side. Wherever possible, include their ideas in your management plans, rather than imposing interventions upon them; explain your reasons for suggesting certain initiatives, and make time to address their questions and worries about management.

You and your patient will sometimes completely disagree on management, e.g. they want you to arrest the Triads; you want to restart their antipsychotic. Acting in someone's best interests by doing something against their will is unpleasant, but ignoring this fact only deepens resentment. Clearly explain your reasoning, be patient, and show compassion, even when your patient hates you or thinks you're part of a plot. Act with a sense of the impact of your behaviour and acknowledge – with them, where appropriate – that detention is frightening, medications can be unpleasant, and your plan may *feel* abusive. You won't always agree, but by recognising your patients' experience, you're better placed to keep your humanity without overriding theirs.

Holistic management

Your formulation table can help you identify bio-psycho-social areas for change in the management (compare Table 9.1 with Table 8.1, p. 43).

Sometimes you'll struggle to think of things for all boxes – and that's OK, so long as you're open to thinking about all areas. You can't do everything yourself, but can share ideas with the patient and those involved in their care, e.g. relatives, GP, CC.

Staff may be used to doctors only prescribing or dealing with physical health problems. That's fine, but can be rather boring. See yourself as more than medical, and colleagues will involve you more creatively with patients.

Table 9.1 Example of bio-psycho-social management.

Timing	Biological	Psychological	Social
Short term **(immediate)**	Medication Prevent access to cannabis Baseline observations/tests Physical health	Psychoeducation	Hospital admission Facilitate family contact
Medium term **(weeks – months)**	Monitor medication response Try different medications Ongoing physical healthcare	CBT for psychosis Motivational interviewing around cannabis use	Liaise with hostel and employer Review benefits Vocational training Input from faith group
Long term **(months – years)**	Withdraw/reduce medications Ongoing physical healthcare	Family therapy Relapse prevention work	Voluntary/ paid employment Cultural support groups/day centres Carer support groups

---

PATIENT VIEW:

I can't just be stuck on this ward necking Olanzapine. Yeah, I agree that when someone's florid like I was, you can't go into in-depth psychotherapy. But, it would have been good to have the medium-term plan acknowledged ... be given some information and not just treated like a nutter. There were some well bits within me they could have tried to get through to.

'Neil'

Further reading

Slade, M. (2013) *100 Ways to Support Recovery*, Rethink Mental Illness, 2nd edn.
Shepherd, G., Boardman, J. and Slade, M. (2008) Making Recovery a Reality, *The Sainsbury Centre for Mental Health*, London.
Rethink: www.rethink.org/100ways

CHAPTER 10

Physical healthcare

Katherine Beck, Stephanie Young, and Juliet Hurn

South London & Maudsley NHS Foundation Trust, London, England

Whether or not you become a psychiatrist, you'll need to recognise and manage psychiatric and physical problems together. Remember:
- One in three patients seeing GPs have mental health problems
- 20–30% of patients on general hospital wards suffer delirium
- People with enduring mental health problems die up to 20 years earlier than expected. Reasons include:
  - High rates of smoking and substance use
  - Social deprivation, sedentary lifestyle, poor diet, obesity
  - Higher rates of physical illness, especially diabetes and cardiovascular disease
  - Psychotropic medication side effects, e.g. metabolic syndrome from antipsychotics.

Healthcare barriers

Mental illness makes it harder to access physical healthcare for many reasons:
- Patient factors:
  - Fear or embarrassment
  - Chaotic lifestyle; forgetting appointments/medication
  - Symptoms, e.g. agoraphobia, negative symptoms
  - Medication side effects, e.g. sedation
  - Communication problems
  - Poor motivation
  - Poor mobility
  - Lack of education.
- Healthcare factors:
  - Diagnostic overshadowing (wrongly attributing physical symptoms to existing mental illness)
  - Insufficient time for assessments
  - Stigma
  - Ignorance of mental illness and its impact on physical health.

CARER VIEW:

Any time she went into hospital, whether it was ear, nose, throat or foot, you know where she pitch up? In the psychiatric unit. When I went in there the last time, I didn't recognise her. I recognise her from her voice. She was like a balloon. She had been on the psychiatric unit and she had a heart problem. She was begging me to be out of there because she was dying and she didn't want to die there ... They come in with a physical problem and the next minute they're on the psychiatric ward and they're not sure why.

'Alberta'

Psychiatry: Breaking the ICE – Introductions, Common Tasks and Emergencies for Trainees, First Edition.
Edited by Sarah Stringer, Juliet Hurn and Anna M Burnside.
© 2016 John Wiley & Sons, Ltd. Published 2016 by John Wiley & Sons, Ltd.
Companion Website: www.psychiatryice.com

Health promotion and illness prevention

You may be the only doctor your patient sees from year to year – but you're well placed to address the barriers and promote healthy living. Always try to:
- Ensure people register with a GP
- Help them access the GP, e.g. liaise with the surgery; ask their CC to accompany them to appointments
- Be alert to *metabolic syndrome* (Table 10.1) – this cluster of cardiovascular risk factors triples the risk of MI/CVA and doubles mortality rates from these.
  - Risks increase with *Severe Mental Illness* (SMI), i.e. people with enduring psychotic/severe affective illnesses and associated disability or risk
  - Psychotropics (particularly antipsychotics) increase the risk
  - Treat proactively (Appendix A1)
- Include a systems review when taking a PMHx:
  - Routinely cover cardiovascular history, risk factors and existing pathology
  - Be alert to new or unexplained symptoms, e.g. weight loss
  - Check health screenings are up to date, e.g. dental, cervical, breast, sexual
- Explore diet, exercise, alcohol, drugs and smoking. Don't lecture people, but consider:
  - Simple psychoeducation.
  - Offering written patient information
  - Signposting, e.g. smoking cessation clinic, healthy living groups
  - Use Motivational Interviewing techniques (p74)
- Prescribe thoughtfully:
  - Think about side effect profiles, drug interactions and physical comorbidity
  - Consider changing to medications less likely to increase vascular/metabolic risk (Appendix B).

TIP: If you're prescribing drugs that affect the ECG, learn how to read an ECG.

Julian Martin Braybrooke Dace, GP

Table 10.1 Metabolic syndrome.

Factor	Value
Central obesity	Waist circumference
	Men $\geq$94cm ($\geq$90cm if Asian)
	Women $\geq$80cm
	Or Body Mass Index (BMI) > 30
Plus any 2 of:	
Raised BP	Systolic $\geq$130mmHg *or*
	Diastolic $\geq$85mmHg
	or treatment for hypertension
Raised fasting glucose	$\geq$5.6mmol/L
	or diagnosed type II diabetes
Hypertriglyceridaemia	$\geq$1.7mmol/L
	or treatment of hypertriglyceridaemia
Reduced HDL	Men < 1.03mmol/L
	Women < 1.29mmol/L
	or treatment of hypercholesterolaemia

Source: Adapted from International Diabetes Federation 2006.

Physical healthcare on psychiatric wards

Admission may enable physical care the GP has been trying to organise for years – so check for GPs' concerns and make the time count. Aim to examine and perform baseline investigations as part of the admission clerking, and certainly within the first 24 hours. See p37 for further details.

RMNs are specialists in mental – not physical – health, so:
- If you panic, they'll panic
- Problems may be more *or* less serious than they initially communicated
- Structured medical handovers help staff focus their thoughts. Use the ones they recognise, e.g.
  - SBAR (Situation, Background, Assessment, Response)
  - SOS (Story, Observation, Signs)
- Early Warning Scoring (EWS) systems for physical observations vary, so check local use, and which scores trigger medical reviews or suggest an emergency
- Check how much staff know about the health condition
- Educate respectfully
- Clearly state:
  - Physical observations: type and frequency
  - When to contact the doctor, e.g. pulse ranges, 'red flag' symptoms
- Place relevant patient information leaflets in the notes or observation chart.

If you're concerned about your ward's physical healthcare, discuss this with your consultant in supervision, and consider providing formal teaching.

> **TIP:** Remember at all times that you have a medical training and your psychiatric nursing colleagues have a very limited one – *you* are the safety net for physical problems.
>
> Roger Walters, CAMHS Consultant

Physical healthcare in the community

Physical investigation and management is usually less practical in the community. When starting your post, check:
- Expectations – supervisor ± Trust physical healthcare policy
  - Which tests are delegated to GPs, and which should you organise?
- Your clinic room – what's available, does it work?
- How to refer locally
  - Investigations (including phlebotomy service venue/times)
  - Specialist medical advice (NB: in some Trusts, referrals are all via the GP)

> **TIP:** Although most patients will be registered with a GP, many never attend. Maintain your physical assessment skills: you may be the one who spots thyrotoxicosis, idiopathic Parkinson's disease, or an early brain tumour. Don't let your stethoscope, tendon hammer, and ophthalmoscope gather dust.

GPs have monitoring targets for patients with severe mental illness (SMI) via Annual Health Checks (Appendix A1), partially mirroring recommended testing for people using psychotropics (Appendix A4-6). GPs should forward results to your team; CCs should chase them if they don't. You can help by:
- Reminding GPs about the Annual Health Check whenever you write
- Covering physical health in CPA meetings (Ch.19)
- Arranging opportunistic testing where possible

- Ensuring consistent documentation of physical health information, e.g. known co-morbidity, latest Annual Health Check results.

> **TIP:** Teams usually welcome physical healthcare audits. Ideas include standards of:
> - Clinic room equipment
> - Physical health monitoring/documentation
> - Offering relevant interventions, e.g. smoking cessation.

Liaising with other health care professionals

Although people will look to you for medical expertise, you're still a junior doctor and shouldn't expect to know everything. Good sources of information for diagnosis and management of common medical conditions include:
- NICE guidelines
- GP Notebook: www.gpnotebook.co.uk
- Oxford Handbooks (Clinical Medicine/General Practice).

Further medical follow-up or management can be arranged via the GP or specialists in the local general hospital. Write a referral letter if routine, but speak on the telephone (e.g. via the hospital switchboard) if urgent.

Letters to medical colleagues

Any referral letter should clearly state:
- Psychiatric and medical diagnoses
- Medications
- Physical findings $\pm$ investigation results
- Your medical concern or question
- Any specific requests for monitoring or follow-up
- Risks to staff (if relevant)
- Thanks for their help
- Your contact details, should they require further information.

Emergency transfers to ED should be succinct, but also include:
- Any treatment given
- Status (informal/detained)
- Whether accompanied by RMN
- What to do if they try to leave
- Contact details: you/liaison psychiatry/home ward.

Routine outpatients: note any engagement problems and suggest solutions, e.g.
- Realistic appointment times, e.g. avoid early mornings
- Informing you/CC of appointments so you can facilitate attendance
- Double-length appointments if communication or anxiety problems
- Patient's contact details (NB: mobile numbers can change frequently).

> **TIP:** You'll quickly learn which medical colleagues are sympathetic and helpful. Their contact details are gold dust.

Medical emergencies

Expect to lead management in any medical emergency in CMHTs or psychiatric units. Preparation is essential: find out which emergency drugs and equipment are available, remind yourself how to use them, and update your Immediate Life Support skills yearly. When called to an emergency:
- Stay calm
- Assess urgency
- Quickly decide whether you need help, e.g. 999/ERT
- Don't be afraid to call an ambulance, sooner rather than later
- Send staff to meet and direct paramedics or medics, as locked doors and restricted access can cause fatal delays.

If transferring someone to hospital, always write a cover letter $\pm$ ring ahead so the medics understand the problem and can contact you if required. Otherwise, the patient may return without appropriate assessment and management. See Ch.65 for management of medical emergencies on psychiatric wards.

References

The International Diabetes Federation (2006) The IDF consensus worldwide definition of the metabolic syndrome.
  ○ http://www.idf.org/webdata/docs/IDF_Meta_def_final.pdf

Further reading

Cormac I. and Gray D. (2012) *Essentials of Physical Health in Psychiatry*, RCPsych Publications, London.
World Psychiatric Association educational module: Physical illness in patients with severe mental disorders (2011) De Hert *et al.*, *World Psychiatry*, **10**, 52–77 and 138–151.
The Abandoned Illness: A Report by the Schizophrenia Commission (Rethink) (2012) Schizophrenia Commission, London. Available at: http://www.rethink.org/about-us/the-schizophrenia-commission
Report of the National Audit of Schizophrenia (NAS) (2012), HQIP and Royal College of Psychiatrists, London.

Health monitoring:

Lester UK adaptation: Positive Cardiometabolic Health Resource, 2014 update
  ○ Available at www.rcpsych.ac.uk
Physical health checks for people with SMI: a primary care guide
  ○ www.physicalsmi.webeden.co.uk/
Cardiovascular Risk Prediction Charts are reproduced in the BNF's Appendices

Health education/resources

www.nhs.uk/smokefree
www.rethink.org/living-with-mental-illness/wellbeing-physical-health
  ○ Resources and patient information leaflets on wellbeing and physical health
  ○ Comprehensive downloadable Good Health Guide.
www.rethink.org/about-us/health-professionals/physical-health-resources
  ○ Physical health resources for professionals, patients and carers.

CHAPTER 11

Medications

Noreen Jakeman[1] and Sarah Stringer[2]

[1] *Lewisham & Greenwich NHS Trust, London, England*
[2] *King's College London, London, England*

PATIENT VIEW:

When they give them medication it's about controlling them.

'Derek'

Don't expect to know everything about psychotropic medications straight away. Before prescribing, speak to your mental health pharmacist and check current guidance:

- British National Formulary (BNF)/Trust formulary
- Maudsley Prescribing Guidelines
- Bazire's Psychotropic Drug Directory
- www.medicines.org.uk

TIP: You can't ask pharmacists a question that's too simple, stupid, or that you 'should' already know – we're happy to answer them all, and you probably won't be the first to ask. I'd much rather you called me first than have to chase you after you've prescribed something you didn't mean to. And we're emotional creatures – we feel left out if you don't show us a bit of love and ask for our input!

Siobhan Gee, Pharmacist

Medicines management

Medicines management includes every step from choosing to discontinuing medication, and involves patients, carers, nurses, doctors and pharmacists.

PATIENT VIEW:

The trouble is, I spend so much of my life being ill … I don't want to spend the rest of my life being asleep.

'Sarah'

Psychiatry: Breaking the ICE – Introductions, Common Tasks and Emergencies for Trainees, First Edition.
Edited by Sarah Stringer, Juliet Hurn and Anna M Burnside.
© 2016 John Wiley & Sons, Ltd. Published 2016 by John Wiley & Sons, Ltd.
Companion Website: www.psychiatryice.com

1. Choosing

The 'right' medication depends on the patient's problems and acceptability; side effect profile; interactions/contraindications; effectiveness and cost. Gone are the days when a doctor prescribes and the patient meekly swallows tablets. Remember:
- Medication won't work if the patient doesn't take it …
  - …They won't take it if they think it's unhelpful, dangerous or unpleasant
- Except in emergencies, all medication must be fully discussed with patients
- Don't withhold information, hoping that ignorance will help adherence
  - Patients will discover side effects and you'll lose their trust
- You can ask your pharmacist to speak with patients
- Your Trust may have prescribing protocols or a formulary of the medications you're *allowed* to prescribe
- Most psychotropics can cause drowsiness – especially with alcohol. People shouldn't drive or operate heavy machinery if affected.
- Except for PRN medications, medications should be taken regularly
  - People commonly use medication 'as and when' they notice symptoms, but this may cause more side effects or relapse.

> **TIP:** Don't accept drug reps' visits or gifts. Their job is promoting their company's product and their information is inevitably biased. If you enjoy drug company perks you'll appear compromised, however strongly you protest immunity to promotional material and activities. Your patients have a right to objective advice, so get your information from the academic literature or your pharmacist.
>
> Nicola Byrne, Consultant

2. Prescribing

Before prescribing anything, check with the patient, their notes and drug chart:
- Current medications
  - Reason for each drug (*still* needed?)
  - Side effects
  - Drug interactions/contraindicated combinations
- Baseline and monitoring tests – completed and OK? (Appendix A4-6)
- PMHx
- Cardiac, renal and liver function
- Allergies and previous side effects
- Substance misuse (including smoking)
- MHA status (can the medication be prescribed under the current section? p101).

Try to avoid medications which will exacerbate existing problems, e.g. if someone's overweight, olanzapine isn't the best first choice. Never multi-task when writing drug charts or prescriptions: you must clearly record the right drug, dose, time, frequency $\pm$ duration. Anything less can cause problems, including death.
- *Start low, go slow* (use low doses and increase slowly, in small increments)
- Continue at the lowest effective dose
- Generally, high doses or polypharmacy add side effects, rather than benefits
- Don't exceed BNF maximum doses without a documented MDT decision, including planned reviews and monitoring
- Abbreviations are dangerous, e.g.
  - Write *chlorpromazine* and *carbamazepine* (*CPZ* and *CBZ* are easily confused)
  - Write insulin *units* in full (not as *iu* or *u*).

3. Dispensing

This is the pharmacy's job. On the ward, check the pharmacy closing time and daily deadlines for discharge medications ('to take out'/'TTOs'). Medications may not be in stock, so ask the pharmacist before prescribing anything unusual.

4. Administration

Nursing staff, carers or patients may administer medication. Syrups and orodispersible tablets can be more acceptable and less easily 'cheeked' or palmed than tablets. Don't crush tablets without first checking suitability with pharmacy.

5. Reviewing

Review medication every time you see a patient:
- Is the person adherent? Can you enhance adherence? (p177–8)
- Can short-term medications be stopped/reduced?
- Should you change the dose? (Are they feeling better or worse?)
- If someone isn't 'responding', check adherence before changing/increasing medication
- Side effects – *proactively* check and use rating scales to monitor side effects thoroughly
- Monitoring requirements? (Appendix A4–6)
- Can you simplify dosing regimens?

6. Discontinuing

Stopping medication is also important, whether due to side effects, patient preference, lack of benefit or swapping to another drug. Find out:
- Will sudden cessation cause problems?
- Should you cross-taper with another drug?
- Has the patient stopped it anyway?

Talking about medications

> **PATIENT VIEW:**
>
> Medication's very important – it's a very responsible thing to have to manage ... But if it's seen without relationship to all other factors then it's just harmful and reduces people to being a disorder.
>
> **'Bill'**

Remember, psychosocial interventions may mean you don't *need* medications, or can use lower doses. Never ignore this when discussing medications.

1. Introducing medication

Medication may be welcomed or rejected, due to insight, past experience, and the person's background beliefs, e.g. biochemists may consider medication more willingly than homeopaths would. The starting point for choosing a medication should be the symptoms or problems troubling the patient. However:
- Patients may not see their symptoms as 'symptoms'
- Distress may be unrelated to their most *obvious* symptoms.

Find out what bothers them, what they think is causing problems, and what might help. Wherever you can agree a problem, you can discuss solutions, which may include medication. When you *can't*

Table 11.1 Example ways to discuss medication.

Patient situation	Possible approaches
Good insight/keen on biological explanations	*In psychosis, brain dopamine levels go very high, making it hard to know what's real. In your case, you've heard the devil speaking. Antipsychotics lower dopamine levels, making it easier to know what's real again. My hope is that this medication will soften or completely remove the voice you're hearing.*
Open to alternative explanations	*As a doctor, I believe that when you hear the devil's voice, it's a sign of mental illness, not a sign that you're a bad person. I think your mind is playing a very frightening trick on you. This medication has helped people with similar problems, and I think it could help you. How would you feel about trying it, to see if it helps?*
Distressed but can't consider alternative explanations	*You're very frightened and distracted, because of what you're hearing. I think this medication will help you feel less stressed and frightened, and better able to cope.*

agree on problems (e.g. with a manic patient, delighted by his 'fantastic libido') – clearly explain the concerns of the team and carers.

Although your approach will change with different patients (Table 11.1), never lie about medication, e.g. giving someone an antipsychotic as a 'sleeping tablet'. Try to let different belief systems co-exist, rather than fighting to make someone accept the medical model. For example, if someone believes that prayer will cure their depression, it won't help to 'prove' them wrong. However, if they'd ever use paracetamol for a headache, you've a starting point for discussion, which needn't undermine their faith.

PATIENT VIEW:

I felt that the drugs were killing me. Nobody acknowledged that they were harmful or that there was the alternative to taking them. In fact they considered it part of my illness that I didn't want to take the medication!

'Pierre'

---

2. Provide information and choices

Wherever possible, offer choices, even when treating under the MHA. Keep a stash of patient information leaflets (PILs) handy in your office – whether from your Trust or the RCPsych website. Some people happily take medication after a brief description; others ask searching questions, so involve your pharmacist when stuck. Patients won't mind if you spend extra time checking something – but *will* mind a quick, wrong answer.

All medications have side effects, but not everyone suffers them. Where side effects do occur, they might be:

• Intolerable
• Tolerable
• Helpful, e.g. sedation for someone with chronic insomnia.

If you can, offer a choice of two to three medications and give written information, documenting that you've had the discussion. Generally speaking, the better your discussions and the greater choice you offer, the more likely they'll *take* their medication – or *tell* you if they stop it. Some will always refuse medications, while others will plead for things you can't prescribe. Try to balance their preferences with the risks/benefits and a clear clinical reason for prescribing.

> **PATIENT VIEW:**
>
> If you report side effects, the typical response is to ignore it. I feel the medication makes me demotivated but my psychiatrist tells me it's not a side effect, but the illness. The least he could do is look at the list of side effects and say if it's on there. I don't feel heard. I'd like to know I've not imagined it.
>
> 'Corina'

3. Team approach

Work closely with patients and their carers as a team: you bring the medical expertise; they bring their in-depth knowledge of themselves. Take their concerns seriously, and check if 'idiosyncratic' complaints are recognised side effects (they often are). People may willingly tolerate transient or non-serious side effects with reassurance and close monitoring.

The usefulness of any drug is determined by:

- Patient and carer views
- Staff observations.

Rating scales can help monitor progress – if using them, share results with the patient.

- Psychosis:
  - The Positive And Negative Syndrome Scale (PANSS)
  - Brief Psychiatric Rating Scale (BPRS)
- Depression:
  - Beck Depression Inventory (BDI)
  - Hamilton Depression Rating Scale (HDRS/HAM-D)
  - Montgomery-Asberg Depression Scale (MDRS)
- Mania:
  - Young Mania Rating Scale (YMRS).

TIP: A *BDI* is not 'a beady eye'.

John Joyce, Consultant

Explaining common psychotropics

Without explanation and choice, you may as well leave the drug chart blank. This section covers basic advice on common psychotropic medications for fit, working age, non-pregnant adults.

1. Antipsychotics

These are dopamine antagonists. First generation antipsychotics (FGAs/*typicals*) are the older drugs, while second generation antipsychotics (SGAs/*atypicals*) are the newer ones. It's a fairly arbitrary distinction, and although side effects differ, they overlap between the two groups.

Except for clozapine, antipsychotics are all roughly as good as each other for positive symptoms, though SGAs *may* be better against negative symptoms. The main difference is side effect tolerability. All antipsychotics can cause extrapyramidal side effects (EPSE), but as a rule of thumb:

- FGAs: worse EPSE and hyperprolactinaemia
- SGAs: worse metabolic syndrome ($\uparrow$ BP, BMI, glucose, lipids).

How we think antipsychotics work

- Dopamine is an important brain chemical, with many functions
- If dopamine levels rise in some areas of the brain, they cause psychotic symptoms
- Antipsychotics lower dopamine levels.

Antipsychotics are also used for mania/bipolar affective disorder, depression, some anxiety disorders, and rapid tranquilisation (p442–444).

Time-frame
- *Oral*
  - NICE suggests a four to six week trial before changing
  - Increasing evidence shows:
    - Psychotic symptoms start to respond within the first week
    - The first fortnight is a good indicator of whether the drug will work
    - If *no* response by week three, likely to need a different drug
  - Consider clozapine in treatment-resistant schizophrenia, i.e. where there's no response to two full trials of antipsychotics (including at least one SGA)
- *Depot:*
  - Injection taken every one to four weeks (depending on medication)
  - Must test tolerability ± efficacy beforehand (i.e. tablets/test dose)
  - Takes longer than tablets to reach steady state and produce effects
  - Good
    - No need to remember to take tablets every day (some people feel they can nearly forget about their illness)
    - Reduced relapse frequency and severity
    - Steady plasma levels
  - Bad
    - Injections hurt
    - Buttock injections are embarrassing
    - Dose changes take weeks to take effect, and side effects are harder to reverse.

PATIENT VIEW:

I was so upset about having been given the injection … That I couldn't now get out of me. Stuck in me.

'Sarah'

Likelihood of recovery
- If a particular antipsychotic has helped before, it's likely to help again
- ~8 in 10 people improve with antipsychotics
- ~2 in 10 are treatment resistant and need clozapine (Ch.37)
  - At least a third of people respond to clozapine; this can double over a year.

Side effects
See Appendix B(1–3) for relative side effect profiles and specific antipsychotic information.
- *Common* (Ch.36)
  - EPSE – stiffness, tremor, dystonia, akathisia, tardive dyskinesia
  - Sedation/feeling sluggish or slowed down
  - Weight gain ± metabolic syndrome
  - Sexual side effects (anorgasmia, erectile dysfunction, amenorrhoea)
- *Serious (though rare) – seek urgent help*
  - Stiff + feverish + confused (neuroleptic malignant syndrome, Ch. 67).

TIP: Two things with antipsychotics … If someone's getting EPSE, they're probably getting too much medication. If the *social worker's* begging you to increase the meds, you probably should.

Phil Timms, Consultant

Monitoring

Careful monitoring helps pick up side effects earlier than the patient might notice them, e.g. BP, weight, ECG and blood tests (Appendices A3-5):
- Before starting medications
- Three to six monthly in the first year
- Then yearly, if everything's OK .

Clozapine has special monitoring requirements (Ch.37).

Duration and stopping

Roughly three out of four people have more than one episode of psychosis; symptoms often come and go.
- If symptoms are likely to return, they'll often arise:
  - Within three to six months of stopping medication
  - When stressed
  - With illicit drug use.
- Recommended duration of use:
  - First episode of psychosis: one to two years (many services now recommend three years)
    - Often best to think in six-monthly blocks, as less overwhelming
  - Multiple episodes of psychosis: longer, e.g. five years (some people need lifelong treatment, though *may* be able to use lower maintenance doses)
- Encourage the patient to tell their CC or doctor before stopping medication. They can organise a relapse prevention plan, then decrease the medication gradually and safely
  - Other treatments (e.g. CBT) should be in place before stopping medication
  - Carers and professionals can help the person monitor for signs of relapse.

TIP: Check switching regimes with pharmacy. You can usually simply stop the first antipsychotic and start the next immediately. An exception is aripiprazole, which should be cross-tapered if used as the second drug (otherwise, symptoms may worsen).

2. Antidepressants

Older and newer antidepressants are roughly as effective as each other, but Selective Serotonin Reuptake Inhibitors (SSRIs) are recommended first, as their side effects are easier to tolerate, and they're less dangerous in overdose. Mirtazapine can help if sedation is needed.

Some antidepressants are used for other problems, e.g. anxiety disorders, bulimia nervosa, chronic pain.

How we think antidepressants work

Medication isn't usually needed in mild depression, though may help with *chronic* mild symptoms (e.g. >2y). The more severe the depression, the more helpful antidepressants are in getting and staying well. Antidepressants reduce the duration of moderate/severe depressive episodes.
- In depression, some brain chemicals become low (e.g. serotonin, noradrenaline), producing the symptoms of low mood, energy, enjoyment, etc
- Most antidepressants increase these chemicals, and may also affect the number of receptors available to register them
- Antidepressants *aren't* addictive (the patient won't need higher and higher amounts or crave them when they stop)
- They don't work unless taken every day. Missing doses or suddenly stopping antidepressants can cause unpleasant *discontinuation symptoms* (p60).

Time-frame
- Start to see antidepressant effect in first one to two weeks
- Most side effects also appear in first one to two weeks
- Gradual improvement over the coming weeks
- If no effect at all by three to four weeks, consider increasing the dose/changing the drug.

Likelihood of recovery
- Six to seven people out of ten get better with their first antidepressant
- If a particular antidepressant has helped before, it's likely to help again
- If the depression doesn't clear, try a different antidepressant. Some antidepressants can be combined with each other, or other drugs (e.g. lithium, antipsychotics).

Side effects of SSRIs (see Appendix B5 for non-SSRIs)
- *Common*
  ○ Early (first two weeks) or to a lesser extent with dose increases:
    - Nausea $\pm$ vomiting, indigestion, appetite/weight loss, diarrhoea
    - Anxiety-type symptoms: agitation, restlessness, anxiety, shakiness, sweating
    - Headache
    - Insomnia
    - Fatigue
  ○ Later/longer-term
    - Sexual dysfunction
- *Serious (seek urgent help)*
  ○ Suicidal thoughts/acts (fairly common, especially in under-30s)
  ○ Serotonin syndrome (Ch.67), e.g. restless, sweating, shaking, muscle twitches, fits, confusion
  ○ Rash
  ○ Hyponatraemia – cramps, nausea, dizziness, confusion, fits (especially elderly)
  ○ Upper gastrointestinal bleeds (especially elderly, alcohol dependent, history of peptic ulcer, or using steroids/non-steroidal anti-inflammatory drugs).

TIP: Take with food and in the morning to reduce indigestion and insomnia.

Monitoring
Most antidepressants don't need specific monitoring (Appendix A4). Consider:
- ECG if using es-/citalopram (or tricyclics), especially where there may be high peak levels, e.g. liver impairment, high doses, electrolyte disturbance, overdose
- Monitoring sodium levels in elderly patients.

Duration and stopping
At least half the people who suffer one episode of depression will go on to have a second; the risk of recurrence increases with each episode.
- First episode of depression: once fully well, continue for six to nine months
- If >1 episode, continue for $\geq$2 years (some people need long-term medication)
- *Discontinuation syndrome* can occur if antidepressants are stopped *suddenly*. If problematic, reintroduce the antidepressant and discontinue more gradually. Discontinuation symptoms include:
  ○ Anxiety, irritability, tearfulness
  ○ Flu-like symptoms – sweats, chills, headache, muscle ache, nausea, dizziness
  ○ 'Electric-shock' feelings
  ○ Insomnia/vivid dreams

- Encourage the patient to tell their CC or doctor before stopping the medication. They can organise a relapse prevention plan, then decrease the medication gradually and safely over at least 4 weeks (NB: due to its long half-life, fluoxetine can often just be stopped)
  - Other treatments (e.g. CBT, sleep hygiene) should be in place beforehand
  - Carers and professionals can help the patient monitor for signs of relapse
  - Mild discontinuation symptoms resolve in a few days, but it can help to withdraw more slowly.

3. Mood stabilisers (see also Ch.25)

Lithium and sodium valproate are the most commonly prescribed mood stabilisers, used for:
- Acute hypomania/mania
- Longer-term prophylaxis if:
  - Diagnosis of bipolar affective disorder (BPAD) *or*
  - One manic episode but significant risk/impact.

They reduce:
- Manic relapses (efficacy: lithium + valproate >lithium >valproate)
- Depressive relapses: less effective, but most evidence for lithium.

Lithium decreases suicide risk, and has a role in resistant/recurrent unipolar depression. It's sometimes used to raise WCC for people using clozapine.

Antipsychotics are also used for mood stabilisation in acute mania or BPAD prophylaxis (e.g. aripiprazole, olanzapine, risperidone, quetiapine). They require the usual antipsychotic monitoring. Some offer IM options and none need drug levels, which can help when people are acutely uncooperative or chaotic.

Never use lone antidepressants to treat BPAD depression, as they can 'switch' the person into hypomania/mania.

> **TIP:** Lithium packs should be issued to all new starters: they give patient information and record blood levels and tests.

How we think mood stabilisers work
- Broadly speaking, they smooth out mood swings, removing the extreme highs ($\pm$ extreme lows) which cause problems, e.g. hospital admissions
- We don't really know beyond this.

Time-frame
- Lithium and valproate usually take at least a week to affect a manic episode
- Depression takes longer (and usually also needs an antidepressant).

Likelihood of recovery
- Roughly half the people given lithium or valproate will recover from mania
- Some people who don't respond to lithium may respond to valproate (and vice versa)
- If a particular mood stabiliser has helped before, it's very likely to work again.

Side effects
See Table 11.2 and Box 11.1. Both lithium and valproate side effects may be helped by slightly lowering doses.

All mood stabilisers are teratogenic, but valproate's the worst.
- Discuss the risks (Table 29.1, p186) with *all* women of child-bearing age before prescribing, remembering that mania may increase the risk of unplanned pregnancy, through sexual disinhibition and chaotic behaviour

- Reliable contraception is essential
- She should alert you/her GP immediately if planning pregnancy or suspects she might be pregnant (Ch29)
- *Avoid valproate in women of child-bearing age.* If valproate (or carbamazepine) *must* be used, prescribe prophylactic folate 5 mg od.

PATIENT VIEW:

Lithium [...] interfered with my mood so there were no ups and downs in my life. Everything was grey and I wasn't actually interested in doing anything. The hours stretched away from me and I could not conceive of ever being interested in anything ever again until I died. It was very frightening.

Janey Antoniou, *Experiences of Mental Health In-Patient Care, p35*

TIP: NSAIDs can trigger lithium toxicity. Tell patients and check their charts!

Monitoring

Pregnancy tests are sensible before prescribing for women of child-bearing age. See Appendices A4 and A6 for baseline and ongoing monitoring.

Duration and stopping

There's no clear guidance on treatment duration in BPAD, but the more episodes there are, the more there are likely to be. Some people need life-long medication.

- Advice is usually from two to five years, depending on psychosocial stressors and the severity and frequency of relapses
  - It's often less overwhelming to think in 6-monthly blocks
- *Suddenly stopping* medication (especially lithium) has a high risk of manic relapse
- Encourage the patient to talk to their CC or doctor before stopping the medication (*or* considering pregnancy, Ch.29). They can organise a relapse prevention plan, then decrease the medication gradually and safely
  - Other treatments (e.g. CBT, sleep hygiene) should be in place before stopping medication
  - Mood stabilisers should be withdrawn over one to three months (especially lithium)
  - Carers and professionals can help the patient monitor for signs of relapse.

Box 11.1 Lithium toxicity (Ch.69)

If salt levels drop, the kidneys can't remove lithium, so levels build up to dangerous levels. Lithium toxicity can kill. Tell patients to:

- Avoid toxicity
  - Check every new prescription is the same *brand* as usual
  - Avoid low-salt diets; keep well-hydrated
  - Tell their psychiatrist *and* GP if new medications are prescribed
  - Check all OTC medications (especially painkillers) with their pharmacist
  - If they forget a dose, take it as soon as possible unless their next dose is due – never take a double dose to 'catch up'
- Stop lithium and contact a doctor urgently if:
  - Nausea, vomiting, diarrhoea
  - Coarse tremor, ataxia, slurred speech, blurred vision
  - Weakness, muscle twitches, paraesthesia
  - Feeling muddled, drowsy
  - Fits.

Table 11.2 Lithium and valproate side effects.

Problem	Lithium	Valproate
Common early	• GI upset • Tiredness • Tremor • Loss of appetite • Nasty 'metallic' taste/dry mouth • Thirst • Urinary frequency	• GI upset • Tiredness • Tremor (usually intention; some develop parkinsonism)
Common later	• Weight gain • Swollen ankles • Skin problems - e.g. worsens acne/psoriasis • Thirst • Urinary frequency • Nephrogenic diabetes insipidus • Hypothyroidism (p163) • Hyperparathyroidism ($\uparrow$ calcium = endocrine referral) • Mild cognitive impairment (poor memory, slowed reaction times)	• Weight gain • Swollen ankles • Irregular periods • Hair loss ($\pm$ curly regrowth) • Blood cell changes ($\downarrow$platelets, WCC; red cell hypoplasia).
Uncommon but severe	• Chronic kidney disease in 1.2% (p163) • Lithium toxicity (Ch.69)	• Liver failure • Pancreatitis • Confusion

In pregnancy (see p186 for detail)	Cardiac malformation (Ebstein's anomaly)	• Foetal malformations, including:
		  ○ Spina bifida
		  ○ Cleft palate
		  ○ Cardiac defects
		• Cognitive dysfunction

4. Common PRNs

PRN medications are commonly used for agitation, aggression or problems with sleep. (You'll also use benzodiazepines in treating alcohol withdrawal - see Ch.40.)

How they work

• Benzodiazepines help the brain's calming chemicals (GABA) make the brain's pathways less excitable, e.g. diazepam, lorazepam, clonazepam
• Z-hypnotics are similar, e.g. zopiclone, zolpidem
• Promethazine is a sedating antihistamine.

Expected time frame for response

Onset varies, e.g.
• Benzodiazepines

  ○ Oral 20–30 minutes
  ○ IM 10–30 minutes
- Promethazine: IM 1–2h; oral longer
- Z-hypnotics ~30minutes.

Likelihood of response

They usually work, except where people are tolerant, e.g. long-term benzodiazepine use or alcohol dependency. In this case, promethazine treats anxiety/agitation better than Z-hypnotics or benzodiazepines, *but* a formal benzodiazepine detoxication may be required.

Side effects

All can cause poor coordination ($\pm$ falls), drowsiness, feeling 'drugged-up'. A morning 'hangover' or sluggishness can occur when given as night sedation, but may be reduced by taking medication earlier in the evening.

Monitoring

No tests are needed, except in rapid tranquilisation (Appendix A8).

Duration and stopping

None of these tablets deal with the underlying problem, so should be seen as short-term interventions. Benzodiazepines and Z-hypnotics are dependency-forming if used daily for >4 weeks. Once tolerant, the patient may feel shaky, panicky and unable to sleep or relax *without* them.

The team should regularly review the need for these medications with the patient, e.g. at each ward round.

References

Taylor, D., Paton, C. & Kapur, S. (2015) *The Maudsley Prescribing Guidelines in Psychiatry*, 12th edn, Wiley-Blackwell, Chichester.

Further reading

Hardcastle, M., Kennard, D., Grandison, S., Fagin, L. (2007) *Experiences of Mental Health In-Patient Care. Narratives from Service Users, Carers and Professionals*, Routledge, Oxford.
www.rcpsych.ac.uk/healthadvice/moreinformation/aboutourleaflets.aspx
www.emc.medicines.org.uk
www.choiceandmedication.org – if your Trust subscribes.

CHAPTER 12

Psychological interventions

Jane Bunclark[1], Natasha Liu-Thwaites[1], Cheryl Kipping[1], Juliet Hurn[1], and Sarah Stringer[2]

[1] South London & Maudsley NHS Foundation Trust, London, England
[2] King's College London, London, England

PATIENT VIEW:

She was a middle-aged Indian lady with quite a strong accent and I thought, "This isn't going to work: culture difference, age difference, everything difference." Anyway, she was amazing. She said, "Look, I'm not going to ask you any routine questions, just tell me." Then for an hour she just listened to me and simply said, "I'm not going to prescribe you any medication. I'm going to go back to my team to discuss your case with them. Then we'll make an appointment for two weeks and decide the best course … Probably some psychological therapy will be helpful." That was actually the last I saw of her, but she referred me to a psychologist who I then saw for 5 years, who basically kept me alive through my thirties. So, she broke all the rules really … She was pretty fantastic.

'Amanda'

CT psychiatrists receive formal psychotherapy training, but you can be psychologically-minded from day one, by:
• Providing psychoeducation
• Explaining psychotherapies
• Using brief interventions
• Understanding the dynamics of an interaction.

Psychoeducation

This is simply helping people – whether patients, carers or colleagues – understand mental health issues. When explaining anything:
• Find out what they already know or think
• Ask what they'd *like* to know
• Prioritise what you'll cover, e.g. write a list of what they want to know, and ask what's most important *today*
• 'Chunk and check': give a small chunk of information, then check for understanding (or questions) before giving another chunk
• Summarise or get the other person to summarise key messages at the end.
This approach will get you further than a rambling monologue, and is good practice for the MRCPsych practical exam (p112).

PATIENT VIEW:

My current psychiatrist doesn't give a big sweeping diagnosis – he just gives little chunks of information and I find that really helpful. He gives me encouragement and tells me what I'm doing well, even when I can't see it, but not in a way that minimises what's going on … When I'm with him I might feel like we have a revelation but then by the time I'm home again, I forget it and I'm back to square one. One day, I said to him as a joke, "I wish I'd written that down." And then he started making notes for me, nothing spectacular but I find it so helpful.

'Alex'

Mental illness is often seen as weird or frightening, and this has a major impact on people with psychiatric problems. Psychoeducation can fight this stigma, especially if you emphasise:
- Everyone has mental health and physical health
- Mental illness is:
  - Simply when the mind becomes unwell
  - Common (one in four people suffer mental health problems each year)
  - Not a sign of weakness
  - Just as disabling as physical illness
  - Deserving of help
  - Treatable.

Medical diagnoses may conflict with a patient's understanding of their problem. Try to understand their view and offer yours as a possible explanation, e.g. *As a doctor, I meet lots of people with problems that seem to me to be like yours. One way of looking at these problems is that they might mean you're depressed. What do you think about that?*

PATIENT VIEW:

We don't know, really, how the mind works. That's the truth. I think it would actually be helpful to say, 'Probably, your symptoms suggest that you're bipolar, but the truth is, there's a lot we don't know. This is what we're going to go with because it's the best fit at the moment so if you can hang with this treatment, we'll see where we are in three months." Basically what they say to each other!

'Martin'

TIP: There's excellent information available for patients and carers (as well as doctors trying to find good ways to explain things):
- www.time-to-change.org.uk
- www.mind.org.uk
- www.rcpsych.ac.uk/healthadvice.aspx

Explaining psychotherapies

TIP: Healing in psychotherapy has nothing to do with psychology; connection, not self, heals.

Samuel Shem, *Mount Misery*

Talking treatments help people understand themselves, their problems and relationships, and can help them make changes. It's easiest to explain therapies once you've observed or practiced them yourself, but a basic understanding of the common types is helpful when suggesting a referral (Table 12.1).

Not all therapies are available locally, so check local provision, waiting times, and referral routes/practicalities of referral. Cognitive Behaviour Therapy (CBT) is most widely available, and some of your teammates may have specialist training, enabling them to offer therapy to CMHT/ward patients. The Improving Access to Psychological Therapies (IAPT) service is a national initiative, providing swift access to CBT for depression and anxiety (self or GP referral).

Suitability for therapy

Don't assume someone can't use therapy, based on their ethnicity, culture or intelligence (Table 12.2). The essential factor across *all* therapies is the relationship between the therapist and the client. Before referring, consider suitability, based on:

- *Past therapy* – experience, engagement, benefits
- *Psychological mindedness* – ability to talk and reflect on thoughts, feelings and patterns of behaviour.
- *Motivation*
    - Do they *want* therapy?
    - *Why?* E.g. 'quick fix'/coping strategies versus understanding how their experiences relate to current feelings/behaviours/problems?
    - Can they commit to regular attendance? For how long?
    - Do they want to make changes?
    - Do they feel they have the capacity/flexibility to make changes?
- *Resilience*
    - Therapy can be frustrating, hard and emotional – could they tolerate this?
    - Evidence of existing functional coping strategies
    - Do they have other supports (e.g. friends) for coping between sessions?
    - Are they likely to increase self-harm/substance misuse to deal with stress?

Your interaction with patients and carers may be their first taste of a therapeutic relationship. If they find their time with you helpful, they may be more willing to try psychotherapy.

Patients sometimes want recommendations for private therapists. Explain that there are many self-styled, unregulated 'therapists' who range from nice but ineffectual to downright dangerous. Crystals and whale music can be surprisingly expensive… Encourage people to find registered therapists through trusted regulatory bodies:

- UK Council for Psychotherapy (UKCP)
    - **www.psychotherapy.org.uk**
- British Association of Counselling and psychotherapy (BACP)
    - **www.bacp.co.uk**
- British Association for Behavioural and Cognitive Psychotherapies (all qualified CBT therapists)
    - **www.babcp.com**

PATIENT VIEW:

There seems to be a discrepancy in who gets referred for talking therapies. If you're from a wealthy background, or perhaps more articulate, you may be offered counselling. Our black counterparts seem to have more problems accessing counselling than non-black people. It's getting better now, but it still needs a lot of work.

'Alice'

Table 12.1 Summary of common psychotherapies.

Therapy	Format	Key ideas	Common uses
CBT	4–16 weekly sessions Group or individual	Problem-focused Collaborative Based in the here-and-now (touches on, but doesn't focus on the past) Thoughts, moods, behaviours and physiology all affect each other. By changing thoughts or behaviour, you can change the other areas and get better. *Behavioural experiments* test new ways of behaving to see what happens The interpretation of a situation is often part of the problem, e.g. seeing a minor failure as evidence they'll always fail. *Thought diaries* identify problems with thinking and alternative ways of thinking. Work happens in sessions and in person's own time ('homework') Patient develops a toolkit of ways to stay well after therapy	Depression, anxiety, psychosis, substance misuse, eating disorders (NB: CBT has an increasingly evidence base in most disorders)
Psychoanalytic psychotherapy	Intensive, individual e.g. 4–5 sessions a week for years	Psychoanalytic follows original Freudian methods; psychodynamic draws more broadly, e.g. from Freud, Jung, Klein, Adler. Both share common ideas: Past experiences leave their mark, creating unconscious motivations and conflicts, which play out in relationships, thinking and behaviour	Less evidence-based than CBT, but harder to study due to duration and varied methods
Psychodynamic psychotherapy	Individual, 1–3 sessions a week for months/years	Clients transfer feelings they have about important people in their lives onto their therapist (transference) Therapists use the therapeutic relationship to understand the unconscious content of the client's mind, providing insight into problems and relieving distress and tension.	Self-awareness, relationship problems, personality disorders
Brief Dynamic Interpersonal Therapy (DIT)	Individual, ~16 weekly sessions	Short version of psychodynamic therapy	Depression, relationship problems
Mindfulness	Nil fixed: may learn in groups and continue individual or group practice	Mindfulness = being purposefully aware of the present moment and experiences (thoughts, emotions, physical sensations). Mindful awareness notices experiences without judging them as 'good' or 'bad'. Most people aren't mindful, functioning on autopilot/blocking-out or ruminating on experiences Concepts are drawn from Buddhist traditions but mindfulness isn't itself religious	Growing evidence base for physical and mental health problems, e.g. chronic pain, recurrent depression, anxiety disorders

Table 12.1 (*continued*)

Therapy	Format	Key ideas	Common uses
Acceptance and Commitment Therapy (ACT)	Group or individual, varied duration	Combines elements of CBT with mindfulness Encourages noticing and acceptance of thoughts and experiences, rather than simply trying to change them Supports people to clarify and pursue things they value in life	Depression, anxiety, psychosis. Increasingly used in liaison settings to help people cope with chronic disease.
Dialectical Behaviour Therapy (DBT)	Combines individual *and* group therapy; varied duration	Emotions can be overwhelming, intense and hard to handle, especially if there was little space for them to be heard or taken seriously in childhood. This might lead to unpredictable outbursts, emotional surges, or self-harm in adulthood. DBT finds a balance between accepting feelings and behaviour, and changing them, e.g. therapist might validate client's urges to self-harm as understandable, whilst remaining clear that self-harm is unhelpful and offering alternatives. Includes mindfulness, distress tolerance (e.g. self-soothing techniques), interpersonal skills (e.g. assertiveness training), and emotional regulation.	Emotionally unstable personality disorder
Cognitive Analytic Therapy (CAT)	4–24 weeks (usually 16).	Combines CBT and psychodynamic principles, focusing clearly on goals for change Client and therapist work together to understand thoughts, feelings and behaviours, and the past experiences that led to these. Focuses on specific problems and the behaviour patterns which perpetuate them. CAT aims to find choices or 'exits' to help the person escape these recurrent patterns.	Mostly personality disorders
Mentalisation-Based Therapy (MBT)	18 months: individual + group sessions, often on a full or partial inpatient basis.	Without attentive and tuned-in parents, people lack teaching around their emotional states and grow up with a reduced ability to mentalise (to *think about thinking*). As a result, they tend to *act*, rather than *think* about thoughts and feelings. They struggle to: • Get perspective on thoughts or emotions • Read other people's mental states • Imagine how their behaviour will affect others	Emotionally unstable personality disorder

(*continued overleaf*)

Table 12.1 (*continued*)

Therapy	Format	Key ideas	Common uses
		MBT aims to improve someone's understanding of their own and other people's mental states. It encourages people to step back from their emotions and think about them more clearly. Crossover with mindfulness, but MBT also helps people make *sense* of mental experiences (not simply accepting them).	
Family therapy/ couples therapy	Variable. May see individuals separately as well as for family/ couple sessions	Therapists work with groups of people (couples, families, housemates) to understand the systems of interaction between them and work out problems together. Emphasis on finding relationship patterns which cause difficulties, rather than pinning the problem on one person. Therapist facilitates conversations between people to bring out the best in them, help them understand each other's feelings, communicate more effectively, and draw attention to difficulties and solutions. NB: Referrals may make relatives feel you're *blaming* them for problems. Explain this isn't the case: everyone in a group affects all other group members. The better the family/couple get on, the better it is for everyone.	CAMHS, psychosis, eating disorders, relationship problems
Humanistic Therapies e.g. Rogerian/ person-centred counselling, Transactional Analysis, Gestalt psychotherapy, Neurolinguistic programming.	Weekly for 6–12 weeks (or open-ended if private).	Focus on insight, self-development, growth and taking responsibility for personal development. Therapists create an empathic and non-judgemental space to help people recognise their strengths, creativity and choices. Helps people get in touch with their feelings, express them, and find new ways of seeing themselves and the world.	Low level mental illness and stress; confidence-building

Brief interventions

The following skills are helpful for patients *and* doctors in numerous situations:
- Relaxation techniques
- Sleep hygiene
- SMART goals
- Behavioural activation
- Motivational interviewing.

Table 12.2 Common therapy exclusion criteria.

Patient factors	Notes
Acute crisis: • Mental health, e.g. actively suicidal • Social, e.g. homeless	Address crises first, then refer
Chaotic Unwilling	Unlikely to engage
Very isolated/unsupported	Need *some* external support, otherwise the patient and the lone therapist hold all the risk (unsafe and impractical)
Significant substance misuse Likely to self-harm/misuse substances if stressed/challenged Violent Psychotic	The exception is therapists specialising in these issues (e.g. motivational interviewing, DBT, CBT for psychosis), *but* they usually only provide therapy as part of a comprehensive care package.

1. Relaxation techniques

If you or your patient already have effective relaxation techniques, use them. Otherwise, try one of the following, ideally *with* the patient the first time, since it shows you believe it's important, and lets you address misunderstandings or problems. Explain that relaxation exercises work best when practiced once or twice a day – this helps with overall levels of anxiety, and makes it easier to relax when actually anxious. Exercises can be done standing, sitting or lying down (in clinics, demonstrate sitting).

Breathing exercises

Useful when feeling anxious, out-of-control or suffering panic attacks.
• Sit comfortably, with hands on legs or in your lap (hands on tummy if lying down)
• Explain what you'll do *before* getting the patient to copy
• Take a slow, deep breath in through your nose: let your chest expand and tummy rise
• Hold for two to three seconds, then breathe out slowly through your mouth, imagining the tension flowing out of your body.
  ◦ Some people like to imagine their lungs as balloons, gently expanding and shrinking down
  ◦ Others may prefer to count silently as they breathe (e.g. *In*, 2, 3 – *hold*, 2, 3 – *out*, 2, 3). If so, encourage them to count slowly, and *don't* give counting exercises to people with counting OCD.

Progressive muscle relaxation

Especially useful when people say they're too tense to relax. *Perfect* relaxation isn't needed, instead, focus on the body (not worries), and *notice* the difference between tensed and relaxed sensations. Don't do anything that causes pain; avoid arthritic or injured areas.
• Sit comfortably, eyes closed, breathing steadily
• Ask them to focus on the muscles you're working on (they can watch you if unsure)
• Tense an area for a few seconds, then relax the muscles as you breathe out, imagining the tension falling away
• Wait a few seconds before moving on
• Remind the patient to keep breathing if they start breath-holding
• The order doesn't matter, but give a memorable pattern, e.g. from toes to forehead

- At the end, allow a few seconds to notice the overall feel of the body before opening the eyes. It may help to imagine a ripple of relaxation up and down the body.

> **TIP:** Some people (especially survivors of childhood sexual abuse) may find the sensation of 'letting go' frightening. Check if they're scared of relaxing before using this exercise. They may prefer to practice alone, somewhere they feel safe, or with their eyes open.
>
> Alison Roberts, Clinical Psychologist

2. Sleep hygiene

These are simply the rules of sleeping well. Check current sleeping habits before giving targeted advice. Following these rules faithfully resets the sleep-wake cycle within a few days.
- Routine: go to bed and get up at set times (whether tired or not)
- Protect the bed: it's for sleep or sex (not studying, eating, watching TV)
- Daytime: wear the body out a little, e.g. exercise (but not just before bed)
  - No naps/lying in bed or on the sofa
  - No caffeine after 4pm (exclude completely if possible)
- One hour before bed: wind-down, e.g. warm bath, soothing music, relaxation exercises
  - Avoid drinks (midnight toilet breaks), smoking, alcohol or drugs
  - Avoid stimulation, e.g. watching a horror movie/studying
- Prepare the bedroom: quiet, dark, and a comfortable temperature
  - If needed, add ear-plugs, eye-visors, curtain linings
- In bed: don't worry about sleeping or not sleeping; the key is *resting* the body
  - Consider doing relaxation exercises
  - If not sleepy after 20–30 minutes, leave the bedroom and be *bored* for 20–30 minutes, e.g. read the telephone directory.
  - Return to bed and repeat this cycle until sleepy (stay in bed) or the alarm goes (get up).

Acknowledge the frustration of not having an immediate fix, but try to dissuade people from using sleeping tablets or alcohol to sleep: they ruin sleep patterns, offer poor-quality sleep, and risk dependency. The exception is patients who've suffered hypomania/mania; sleeping tablets are often essential as insomnia can trigger relapse.

3. SMART goals

Big, complicated or chronic problems are hard to solve. We go round in circles, distractedly chipping at different bits of the problem, achieving only a sense of failure. It's easy to feel as overwhelmed by your patients' problems as they do, but all problems can be prioritised and then broken down into steps; these steps can be made into *SMART*
Goals:
- **S**pecific
- **M**easurable
- **A**chievable
- **R**ealistic
- **T**ime-limited.

Explain that SMART goals are more likely to succeed. Start with something short-term, to get a swift impact:
- *If you could change one small thing over the next week or two, what would it be?*

Whatever they suggest, help them to think about the logical steps to achieve it. Where multiple steps are needed, each can be a SMART goal, but don't overload with goals, as this undermines the overall Achievability. A non-SMART goal might be, "I'll sort out my debts". Don't dismiss it – just try to SMARTen it up, e.g.

- *When can you do that?*
- *Is that realistic for this week?*
- *How can you make sure you'll manage that?*
- *What's the* first *step towards that goal?*

The SMART goal might be, "By Friday I'll book an appointment with Citizen's Advice Bureau to discuss my debts".

Focus on a short-term SMART goal in the one-off assessment or the start of your outpatient work with someone. You or the CC should check progress, give praise, and support someone to address obstacles. Medium and longer-term goals are also important, but need continued support, e.g. by GP, CC, carers.

4. Behavioural activation (BA)

BA uses behaviours to encourage positive change. It's a key first-step in CBT for depression and anxiety, and can help with negative symptoms of psychosis. In all these states, people tend to withdraw and do less; life becomes boring and problems take centre-stage. Like a car left in a garage, doing nothing drains a person's battery, until they grind to a halt. Well-meaning carers may see withdrawal as laziness, and depressed people may feel they don't *deserve* to enjoy themselves. Therefore, *prescribing* activity legitimises it as an important thing to do, rather than an undeserved or selfish treat.

Suggest people do *one activity a day*, which is purely for them. Activities should either be enjoyable or give a sense of achievement ('mastery'). Find out what they *used* to enjoy or how they filled their time before problems started. They may prefer to do the same thing every day, plan different activities across the week, or choose from a daily 'menu', e.g.

- Call Mum
- Walk dog
- Coffee with Lisa
- Cinema
- Bike ride
- (Free) art gallery with Rakeem
- Soak in the bath, listening to music.

> **TIP:** One option is creating a list of treats for each sense, e.g. listen to music/phone a friend, smell a flower or remember a favourite spice, eat a favourite fruit or meal, a hug with a loved one, look at photos or a magazine or take a walk in the park.
>
> **Penny Henderson, psychotherapist**

Gently discourage activities which are:
- Not SMART
- Likely to worsen problems, e.g. calling an abusive ex-partner for a chat; expensive activities when struggling with debt
- Self-destructive, e.g. involving alcohol, drugs, comfort eating, self-cutting
- Self-punitive, often characterised by *should* or *must* statements, e.g. I *should* visit my sick mother-in-law.

Where possible, involve carers in the behavioural campaign, but be clear that this must be done gently, not by bullying. Encourage the person to follow their plan, rather than their mood (do what the plan says, even if they don't feel like it). People often predict they won't enjoy things at all. If so, offer a printed table (e.g. Table 12.3) for them to complete and test this belief.

You or the CC should review progress weekly, helping the patient to reflect on it, e.g. *What helped most? What do you think [your enjoyment of that] means?* Everyone involved should praise effort, and delight in improvements, however small – it's all evidence that the person can change their situation.

Table 12.3 Example behavioural diary.

Day	Activity	Predicted enjoyment	Mood before	Actual enjoyment	Mood afterwards
Monday	Walk dog	0/10	Depressed 10/10	3/10	Depressed 6/10
Tuesday					

TIP: People often say there's no point doing small things – or think it proves how pathetic they are. I often use the analogy of physiotherapy, explaining their recovery is like the small, repetitive strengthening exercises they might do if they'd broken their wrist.

Alison Roberts, Clinical Psychologist

5. Motivational interviewing (MI)

Did your parents ever try to tell you what to do?
- *Don't do that!*
- *That's really bad for you …*
- *I wouldn't do that if I were you …*

Unless you were abnormally compliant, you probably *didn't* always obey them. In fact, nagging may have triggered a strop or made you do the opposite – either overtly (to spite your parents), or secretly (to shut them up). Maybe you smoked, got drunk, dated the 'wrong' people, wore ridiculous clothes… Maybe you still do. If you changed, you'll have found your own reasons for this, *despite* their lectures and disapproving looks.

For some reason, doctors feel compelled to tell patients what's best for them, even though it doesn't work. In psychiatry, you'll meet people who can't or won't change behaviours which could improve their health and wellbeing, e.g. substance misuse, exercise, medication adherence, or leaving an abusive partner. Understand that the behaviour provides them with significant benefits – if not, they'd have changed ages ago. Remember:
- Change is difficult
- People have to *want* to change
- You've no responsibility to *make* anyone change
- Ambivalence about change is normal (i.e. conflicting feelings for and against change)
- When someone has capacity, they can make unwise ('bad') decisions.

Motivational interviewing (MI) is an evidence-based alternative to nagging and lectures.
- MI is an *approach* which build readiness for change by:
  - Developing collaborative relationships
  - Structuring conversations
  - Helping someone explore and resolve ambivalence about change
- Core principles include:
  - Empathy, optimism, reflective listening
  - Respecting the person's autonomy to identify their *own* values and motivation to change.

MI recognises the *stages of change model* (Prochaska and DiClemente, 1982) and helps people work through the stages at their own pace:
- *Precontemplation:*
  - Not yet acknowledging a problem (no matter how obvious it seems to others)
- *Contemplation:*
  - Acknowledging a problem and *possibility* of change – but unsure what to do
- *Preparation:*
  - Making plans to change, e.g. looking at logistics, setting a date
- *Action:*
  - Trying out a change, e.g. cutting down alcohol

- *Maintenance:*
  - Successfully continuing the change
- *Relapse:*
  - Returning to the old behaviour.

You can learn to incorporate basic MI techniques into your daily work.

Take a non-judgmental, supportive stance:

- Use open body language; look interested, not anxious/disapproving
- See yourself as team-mates, not opponents
- Don't push your own view/leap to problem-solve
- Build confidence: be positive and encouraging about the person's strengths and ability to change
- Avoid lectures/monologues. Before offering *any* information (e.g. on risks of smoking), ask:
  - What they know
  - What they'd like to know
  - Whether they'd like *you* to explain it
- If the person becomes defensive, you've pushed too far. Back off ± apologise.

Empathise

Understand the world through your patient's eyes. What are their views, goals and ideas? From here you can help them:

- Discover *their* reasons for change
  - When they do, they'll talk themselves into change
- Work out where they want to be in life
  - When there's discrepancy between this and where they are now, there's a greater chance they'll decide to change.

Ask open-ended questions

This encourages people to explore issues themselves, rather than being herded down the path you want them to take, e.g.

- *Thanks for coming today. What would you find it useful to talk about?*
- *What do you like best about smoking cannabis?*
- *Have you noticed any drawbacks?* (Only *after* establishing positives)
- *What would life be like without cannabis?*

Practice reflective listening

Rather than jumping in with more questions or advice, listen to their ideas, make a guess at what they mean and reflect this back to them. Early on, keep positives and negatives together, rather than taking sides:

- *So you like how cannabis relaxes you* and *you notice the voices get worse when you smoke?*

Encourage 'change talk'

Let them build their *own* case for change, and help them resolve ambivalence about this.

- Notice, paraphrase and amplify statements about change:
  - *So because your girlfriend hates cannabis – and you really want to stay with her – you've thought it might help to cut down?*
  - *So you feel you need to stop smoking because of your debt?*
  - *How did you manage to cut down before?*
- Explore change:
  - *How important is it for you to change?*
  - *How confident do you feel about changing on a scale of zero to ten?*

- • *... What made you give three rather than zero?*
- • *... What would you need to be doing to make this a four?*
  - ◦ *What changes would make most sense to you?*
  - ◦ *How might things be different if you did this?*
- • Help them think of first steps. Small steps are fine, and usually more realistic than monumental changes.
  - ◦ *What one thing could you start by doing?*
  - ◦ *Talk me through how you'd do that.*

See obstacles as opportunities

When people raise obstacles to change, don't get annoyed – they're just highlighting how hard change will be. Help them think about tackling obstacles, e.g.

- • *What else could you do to cope with the voices?*
- • *What could you say to your friends when they come round to smoke?*
- • *How could you cope with the dealers?*

Be optimistic

Therapeutic optimism is essential, regardless of how unlikely or difficult change may seem. Even the most challenging patients can make sustained changes.

- • If you don't believe the person can change, why should they?
- • When people relapse, all is not lost. They may have gained useful insights and experience for next time around.
- • They may not want to change now – but they may, later.

> **TIP:** How many psychiatrists does it take to change a light bulb? None. The light bulb will change when it's ready.

Understanding the dynamics of an interaction

> **TIP:** The unconscious can get you every time. But it's OK if you eventually work this out.
>
> Elizabeth Venables, Consultant

There are many ways of understanding your interactions with people, and you don't need to stick to one theory and reject the others. Some will make sense of a particular person at a particular meeting, but may not be so helpful at other times. Be open to understanding your *own* behaviours through these theories, too – they can offer useful insights into your reactions in different situations. *Motivation* is a useful concept for understanding interactions with patients, carers and staff, whether you take a functional or more dynamic approach.

1. Functional approach

Operant conditioning states that behaviours which are reinforced will continue, while behaviours which aren't reinforced will eventually cease. In other words, people are motivated to repeat behaviours which gain rewards or avoid unpleasant experiences.

Any behaviour can be broken down into an ABC approach, identifying the:
- Antecedent (trigger)
- Behaviour
- Consequence.

Here's an example: *Sarah is an 18-year old inpatient with psychosis. As you tried to leave the ward, she approached you to discuss medication side effects. When you said you couldn't do this immediately, she swore and threw a plate of food across the floor.*

The *behaviour* is swearing and throwing food. By identifying *antecedents* you may understand *why* and *when* a behaviour happens. This gives you ways to *prevent* it, e.g.
- If Sarah has been trying to get your attention politely for hours, her frustration is understandable. Looking back, you might have prevented this situation by noticing her needs earlier, setting a time to speak to her, and sticking to it.
- Smoking cannabis can increase irritability, so if relevant, it may help to prevent access, e.g. searching Sarah's room or temporarily suspending unescorted leave.
- Ward dynamics can increase tension, e.g. taunting by another patient. Here, you might help by mediating between Sarah and the other patient, or ensuring staff are alert to the problem.

Consequences are the other part of the ABC equation: what happens in response to the behaviour? Table 12.4 shows the result of different responses.

Table 12.4 Operant conditioning.

Sarah swears and throws food …	
… *you immediately spend an hour with her, discussing medication.* = **Positive reinforcement**: something *nice* is *given* in response to the behaviour • Behaviour *more* likely to be repeated.	… *staff restrain her and give IM medication.* = **Punishment:** something *unpleasant* is *given* in response to the behaviour • Behaviour *less* likely to be repeated.
… *you stop the medication, removing side effects* = **Negative reinforcement:** something *unpleasant* is *removed* in response to the behaviour • Behaviour *more* likely to be repeated.	… *Sarah's leave is suspended.* = **Cost response:** something *nice* is *removed* in response to the behaviour • Behaviour *less* likely to be repeated.

Remember that multiple consequences may happen at once, complicating the picture, e.g. you stop medication *and* Sarah's leave is suspended. Additionally, people may have different views of what is pleasant or unpleasant, e.g. rather than being disappointed at losing leave, Sarah might be glad of an excuse not to visit her overbearing family. With any behaviour, ask yourself:
- What does this person hope to gain or avoid by doing this? (the *function* of the behaviour)
- Do I *want* to reinforce this behaviour?
- Can I offer other ways for them to get what they want?

In Sarah's case, she may have learned that her needs are only met when she shouts and throws things. You can decide how to respond, e.g.
- Explain you feel unsafe and will leave the room if she keeps shouting (cost response – removal of your attention)
- Offer to talk once she stops shouting (offer choice)
- When Sarah discusses her needs calmly, you give full attention, try to meet her needs *and* praise her for her self-control (positive reinforcement).

Most people would prefer doctors to reward, rather than punish them. Ethically, you shouldn't punish patients, though it's easy to do, e.g. scolding or increasing medication in response to 'bad' behaviour, rather than for clinical reasons. Additionally, aspects of management can be *perceived* as punishment, even if that's not your intention. If you're aware of these issues, and use rewards wherever possible, you'll get on better with people.

Some final points about reinforcement:

- *Immediate reinforcement* is most effective for encouraging the repetition of a behaviour, e.g. praise someone immediately, not a week later
- *Vicarious learning*: other patients will copy behaviours which are reinforced; this can hugely affect ward dynamics
- *Intermittent reinforcement* is when rewards come at *some* point, but not every time. It's particularly important when you're trying to cause extinction of unwanted behaviours, e.g. a patient who threatens violence to gain benzodiazepines. Although you might refuse to prescribe benzodiazepines, it only needs one person to buckle at some point, and the reinforcement is powerfully maintained. The patient learns that it might take 15, 21 or 35 threats, but at some point, they'll get what they want, so should keep making threats.

Careful use of reinforcement can help people learn and test out new behaviours, making it easier for them to work with you and get on with friends and family. A shared team response and clear boundaries ensure that everyone knows the rules of expected behaviour, and people don't have to guess the outcome.

> **TIP:** Remember that patients reinforce *us* (e.g. through praise) and that reinforcement is just as relevant in your relationships with colleagues, family and friends as it is with patients. Never underestimate the reinforcement of smiling and thanking people.

2. Psychodynamic approaches

You don't need to be a therapist to use psychodynamic principles. These are *theories*, which help understand and explain behaviour, and are generally best held in your head or discussed with your team, rather than presented to a patient as 'the truth'.

Transference and counter-transference

You've probably had lots of communication skills teaching, but may not have come across the ideas of transference and counter-transference. These are the invisible collection of thoughts, memories and feelings, which travel between you and your patient in an interview, affecting how you get on with each other. It helps to think about the 'vibe' or emotional atmosphere you experience from a patient, remembering that you give off a 'vibe' yourself.

- Your patient's emotional atmosphere comes from their past experiences, expectations, *and* what they feel when they relate to you (transference). They're essentially *transferring* part of a previous relationship to the one with you now.
- Yours comes from your past experiences *and* what you feel when you relate to them (counter-transference).

Transference and counter-transference affect the interview, whether they creep about stealthily or ricochet around the room like fireworks. You'll probably remember patients who hated or became particularly attached to you (transference). Likewise, there will have been some *you* saw as extra 'special' or extremely 'difficult'; they 'got under your skin' or 'pushed all your buttons' (counter-transference). The reason may have been obvious, e.g. a lovely elderly woman who reminded you of your gran. Other times, you may not have understood *why* certain patients affected you, and only noticed you were behaving in a mysteriously out-of-character way.

Emotionally-charged interviews can become confusing, and – consciously or not – we tend to do one of two things with these tricky emotions:

- React to them
- Ignore them.

Reacting in a knee-jerk manner runs the risk of unprofessional behaviour or conflict, e.g. getting angry, dismissing or becoming over-involved. You'll tend to re-enact patterns from the person's usual relationships, and since they've had these responses all their life, it won't help to recreate them with you, but may prevent you engaging and helping them.

Ignoring emotions might therefore seem a good idea, but causes different problems. It effectively sweeps feelings under your subconscious rug, where they'll build up until you trip over them and have to react to them later – with this patient, another patient, or your family and friends. Ignoring the emotional atmosphere also amputates your clinical antenna; without tapping into the feelings, it's hard to empathise or help someone.

So, there is a third way: *noticing*. It's normal to feel emotions: anger, fear, helplessness, exasperation, etc. Deliberately take your own emotional temperature: notice how you feel, and *allow* yourself to privately feel this way for a moment, even if you need to take a break from the interview. Don't rise to the emotions; don't fight them; and don't try to judge whether they're 'good' or 'bad' – simply notice them. They'll feel easier to handle, and you'll be able to think more clearly. Now ask yourself:

- *Why are they feeling this way?*
- *Why am I feeling this way?*
- *What does this tell me about them?*
- *What's the most helpful way to respond, with these things in mind?*

Tapping into transference and countertransference helps you understand someone's motivations for saying and doing things. It'll also ensure that you don't pathologise behaviour: just because someone's silent, suspicious, rude or hostile, doesn't mean they have a psychiatric diagnosis, but may offer insights into their experience of life and other people.

Not all staff talk about *transference* and *countertransference*. That's OK, and you can simply talk about how the patient feels and how you or the team feel in return.

TIP: One thing you're never told is this: each meeting demands its own particular emotional responses. It's natural to feel anxious with the anxious; to feel low with the depressed; and if you feel split and confused in the face of psychosis – that's natural too. My advice to my former, more troubled self, is not to worry about these feelings. Let them come. Let them be. And let them go again. You'll have the odd disturbed night, what with all these emotions beyond yourself – but by the morning, you'll be a few steps closer to everything important and humane.

Ben Robinson, CT1

PATIENT VIEW:

I was talking to a psychiatrist, and I just had the clothes I came in with, I had a short skirt on ... I could see him looking at my legs and making judgements – he just thought I was a tart or something ... Like those textbooks that say, *if a woman's playing with her hair it means she fancies you* ... And then you get into this battle: he was feeding off my body language – which was inaccurate – and then I was feeding off his hostility.

'Chloe'

Ego defence mechanisms

These are the *unconscious* strategies we all sometimes use to protect ourselves against anxiety, low self-esteem or life's harsh realities. We're motivated to minimise emotional discomfort, and these strategies tend to distort or deny reality in some way, making it easier to cope when we'd otherwise feel overwhelmed or threatened. We usually learn a range of defence mechanisms in childhood or adolescence, then outgrow the ones which aren't useful anymore. However, we can get stuck, and use them excessively or inappropriately, causing problems in adult life. Common defences are shown in Table 12.5.

Table 12.5 Common ego defences.

Ego defence mechanism	Explanation	Example
Acting out	Expressing difficult thoughts or feelings through behaviour rather than words.	Your sister's husband cheats on her. Rather than saying she's angry, she cuts herself and punches a wall.
Denial	Refusing to accept the uncomfortable truth about something.	You refuse to believe you have a drinking problem, despite starting each day with vodka.
Humour	Expressing unpleasant or upsetting thoughts and feelings in a witty or funny way; this acknowledges the issue whilst cushioning the impact.	After gaining weight from using steroids, your aunt makes lots of 'fat jokes'.
Intellectualisation	Thinking about an issue in a detached way to avoid the emotional aspects.	Having been diagnosed with cancer, your father spends hours researching his diagnosis, feeling neither sad nor scared.
Passive aggression	Showing disagreement or anger through passive resistance or a negative attitude, rather than verbalising the problem.	Your consultant seems annoyed, but denies anything is wrong. He coughs and fiddles with his mobile when you talk in team meetings, and keeps 'accidentally double-booking' your supervision slot. He owes you a WPBA, but keeps procrastinating and 'losing' his password to the website.
Projection	Misattributing thoughts, feelings or impulses to another person, rather than accepting that they're yours.	Your partner accuses you of being angry with them, when you're not. You suspect they're actually angry with you.
Rationalisation	Justifying an unacceptable behaviour, emotion or experience with logic, avoiding the real (painful) reason.	A colleague fails the MRCPsych practical exam because the actors were 'unrealistic'. You suspect her terrible communication skills might have something to do with it.
Regression	Reverting to an earlier developmental stage to cope with a difficult situation.	Upon hearing his wife has died, a man curls up in bed, refusing to speak or self-care.
Splitting	The inability to see both good and bad aspects of someone/something as a cohesive whole. Extreme views are held, idealising or denigrating those around them. This results in extreme reactions and unstable relationships, since the unavoidable discovery of a fault can switch someone from hero to villain.	A patient tells you, "You're the only doctor who understands me … The rest were idiots." NB: In teams, splitting polarises staff reactions towards a patient: some love them; others loathe them. This splitting destroys a team's ability to work together for the patient's benefit.

Defences protect someone's sensitive or painful areas, much like an antalgic gait or crutches minimise pain when walking. As a doctor, you would:
- Know there was a problem, even if you couldn't diagnose it from observation alone
- Not expect a miracle cure by saying, *"You walk funny!"* or removing their crutches
- Recognise the gait isn't ideal, but their *best* way of coping with their discomfort
- Try to help them trust someone enough to examine the problem, deal with the pain, build muscle strength and find a better way of walking.

Similarly, you wouldn't get far by pointing out ego defences directly (*You're being passive aggressive!*) or ordering their removal (*From now on, express your anger verbally!*). When you spot a possible defence, think to yourself:

- *What triggered this?*
- *What's the defence?*
- *What does it defend against?* (E.g. shame, guilt, rejection, criticism, failure)
- *What does this suggest about:*
  - *… their past experiences?*
  - *… how they interact with other people?*

By building a trusting relationship, you can help someone examine and deal with their underlying problems, and find more functional ways to cope and relate to people, *before* dropping their defences. This might require formal psychotherapy, or simply a reliable relationship with clear boundaries, compassion and encouragement while they try out new strategies. Defences may still flare up at stressful times, but at least the person has self-understanding and options. This can help them get more out of life and avoid making the same mistakes, over and over again. Attend your local Balint group (p112) to explore this further.

TIP: Get used to being both good cop and bad cop – don't become too wedded to one role or the other. To your patients you'll be both, even if (or particularly if) you're doing your job well.

Marcella Fok, ST5

TIP: Personal therapy is mandatory for higher trainees specialising in psychotherapy, but can help you explore and understand your responses and feelings towards people in your life. Some psychotherapy is useful as a means of calibration, and of realising that we are often just as troubled as our patients, despite our doctor-costumes.

Elizabeth Venables, Consultant

TIP: Have several patients told you the same thing? Perhaps, "You don't listen"/"You're patronizing"/"You don't believe me". There can be a real arrogance amongst psychiatrists that it's always our patients who have the problem – and a lack of appreciation that sometimes *we* have a bad attitude. Reflect on whether they are correct and make a conscious effort to change your manner.

Lizzie Hunt, ST4

References

Prochaska, J.O. and DiClemente, C.C. (1982) Transtheoretical therapy: Toward a more integrative model of change. *Psychotherapy: Theory, Research and Practice,* **19** (3), 276–288.

Further reading

Rollnick, S., Butler, C., Kinnersley, P., Gregory, J. and Mash, B. (2010) Motivational interviewing. *British Medical Journal,* **340**, c1900.

Information on therapies:

Overview and free tools: www.psychology.tools
CBT: www.rcpsych.ac.uk/healthadvice/treatmentswellbeing/cbt.aspx
CAT: www.acat.me.uk
DBT: http://www.mind.org.uk/information-support/drugs-and-treatments/dialectical-behaviour-therapy-dbt
MI: www.motivationalinterviewing.org

Bateman, A. and Fonagy, P. (2006) *Mentalization-Based Therapy for Borderline Personality Disorder: A Practical Guide,* Oxford University Press, Oxford.

Self-help materials for patients, and simple (mostly CBT-based) interventions:

Wheel of Wellbeing: www.wheelofwellbeing.org
Moodgym: www.moodgym.anu.edu.au/welcome
Living life to the full: www.llttf.com/
Overcoming: www.overcoming.co.uk
Get self-help: www.getselfhelp.co.uk/
Useful tools: www.psychologytools.org/behavioural-activation.html

Mindfulness

William, M. and Penman, D. (2011) *Mindfulness: A Practical Guide to Finding Peace in a Frantic World.* Piatkus.
Sengal, Z, Williams, M. and Teasdale, J. (2010) *Mindfulness-based Cognitive Therapy for Depression,* 2nd edn, Guildford Press.
www.mindfulnessexperience.org – monthly update summarising mindfulness research

CHAPTER 13

Social interventions

Christina Barras[1], Rory Conn[2], Laurine Hanna[3], Abigail G Crutchlow[3], Juliet Hurn[3], Rachel Thomasson[4], and Anna M Burnside[5]

[1] *South West London & St George's, Mental Health NHS Trust, London, England*
[2] *Tavistock and Portman NHS Foundation Trust, London, England*
[3] *South London & Maudsley NHS Foundation Trust, London, England*
[4] *Manchester Royal Infirmary, Lancashire, England*
[5] *East London NHS Foundation Trust, London, England*

PATIENT VIEW:

I met this most fantastic nurse ... She was completely on my wavelength ... She gave me a whole list of things: a website which did CBT on it; the college where you can go and do courses for recovery; [a contact] where I could go and get help maybe getting a job or doing volunteering. She was the first person who was actually resourceful, and gave me something to work on. So then from that, I started doing some things, I could get my confidence up ... She was the first person who'd ever given me hope.

'Ed'

Much of your most useful work tackles social issues. Put another way, people rarely ask you to top-up their serotonin or lower their dopamine; they usually want help with social stressors. Maslow (1954) suggested that people must usually satisfy their more basic needs in order to relax and focus on meeting their full potential (*self-actualization*), e.g. being creative, moral, problem-solving (Figure 13.1). So, you can't expect people to be 'well' – whatever that means – without addressing basic needs.

PATIENT VIEW:

I've felt creativity make a huge difference – it's something you can bring to whatever you're doing. Step outside of the curriculum, step outside of your job description.

'Angela'

General points

Though you can probably list social risk factors for illnesses, you may feel helpless to tackle them. Fortunately, you simply need to be *aware* of social issues, and address them with the help of expert colleagues (Table 13.1). Good CCs of any background usually draw social interventions together as part of the Care Plan, and take the lead when there's no team specialist.

Psychiatry: Breaking the ICE – Introductions, Common Tasks and Emergencies for Trainees, First Edition.
Edited by Sarah Stringer, Juliet Hurn and Anna M Burnside.
© 2016 John Wiley & Sons, Ltd. Published 2016 by John Wiley & Sons, Ltd.
Companion Website: www.psychiatryice.com

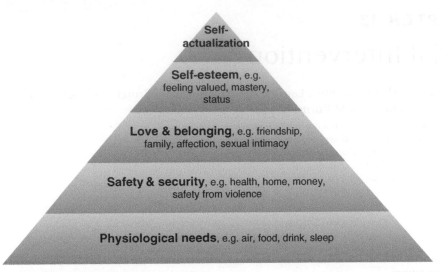

Figure 13.1 Maslow's Hierarchy of Needs (1954).

- Be interested in social issues. People will warm to you when you ask about that music project they're working on, rather than focusing purely on medication.
- Routinely identify areas for social interventions, e.g.
  - *How do you spend your time?*
  - *What did you do before these problems started?*
  - *Who do you see over the week?*
  - *What would you like to do? What stops you?*
  - *What's your home like? Any problems?*
  - *If you could change one area of your life, what would it be?*
- Build a resource file to quickly signpost people to helpful charity websites, support groups, legal advice services, etc
- In CMHTs, accompany CCs when meeting patients in informal surroundings, e.g. home, coffee shops, sports clubs
- On the wards
  - Attend or co-facilitate groups, e.g. music, art, OT. This builds your skills and relationships with patients.
  - Whilst people may not relish a 'mental state review', they may chat comfortably over, for example, a game of pool (confidentiality allowing).

PATIENT VIEW:

A man told me about how he'd worked on a film and music project with a woman who had terrible schizophrenia. They worked together for fourteen months, during which time she had no relapses – longest time since she was diagnosed. It's the power of connection and being alongside another human being and putting your mind in a place which is restorative somehow.

'Amanda'

Advocacy

Advocacy means helping people express their views, explore options, and access information/services, as well as supporting and speaking on their behalf. As a doctor, you may – rightly

Table 13.1 Social management options.

Need	Usual lead	Possible interventions
Education/work	VW/CC	• Access courses, e.g. literacy, numeracy, IT, English, NVQs, apprenticeships, GCSEs, A-Levels, university • Study skills advice or training • Liaise with school/college/university/work, e.g. explain poor attendance or exam performance; advocate for extra support • Help write CVs/interview practice • Facilitate sick leave • Voluntary work/work experience/paid work • Support graded return to work, e.g. part-time/light duties

Housing	SW/OT/ CC	• Liaise with local council/landlord/utility providers to address problems
		• Assess for suitable accommodation ± care package
		• Advocate if threatened eviction
		• If homeless:
		  ○ Advise on day centres/free services/night shelters
		  ○ Direct to homeless person's unit (HPU)
		  ○ Liaise with homeless outreach teams (medical/psychiatric)

Activities	OT/VW/ CC	• Assess and support skills and interests, e.g. evening classes, cookery classes, voluntary groups, time banks, gym referrals
Finances	Benefits advisor/CC /SW	• Benefits review/apply for missing benefits • Medical certificates or reports in support of benefits • Grants/emergency funds, e.g. via charities/occasionally CMHT • Application for free bus pass/disabled parking permit • Signpost to advisory services, e.g. benefits, debt, housing, employment, legal advice • Budgeting/personal allowance advice
Relationships	CC/SW/ OT	• Help develop social networks • Liaise with family/friends, e.g. mediate/explain things • Facilitate ward visits (family/friends) • Assertiveness/social skills training • Carer support/training/respite • Parenting skills training, childcare support, kindergarten, etc • Buddying, mentoring • Charity/service user groups, e.g. sports, discussion, creative arts • Day centres
Identity	CC	• Service user groups • Minority support groups/advocacy, e.g. around culture or sexuality • Support to engage with faith groups • Hospital chaplains (visit while an inpatient; may also see at home)

Key: CC = Care Coordinator; VW = Vocational Worker; SW = Social Worker; OT = Occupational Therapist

or wrongly – wield far more influence than your patient. Use this power to advocate if they're struggling to fight their corner, especially if socially isolated.
- Always seek signed permission before releasing medical information to third parties
- Never underestimate the power of a well-thought-out letter. For example, if someone's threatened with eviction due to rent arrears, *you* might delay eviction or obtain emergency interim funding by writing to the housing provider, explaining how:
  - Psychiatric symptoms have disrupted rent payments
  - Eviction would impact on mental health
- If unsure whether you *should* advocate discuss with your consultant, e.g. providing a job reference
- If someone needs advocacy beyond your ability or scope, signpost to experts (p94).

TIP: If a colleague asks you to write a letter, please do it – the authorities may take more notice of the 'Doctor' title, so use it when you can.

Christopher Wheeler, AMHP

PATIENT VIEW:

They don't offer resources, like there's a service users' cafe, you could go there. They have no idea about all these resources! I know more about all of that than they do.

'Theresa'

Housing and support options

People may find themselves homeless, or in unsafe/uninhabitable accommodation. Their CC or team social worker are best placed to advise on options, and can request that social services complete a *Community Care Assessment* to determine appropriate housing and support.

The council *Housing Department* can register people with the local *Homeless Person's Unit (Housing Welfare)*, and are legally obliged to help those in 'priority need'. They also hold a database of hostels you can share with patients. Other options include:
- *Private rental/council housing* – unsupported; greater independence
- *Bed and breakfast* – temporary measure
- *Short stay hostel* – single/shared room ± access to keyworker. May have rules e.g. regarding alcohol, curfews.
- *Supported living* – often has a rehabilitation role, aiming to move people towards independent living. Terminology can vary, but typically ...
  - 'Low support' – self-contained/group flats with support staff based offsite
  - 'Medium support' – staff onsite, in office hours
  - 'High support' – staff onsite 24 hours a day ± medication supervision.
- *Wet Houses* – for patients with alcohol dependency ('dry' houses are alcohol-free placements).
If someone needs support in their accommodation, statutory services can provide:
- *Floating support* – in-reach to private rental/council tenants, e.g. twice-weekly support worker for help with practical tasks/developing independent living skills
- *Domiciliary Care* – care workers specialising in health and personal care
- *Practical Services* – e.g. laundry and meals-on-wheels schemes; 'blitz clean' if squalor ± hoarding.
Remember that people who've been detained under certain sections of the MHA in England and Wales (3, 37, 47 or 48) have a *right* to Section 117 aftercare (p99), including supported housing. This is a duty of care from health and social services, unless formally discharged because the person *no longer needs* these services (i.e. not because they've disengaged).

People with sufficient social care needs are entitled to *personal budgets*, as part of the Personalisation agenda. The idea is increased autonomy: they can choose to spend money on activities which might not have been traditionally funded, e.g. buying a laptop, alternative therapies.

Employment

The Equality Act 2010 strengthened protection against discrimination by employers; the Mental Health (Discrimination) Act 2013 extended this by allowing people with mental illness to serve as MPs, jurors, and company directors. Nevertheless, many factors (including stigma) make it hard for patients to find, manage, and retain work (Table 13.2). Research conducted by MIND's 'Taking Care of Business' campaign showed that 20% of people who disclosed mental illness were sacked or forced out of their jobs (2011).

Your role includes:

- Discussing work: past, present and aspirations
- Understanding relevant legislation
- Proactively referring to specialist colleagues, e.g. vocational workers, benefits advisors.

Table 13.2 Employment issues.

Situation	Legalities	Notes
Sick leave	Nothing formal needed for the first 7 consecutive days of sick leave (including non-working days). Courtesy dictates they call work to say they're ill! Their employer may ask them to complete a 'self-certification' form upon return. After 7 consecutive days off, they need a doctor's 'fit note' (previously called 'sick note') to allow ongoing sick leave *or* a benefit claim.	Complete Revised Form Med 3. Check your patient's preference for wording their diagnosis. For guidance see Resources, and discuss with seniors if: • Frequently completing fit notes for someone • Feeling pressurised • Unsure whether to state they *may* be fit for work.
Applying for work: whether to disclose mental illness	Under The Equality Act, prospective employers can only ask about health/disability during the application/ interview process for certain reasons, e.g. checking performance of a function intrinsic to the job, national security vetting. They may ask *after* a final job offer is made, to provide occupational health input and make reasonable adjustments. The employer must explain if disclosure of a disability is *obligatory* due to occupational risks, e.g. working with machinery, children. The Disclosure and Barring Service (DBS) has now replaced Criminal Records Bureau (CRB) checks. They don't ask for information on mental illness or previous detentions – only convictions, cautions and warnings.	It's up to your patient to decide whether to disclose. This may be influenced by the type of work and whether their health or medication might affect it. Help them weigh the decision and consider involving a vocational worker. *Disclosure 'pros':* • Protected by equality legislation and may be able to claim support for their disability • Honesty can feel a relief • Sense of being 'in control', e.g. not worrying about involuntary disclosure if they become unwell/someone finds out *Disclosure 'cons' (despite legislation)* • May be less likely to *get* the job (and hard to prove discrimination) • May encounter prejudice or discrimination, e.g. unfriendly colleagues; micromanagement by boss; being passed over for promotion

(continued overleaf)

Table 13.2 (*continued*)

Situation	Legalities	Notes
In work, but taking lots of sick leave ± underperforming	Occupational Health should be involved. Legally, their employer must make 'reasonable adjustments' – for known disabilities, e.g. flexible hours, quiet environment, time off for appointments. After a period of illness, a phased return to work may be helpful. Statutory Sick Pay (SSP) is paid after four weeks of sick leave, and for up to 28 weeks.	Review ± provide fit note. You may be asked to provide letters to employers/Occupational Health, e.g. • Impact of diagnosis • Support needs/suggestions on reasonable adjustments Write if possible, but remember you're not an occupational physician. Consult your senior if unsure, and gain your patient's signed permission for disclosure. Offer to go through the letter before it's sent. It's occasionally helpful to meet with the patient and their employer/Occupational Health professionals.
Long-term unemployed, and: • **Benefits being reviewed/ stopped** *or* • **Asked to attend a Fitness For Work assessment**	>4 weeks off work sick = 'long-term sickness' Returning to work can be very positive, but the prospect of being 'forced' to return can feel overwhelming ± trigger relapse. Fitness For Work assessments can feel stressful and stigmatising.	The Department of Work and Pensions is only contracted to write to GPs when assessing people for benefits, so may miss current psychiatric issues. A brief letter from you may: • Place patients into a higher benefit category • Support an appeal against a loss of benefits • Prevent the need for an assessment interview Your letter should include: • Psychiatric ± medical diagnoses • Current symptoms • Risk • Medication • Level of function • Need for support/mental health input • Specific problems, e.g. communication, interaction, concentration, planning, motivation, fatigue If you think work/work-related training may stress or destabilise your patient, say so in the letter. If a Fitness For Work interview is required, ensure their CC accompanies them.
Discriminated against/fired	The Equality Act 2010 covers discrimination on grounds of disability *or* race, age, gender (or transsexuality), sexual orientation, religion, pregnancy/ children, marriage or civil partnership. This legislation covers unfair dismissal as well as *indirect discrimination*, where there is an unjustifiable policy or practice affecting all employees, but placing someone with a disability at an unfair disadvantage, e.g. changing shift patterns in a way which makes someone with depression work less effectively.	Sources of free legal advice/ employment advice (see Resources) You might offer to provide supporting medical evidence if they're pursuing a case of unlawful dismissal

Benefits

Don't assume people are receiving the right benefits! Table 13.3 outlines the common benefits you'll come across, but this is a constantly changing area, so seek advice through your service's *benefits adviser* (if available) and check resources on p94.

Table 13.3 Common benefits.

Benefit	Basic details
Job Seeker's Allowance (JSA)	If unemployed, but capable of work Requires fortnightly Jobcentre attendance to demonstrate active job search
Employment and Support Allowance (ESA)	If *can't* work due to sickness/disability, and not on Statutory Sick Pay Requires medical examination to show limited capability for work.
Personal independence payment (PIP)	If long-term health condition or disability (whether working or unemployed) Health professional assesses ability to live independently Has daily living + mobility components (replaces Disability Living Allowance)
Housing Benefit	Local council can pay for all/part of someone's rent if on a low income Working and unemployed people can apply
Attendance allowance	Helps provide personal care for over-65s with a mental/physical disability Can also increase the amount of some other benefits
Carer's allowance	For over-16s providing >35 hours of informal care a week to someone with substantial care needs
Universal Credit	Means-tested benefit for those of working age (otherwise Pension Credit) For those on low income (including sickness/disability) **Due to replace many of above benefits from 2015 onwards**

Stigma and discrimination

We often forget how deeply and pervasively stigma affects people with mental health problems. One model views stigma in terms of:
• Ignorance about mental illness
• Negative attitudes, including emotions such as shame or fear
• *Discrimination* – behaviour enshrined by individuals or institutions (Thornicroft, 2006)
The impact may be obvious or subtle:
• Depression, low self-esteem, poor quality of life
• *Self-stigmatising*, e.g. *People like me don't get jobs so there's no point trying …*
• Feeling judged as incompetent or unreliable
• *Social distancing*: friends or acquaintances withdraw
• Relationship breakdown ± loss of parenting role
  ◦ Relatives' responses, e.g. minimising, criticising, withdrawing
  ◦ Families also experience *stigma by association*
• Employment difficulties; loss of income
• Problems accessing housing, benefits, medical care
• Negative media portrayal
• Verbal abuse and victimisation
  ◦ Perjorative terms, labelling, e.g. 'dangerous', 'out-of-control', 'weak', 'scrounger', 'mad', 'crazy', 'psycho' …
• Medication
  ◦ Causing stigmatising side effects, e.g. weight gain, sexual dysfunction, tremor
  ◦ Taking medication can be intrinsically stigmatising, and patients may want to conceal medication from family/friends.

PATIENT VIEW:

No one's saying medication is something people shouldn't get, because some people need medication, but when they become better I wonder if they could reduce the medication, so they don't get all the side effects and don't get ostracised for being too big or because they start dribbling or their hands are shaking.

'Rob'

People cope with stigma in different ways, e.g. concealing a diagnosis, withdrawing from social contacts, distancing themselves from other patients (*I'm not like other people with mental illness*). Some people cope by challenging stigma or educating others – but this isn't easy, usually requiring a degree of self-disclosure, and a great deal of courage and self-belief.

You can combat stigma. But first, you must recognise that psychiatrists are by no means immune. Be honest with yourself: do you treat people differently because of their illness? You won't be able to address your own stigma while you see patients as 'them' and you, your friends, family and colleagues as an invulnerable 'us'. Just recognising that you may hold prejudicial views is a first step to challenging them; next comes a clean-up of stigmatising language, and a willingness to change (see p94). Recognise that many excellent doctors have suffered mental illness.

You can address stigma with patients by:
- Asking about their experiences of stigma
- Asking whether they've disclosed to friends/family. How did this go?
- Discussing how they might talk about their illness with others
  - One way is developing a 'narrative' or 'message' about their illness that they'd be happy sharing with others, e.g. "I was under a lot of stress … but I'm better now and coping in these ways … "/"I have an illness called bipolar disorder, but I'm still *me*, and these are the things I want to do … "
  - A psychologist may help develop this narrative, and work through feelings of shame or embarrassment
- Offering psychoeducation and information about resources/user groups
- Using recovery principles (p45)
- Promoting self-management and active participation in treatment plans
- Encouraging their involvement in education initiatives. (Contact between people with mental illness and those without is an effective anti-stigma strategy.)

When working with a person's family and friends, you can mediate, psychoeducate and signpost to carers' groups.

Society is arguably the hardest thing to change, but you can chip away at stigma by:
- Advocating for your patients (p84)
- Educating, dispelling myths and de-stigmatising – whether at work or in your personal life
- Role-modelling a compassionate stance
- Getting involved with anti-stigma campaigns, e.g. Time to Change
- Offering educational initiatives, e.g. teaching hostel staff or police; visiting schools to talk about mental health.

Anti-stigma work is an essential social intervention, and will enhance patients' quality of life – even if it doesn't neatly fit into their management plans.

PATIENT VIEW:

I had a transient episode of bipolar disorder (which involved quite serious psychosis). I got better, but as I was on my road to recovery, my psychiatrist encouraged me *not* to apply for medical school as she didn't think I'd get in or cope. Well, she could not have been more wrong; I've nearly graduated from med school and my mental health is fine. Just a message out there to give patients hope: sometimes mental illness is *not* permanent, and you can aspire to things and lead a normal life.

'Tilda'

Cultural issues in psychiatry

> **CARER VIEW:**
>
> I had to represent a woman ... She said the spirit was coming across from the Caribbean and biting her. The consultant asked me, "What do you think, could that be true? Does that happen within her culture?" He was trying to understand if this woman was psychotic, or going through a spiritual crisis. The spiritual element needs to be discussed because lots of black people coming to psychiatric services turn to God or to Allah, and they believe that's what's going to get them through.
>
> **'Suzanne'**

Culture can be thought of as a suitcase, into which we cram everything making up our social and cultural identity. Like the contents of a suitcase, these factors can change with time, e.g. as people add things from the cultures around them. Due to the complexity of culture, you can't assume you understand it without exploring it, even if you were born in the same street, attend the same place of worship, and have overlap in your music collections. If you don't know, simply *ask*.

TIP: Culture isn't something only others have. Your patients have attitudes and beliefs influenced by it – so do you.

John Joyce, Consultant

Nine (culture-related) characteristics are protected from discrimination under the Equality Act 2010:
- Age
- Sex
- Disability
- Gender reassignment
- Marriage and civil partnership
- Pregnancy and maternity
- Race
- Religion and belief
- Sexual orientation

Other factors contributing to culture include:
- Language and communication
- Ethnicity and nationality
- Political, family, peer, occupational and societal values
- Socioeconomic class
- Educational experience
- Interest and involvement in music, art, clothing, food, books, hobbies, etc.

Acknowledging and exploring cultural issues in psychiatry helps you to:
- *Contextualise someone's 'psychiatric' presentation*
  - Decide which elements are culturally congruent or possibly pathological
  - Recognise the *meaning* of this to the person and their social group. For example, spiritual possession may be a culturally congruent belief in many countries and faith groups (including Islam, Judaism, Christianity, Hinduism and Buddhism) – but the *meaning* may vary widely, and there will be times when this is understood as a 'normal' or purely spiritual experience, and other times when it's viewed as abnormal.
  - Improve your understanding of predisposing, precipitating and perpetuating factors for this person's illness/recovery.

- ○ Spiritual beliefs and thoughts about suicide may be deeply entwined and should be considered during risk assessments
- *Recognise similarities and differences between your and your patient's cultures*
  - ○ These might make sense of a particular presentation, or reasons for treatment refusal/non-engagement
- *Combat discrimination, especially for groups experiencing recurrent discrimination*
  - ○ Some groups receive very different treatment by the 'system', e.g. Black and Minority Ethnic (BME) groups have higher rates for diagnosing schizophrenia, MHA detentions, hospitalisation, seclusion and fewer referrals for psychotherapy (McKenzie and Bhui, 2007).
  - ○ Discrimination not only affects the treatment offered, but people's willingness to access care or accept help due to previous negative experiences, risking later presentations/engagement difficulties.
- *Understand cultural issues around stigma, shame, rejection*
- *Involve appropriate support networks, depending on the patient's cultural membership(s).*

To best support your patients, you need to understand their (sub)cultures, using all available resources, e.g. patients, carers, interpreters, colleagues, religious leaders, reputable internet sites. It may seem unimportant when time's scarce and your bleep's on fire, but exploring cultural concepts will highlight key issues needing further thought, and encourage colleagues to prioritise these. A note of caution, though: 'cultural norms' should never override human rights, e.g. female genital mutilation is *abuse*, no matter how culturally acceptable it is to some people.

PATIENT VIEW:

These doctors are coming from a different background and they don't understand the problems we face in the black community. They haven't experienced no racism 'cos they're white, most of them. Even though you see a black doctor, he wouldn't relate to me and what I'm saying about racism, because once you become educated sometimes you don't see racism.

'Olufemi'

CARER VIEW:

My mum will say, "I'll talk to the Lord." Does that mean she's got mental health problems? They did a test on my mum thinking she's mentally ill. There's nothing wrong with the woman! But, because she talks like that, because she's a Caribbean woman, she says things that we understand, but the doctors don't, so they referred her for mental health.

'Adam'

Finally, be aware of your own culture, but don't impose it upon patients or colleagues; your job is to provide healthcare to people in need, regardless of their background. If you're uncomfortable with an element of someone's culture or lifestyle, try to understand it better, rather than trying to ignore or change it. A topical example is homophobia, which remains evident in society, including healthcare settings (ILGA-Europe, 2013). See also Box 13.1.

Box 13.1 The Gender Recognition Act (GRA) 2004 – what you need to know

- The GRA allows people with gender dysphoria to live in their preferred gender and obtain a birth certificate with the 'acquired' gender
- Their prior gender and application for/receipt of a Gender Recognition Certificate then become protected information

- In your professional capacity as a doctor, you can be prosecuted for disclosing this information without the patient's explicit (ideally written) consent, e.g. by telling other professionals or including it in medical records.
- If the person lacks capacity, disclosure should be considered under the usual framework of the MCA, and information only shared with specific people when absolutely necessary.

Working with friends and family

> **PATIENT VIEW:**
>
> Doctors have to make decisions whether families can be included or not and how much. They could ask, "Does that person feel more empowered if their family is around and how do we respect their wishes if they say they don't want to see their families?" So it's getting that balancing act and helping the family through that.
>
> 'Faith'

Carers often stoically advocate and support patients, though some need support or education, and a few bring more stress than they relieve. Find out if you have a family (intervention) worker who can undertake targeted support/therapy with families. Always check what someone is happy for you to share *before* talking to their carers. Then:

- Give realistic timeframes, e.g. *I've half an hour free now, but if we don't get through everything, we can meet again*
- Check questions and concerns
- Don't feel pressured to have all the answers – just note down and find out the things you don't know
- Spot signs of carer stress, and offer carers' assessments or local carer's groups if appropriate, via the CC
- *Receive* information without worrying about confidentiality
- If carers disclose something they say you mustn't tell the patient, discuss their reasons. Try not to keep secrets from patients, but if unavoidable (e.g. due to risk), record it in the 'third party' section of the notes.

If you've spoken to the family in private, see the patient afterwards. They may be worried about your meeting (especially if suffering from paranoia), so reassure where possible.

> **CARER VIEW:**
>
> One minute you're somebody's partner and the next minute you're somebody's carer. Part of learning the role is having to learn to be vulnerable, having to learn to ask for help and accept help. This isn't something that seems to be taught in medical training – how to be vulnerable. It seems a very macho environment, survival of the fittest and hundred-hour weeks for junior doctors – it seems opposite to the way service users experience mental health difficulties.
>
> 'Mike'

> **TIP:** Ask every patient who is their carer – or the most important person in their life – and meet them face-to-face to thank them for their support.
>
> Yasir Hameed, Consultant

References

Maslow, A.S. (1943) A theory of human motivation. *Psychological Review*, **50**(4), 370–396.
McKenzie, K. and Bhui, K. (2007) Institutional racism in mental health care. *British Medical Journal*, **334**: 649–650.
Mind (2011) *Taking Care of Business: Employer Solutions for Better Mental Health at Work. A Report of Mind's Business Summit*. Mind, London.
The Equality Act 2010, UK. Available from: http://www.legislation.gov.uk/ukpga/2010/15
The Gender Recognition Act (2004), United Kingdom. Available from:http://www.legislation.gov.uk/ukpa2004/7/contents
Thornicroft, G. (2006) *Shunned: discrimination against people with mental illness*. Oxford University Press, New York.

Further reading

ILGA-Europe (2013) Annual Review of the Human Rights Situation of Lesbian, Gay, Bisexual, Trans and Intersex People in Europe. ILGA-Europe, Brussels.
Lockwood, G., Henderson, C., Thornicroft G. (2012) The Equality Act 2010 and mental health. *British Journal of Psychiatry*, **200**: 182–183.

General/legal advice

Citizens' Advice Bureau 08444 111 444
Civil Legal Advice: free independent, confidential advice on debt, benefits, employment and housing problems; service paid for by legal aid
   o 0345 3454345
   o www.gov.uk/civil-legal-advice
Mind's Legal Advice Service. Tel: 0300 4666463

Personalisation

Social Care Institute for Excellence has information for professionals on personalisation:
   o www.scie.org.uk/topic/keyissues/personalisation

Advocacy

Action for Advocacy – provides details of local advocacy groups/ organisations
   o www.actionforadvocacy.org.uk
   o 020 7921 4395
Voiceability – work with marginalised/vulnerable members of society
   o www.voiceability.org.uk

Accommodation

Shelter including local drop-in services and 24-hour advisory helpline 0808 8004444

Employment/benefits

Check www.gov.uk for latest benefits guidance information
Government's *Online Benefits Advisor* (estimates how much someone's eligible to receive)
   o www.gov.uk/benefits-adviser
Disability Benefits Helpline 0845 7123456
Guidance for doctors on completing fit notes.
   o www.rethink.org/living-with-mental-illness/money-issues-benefits-employment/work-and-mental-illness
   o https://www.gov.uk/government/publications/fit-note-guidance-for-gps

Stigma/discrimination

www.time-to-change.org.uk

Cultural issues

RCPsych leaflets on spirituality and religion
- www.rcpsych.ac.uk/healthadvice/problemsdisorders/leafletformuslimsonstress.aspx   (available   in   Tamil, Urdu, Farsi and Arabic)
- www.rcpsych.ac.uk/mentalhealthinformation/therapies/spiritualityandmentalhealth.aspx

CHAPTER 14

Handovers

Rachel Thomasson

Manchester Royal Infirmary, Manchester, Lancashire, England

The interfaces between services are common places for plans to warp or disappear. It may sound obvious, but the CMHT *won't* magically read a note you scribbled in the ED notes, and the GP won't usually have access to your electronic patient records. Check:
- Can everyone involved in this plan read it?
  - If so, should you prompt them to look? (Verbal handover, e-mail or fax)
  - If not, should you send a copy? (E-mail/fax; post if non-urgent)
- Does the patient need/want a copy?

Don't be a ghostly scribe, secretly writing letters or notes, then silently wafting away. Maximise your impact. People often want to *hear* what you think – so consider personally handing over to CCs, named nurses, or medical colleagues. They may offer additional ideas or spot problems you've overlooked, so verbal handovers can strengthen plans. See p312 for on-call handovers.

Patients are usually copied into correspondence, and can apply to see their notes: always write clearly and respectfully.

> **TIP:** Many Trusts use electronic records, and it's tempting to 'cut and paste' information (e.g. personal history). We'd suggest avoiding this, but recognise you may need to when under pressure. If you do, state that you're quoting an earlier assessment and check the information isn't out-of-date.

> **TIP:** Think twice before sending copies of detailed psychiatric assessments to the GP containing lots of personal information – it'll stay on a patient's record for life and many people will have access to information which the patient thought they were giving you in confidence.
>
> Lucinda Richards, CT3

Psychiatry: Breaking the ICE – Introductions, Common Tasks and Emergencies for Trainees, First Edition.
Edited by Sarah Stringer, Juliet Hurn and Anna M Burnside.
© 2016 John Wiley & Sons, Ltd. Published 2016 by John Wiley & Sons, Ltd.
Companion Website: www.psychiatryice.com

CHAPTER 15

Mental health legislation

Penelope Brown[1], Peter Hindley[1], and Anna M Burnside[2]

[1] South London & Maudsley NHS Foundation Trust, London, England
[2] East London NHS Foundation Trust, London, England

The United Kingdom has three distinct legal systems, covering England and Wales, Scotland, and Northern Ireland. We'll focus on English law (England and Wales), which is based on a *common law* system, and comprises:

- *Statutes:* Acts of law passed by Parliament, which must be obeyed, like a rule book
- *Case law:* principles derived from judges' decisions on individual court cases.

The Mental Health Act (MHA) and Mental Capacity Act (MCA) are statutes, and both have Codes of Practice (CoP) to guide their use. For an overview of the law in Scotland and Northern Ireland, see Appendices E1 and 2.

> **TIP:** Don't underestimate the tension of your dual role: whilst trying to develop a therapeutic relationship, you'll do things patients don't want, e.g. detention, enforcing medication. You'll often feel ambivalent, frustrated or upset. There may not always be a resolution or a 'right' answer – but you must share this in supervision or with involved colleagues to maintain your humanity.
>
> **Juliet Hurn, Editor**

The Mental Health Act 1983 (amended 2007)

The first MHA was passed in 1959, bringing together various statutes and case law. This allowed both voluntary and compulsory admission, and treatment of patients in psychiatric hospitals. It was replaced by the MHA 1983, which remains in force, adding statutory powers to manage patients in the community.

The MHA is divided into chapters (*Parts*), consisting of sections and subsections. The Parts are:

- I: defines mental disorder and who can be subjected to the MHA
- II: sections for civil detention and community treatment
- III: courts' powers to detain and treat patients involved in criminal proceedings
- IV: consent to treatment
- V: mental health tribunals
- VI-X: other powers.

Table 15.1 summarises the most common civil sections; Appendix E3 outlines forensic sections. The type of section doesn't necessarily determine the ward; forensic section patients may be on general wards, and civil section patients may be on forensic units.

Psychiatry: Breaking the ICE – Introductions, Common Tasks and Emergencies for Trainees, First Edition.
Edited by Sarah Stringer, Juliet Hurn and Anna M Burnside.
© 2016 John Wiley & Sons, Ltd. Published 2016 by John Wiley & Sons, Ltd.
Companion Website: www.psychiatryice.com

PATIENT VIEW:

I hated how [the MHA assessment] happened but I also think someone should have helped me before they did. No, I wouldn't have accepted help. But, yeah, I think they should have got it over and done with. That would have given me some of my life back. I do see a good point of the MHA.

'Sarah'

---

1. Guiding principles of the MHA

Use of the MHA requires that patients must be:

- **Protected** from harm and have their human rights recognised
- **Respected** for their qualities, including background, race, religion, gender and sexual orientation
- Treated in the **least restrictive** setting
- Communicated with, and enabled to **participate** in care-related decisions.

2. MHA 2007

In the 1990s, a number of high profile cases (e.g. Zito and Stone, Box 8.2, p42) triggered a review of the MHA, leading to the MHA 2007. This amends (but doesn't replace) both the MHA and MCA. Some of the key amendments were:

- *Definition of mental disorder*
  - Mental disorder was previously defined as mental illness, mental impairment (learning disability) and psychopathic disorder
  - It's now defined as *any disorder or disability of the mind*, more clearly including personality disorders.
- *'Appropriate Treatment' test*
  - Mental disorder previously needed to be 'treatable' in order to detain someone under s3 or s37.
  - Now, *appropriate* treatment must be available to alleviate or prevent the condition worsening – including nursing care, medication and psychological treatment. It's thought this also makes it clearer that people with personality disorders can be detained for treatment.
- *Nearest Relative (NR):*
  - Patients can now displace their NR if that person is unsuitable, e.g. estranged or abusive
- *Community Treatment Orders* (CTOs)
  - Can be applied to patients detained under s3 or s37, enforcing ongoing community treatment
- *Professional Roles:* see below.

3. Responsibilities under the MHA

There are many formal roles under the MHA (* indicates 2007 amendments)

- *Registered Medical Practitioner* (RMP)
  - Any doctor with a full GMC license to practice (i.e. *not* FY1 doctors)
  - RMPs can complete a s5(2).
- *Section 12 approved doctor*
  - RMP with extra MHA training, and approved as having special experience in the diagnosis and treatment of mental disorder
- *Second Opinion Appointed Doctor* (SOAD)
  - RMP appointed by the Care Quality Commission (CQC) to provide a statutory second opinion on medical treatment for detained patients
- *Approved Clinician** (AC)
  - Mental health professionals with specific competencies and AC training
  - Most commonly, consultant psychiatrists; increasingly nurses, psychologists, OTs or social workers

Table 15.1 Common civil sections.

Section	Purpose	Who does it apply to?	Who authorises it?	Do consent to treatment provisions apply?	Duration
s2	Compulsory detention in hospital for assessment (± treatment)	Person suffering from mental disorder of a nature or degree warranting detention in hospital for own health/safety, or risk to others	AMHP + 2 RMPs (1 must be s12 approved; 1 should have prior knowledge of the patient)	Yes: treatment can be given, even without consent.	Up to 28 days
s3	Compulsory detention in hospital for *treatment*	Ditto	Ditto	Yes	Up to 6 months; can then be renewed
s4	*Emergency* admission for assessment when a second RMP is unavailable	Ditto	AMHP + RMP	No	72h, during which time another RMP must assess for conversion to s2
s5(2)	Doctor's holding power of a previously informal inpatient (see p244). NB: Applies to inpatients on psychiatric or general hospital wards, but *not* ED or outpatients	Ditto	Ideally, the AC, though often a junior doctor (the AC's *nominated deputy*)	No	72h, to allow assessment for s2/s3
s5(4)	Nurse's holding power (equivalent of s5(2), but when a doctor is unavailable)	Ditto	A qualified mental health or LD nurse	No	6h, to allow assessment for s5(2)
s7	Guardianship A named guardian, either from the local authority or another person (e.g. a relative), can enforce conditions, including where the patient lives and *attendance* for medical treatment (but treatment can't be *enforced*).	Person aged 16 or over, with a mental disorder warranting reception into guardianship for their own welfare or the protection of others	AMHP + 2 RMPs (1 must be s12 approved)	No	Up to 6 months; can then be renewed
s17	Leave from hospital for detained patients. Conditions can include duration, whether escorted/ unescorted, and other things, e.g. adherence with drug testing.	Person detained under s2 or s3	RC	N/A	As long as someone is detained in hospital. A CTO must be considered for leave >7 days

(continued overleaf)

Table 15.1 Common civil sections. (*continued*)

Section	Purpose	Who does it apply to?	Who authorises it?	Do consent to treatment provisions apply?	Duration
s17A	Community Treatment Order (CTO) A community version of s3 or s37, requiring the patient meets specific conditions, e.g. home address, taking medication, attending for drug and alcohol testing. Patients *must* make themselves available to meet their RC (± SOAD) to consider extension of the CTO. Medication can't be *forced* in the community – but if the patient presents risk and needs to receive treatment, they can be recalled to hospital.	A patient detained under s3 or s37 (not s37/41) who doesn't need to be in hospital but continues to meet criteria for detention and is liable to be recalled.	RC + AMHP	Yes	6 months. A CTO only lasts as long as the patient's liable to be detained under s3, and can be renewed.
s135	Warrant allowing a police constable, accompanied by an AMHP and RMP, to enter an address and remove a person to a place of safety for further assessment. NB: The assessment often happens at the address where the warrant is executed.	Concerns that someone is suffering from a mental disorder and may be a risk to self or others	Magistrate (AMHP makes application)	No	Up to 72h in the place of safety
s136	A police constable can remove someone from a public place to a place of safety for assessment (see Ch.48) NB: s136 doesn't allow entry to a private address.	Someone who appears to be suffering from a mental disorder in a public place, and is thought to pose a risk to self/others.	A police officer	No	As per s135, but the assessment always occurs in the place of safety
s117	'Aftercare': a joint legal obligation for health and social services to provide free aftercare to people who've been detained under certain sections. This might include free accommodation, day centre support and prescriptions.	Anyone detained at anytime under S3, 37, 45(A), 47 or 48.	N/A	No	As long as support is needed around mental health problems (can be life-long).

- *Responsible Clinician* * (RC)
  - ○ AC responsible for a patient detained under the MHA or a CTO
  - ○ Informal patients don't have an RC
- *Approved Mental Health Professional* * (AMHP)
  - ○ Someone with appropriate mental health training and approved by the local authority
  - ○ Pronounced '*amp*'
  - ○ Usually social workers; sometimes nurses, psychologists or OTs
  - ○ Never doctors
- *Nearest Relative* (NR)
  - ○ Relative or friend with legal responsibilities under the MHA, e.g. the power to object to s3, or even discharge them from some sections
  - ○ Not necessarily the next-of-kin or a blood relative, e.g. includes six months as cohabiting partners; 5 years living together as flat mates; someone providing 'substantial care' but not living with the patient.
  - ○ Determined by a hierarchical list, starting with the patient's spouse/civil partner, then eldest adult child, eldest parent, sibling, grandparent ... Ask the AMHP!

TIP: The AMHP carries great power; the only other authorities that can remove someone's liberty are the police and courts – so carrying out the role lawfully with regard to the Mental Health Act and Human Rights Act isn't only crucial, but involves acting with moral integrity, considering the patient's best interests. The first and foremost safeguard of patients' rights is the AMHP's duty to consider the least restrictive alternatives to detention.

Amanda Foakes, AMHP

---

4. Consent to treatment

Consent to treatment law is complex and overlaps considerably with the MCA. In the MHA, consent to treatment issues are covered in Part IV and apply to patients detained under s2, 3, 37 and other forensic sections, but not the very short sections, e.g. s4, 5(2), 136 (Table 15.1). The following rules apply:

- Attempts must always be made to gain consent before giving any treatment
- Treatment can't be given to an objecting, informal patient who has capacity
- The MHA can't enforce treatment for a medical condition unless the condition is a cause or consequence of the mental disorder, e.g. feeding for anorexia nervosa; more controversially – treatment for self-harm. It also allows investigations relating to the mental disorder, e.g. clozapine blood tests.
- Patients covered by Part IV can be given appropriate medical treatment for their mental disorder for the first three months without their consent (or if they lack capacity to consent). Treatment can then only continue in 3 situations:
  - ○ *The patient consents and has capacity to do so.* If so, the RC documents this and completes a form T2, listing all agreed medications. A new T2 must be completed if medication is changed (including dose or route).
  - ○ *A SOAD is consulted and agrees the treatment is necessary.* The SOAD must examine the patient and discuss the case with a nurse and another involved, non-medical professional. The SOAD completes a form T3, specifying allowed treatment and doses. The RC can't override this.
  - ○ *It's an emergency.* Any RMP can authorise treatment *immediately necessary* to save the patient's life, prevent serious deterioration/suffering/violence. The RC should complete the s62 form, and ideally request a SOAD's review before starting emergency treatment.
- Certain treatments can only be given with the patient's consent and a SOAD's agreement, e.g. psychosurgery.

Before changing any medication (including PRN), check the patient's MHA status and whether their treatment is under T2 or T3. Document a capacity assessment and try to gain consent before starting new medication. If you're ever unsure, check with a senior doctor before prescribing.

Consent to treatment also applies to patients under CTOs. If consenting, the RC completes a CTO12 form; a SOAD's permission is needed to treat if objecting or lacking capacity. Note that they occasionally self-present to hospital and can be admitted informally, but if requiring detention, the RC must attend and recall them to hospital (up to 72h). If needing further treatment, the RC can revoke the CTO (with an AMHP's agreement), effectively restarting the previous inpatient s3 or s37.

PATIENT VIEW:

I remember when I was first sectioned. They said, "We need to put you in hospital." I said, "Not going!" Then they called the police. I said, "I'll go in voluntarily," and when I went into hospital and saw the doctor they put a Section 2 on me. I wasn't allowed out. I was so angry. It was the first time I'd ever been into hospital. Completely terrified. I didn't know why I was there or what was wrong with me.

'Fidel'

TIP: I sometimes feel frustrated by doctors using language which sounds as though the outcome of an MHA assessment is already decided, e.g. "Can you come and section Mr X?" It's only a little thing, but saying, "Could you come and complete a MHA assessment?" is much more appropriate.

Adella Habib, AMHP

The Mental Capacity Act 2005

The MCA provides a legal framework for treating people aged 16 or over, and lacking capacity to consent to treatment. It's generally viewed as empowering people, compared to the MHA, which is more restrictive. The MCA's guiding principles are:
- Mental capacity should always be **presumed** unless proven otherwise
- People should be **supported** to make their own decisions
- An **unwise decision** does not mean someone lacks capacity
- Anything done on behalf of someone lacking capacity must be
  ◦ In their **best interests**
  ◦ The **least restrictive** option with respect to their basic rights and freedoms.

The MCA provides a statutory test for mental capacity, and clarifies other issues, including:
- How to determine best interests
- Advanced decision making
- Lasting powers of attorney
- Powers of the Court of Protection
- Role of IMCAs (independent mental capacity advocates).

AMHPs are usually MCA experts and can advise in complicated situations.

1. Assessing capacity
To assess mental capacity, you must:
- Establish an impairment of, or disturbance in, the functioning of the mind or brain
- Check whether the person can:
  ◦ **Understand** the information relevant to the decision

- **Retain** that information
- **Use or weigh** that information as part of the decision-making process
- **Communicate** their decision (in speech, sign language or any other means).

Capacity isn't an all-or-nothing phenomenon but *is* decision and time specific. Detention under the MHA doesn't mean someone lacks capacity. Capacity assessments should be repeated at frequent intervals, and whenever offering a new treatment. See Ch.76 for details.

2. Deprivation of Liberty Safeguards (DoLS)

This is one of the most complex areas of the MCA, relating to authorised deprivation of liberty, e.g. being in hospital without leave or living in a care home and being restricted or receiving certain treatments. DoLS allows someone to be detained in hospital *or a care home* (unlike the MHA which only applies to hospitals). The following rules apply:

- The person must:
  - Not be detained (or liable for detention) under the MHA
  - Be 18 or over
  - Lack capacity with respect to the deprivation of liberty decision
  - Be under 'continuous supervision and control' *and* not free to leave, *if* they tried
- It must be in their best interests to be deprived of liberty

If it's appropriate to use the MHA, this should be used instead of the MCA – and this is the reason why relatively few people are detained in psychiatric hospitals under DoLS. Numbers may rise as the law becomes more familiar.

In order to detain someone under DoLS, a Mental Health Assessor (doctor) and Best Interests Assessor (usually an AMHP) must agree that the deprivation of liberty is necessary. Anyone subject to DoLS must have a representative, which can be an IMCA if they don't have a relative or carer. DoLS can remain in force for up to one year.

> **TIP:** Don't assume the patient wants what you want for them. 'Doctor knows best' – no matter how old fashioned in physical medicine – is especially unappreciated by patients in psychiatry. Far, far more of them have capacity to make decisions than we think on first impressions, and they are the experts in their own experience.
>
> Alex Langford, CT3

Treating children and young people

The law on treating young people is complex, so always involve CAMHS and AMHPs.
There are three important areas:

- Capacity
- Competence
- Parental Responsibility.

1. Capacity

The MCA applies to 16–17 year olds (excluding advance decisions or DoLS). Assessing capacity to make decisions around healthcare is the same as for adults.

2. Competence

Under-16s *can* make healthcare decisions, if Fraser/Gillick *competent.*

- Competence is assessed similarly to capacity, but under-16s are *not* automatically assumed to have competence, and it requires sufficient intelligence to fully understand a decision
  - Under-12s often don't have competence (unless they've significant experience of their health condition)
  - Over-14s are more often competent, depending on their cognitive and emotional maturity
- Decisions to refuse treatment are treated more seriously than those to accept, and the threshold for children to refuse may be higher than for adults

3. Parental Responsibility (PR)

In certain circumstances, people with *PR* can consent to treatment or informal admission for under-16s lacking competence (or 16–17 year olds lacking capacity).

- Consent through PR applies only within the *Scope of Parental Responsibility*, i.e. what a parent would reasonably be expected to do if acting in their child's best interests
  - A parent might reasonably set boundaries that their young child couldn't leave the house. So, you *could* keep a child on a ward under parental consent with reasonable methods, e.g. persuasion, distraction, or locking the door
  - One-off emergency rapid tranquilisation *might* be considered acceptable, but parental consent wouldn't be appropriate for repeated restraint, giving medication against a child's wishes, or holding them against their will for long periods
- Where the child can't make the decision *and* it falls outside the Scope of PR (e.g. decision isn't one a parent could reasonably make; parents lack capacity, or aren't acting in child's best interests):
  - Mental health treatment or admission to psychiatric unit: consider detention under the MHA
  - *Safety and protection (but not treatment):* provision of secure accommodation under Section 25 of the Children Act 1989
  - *Physical health treatment:* you can act in the child's best interests in emergencies, but may otherwise need to involve the courts.

The Human Rights Act 1998

The Human Rights Act (HRA) has 18 Articles, of which some are absolute, and some conditional on an absolute right also being engaged. Articles 2, 3, 5 and 8 have been the main focus of cases influencing mental health law, but the entirety of the Act must be considered in drawing up any new legislation. Table 15.2 summarises how legislation interacts, and how human rights are monitored in a system where people with mental illness are commonly detained.

PATIENT VIEW:

They sectioned me on the ward, then they said, "You stink" and they forcibly put me in the bath. Three female nurses, but as far as I was concerned, that was a sexual assault. They didn't give me a choice. Yeah, I probably did stink but if they'd have said to me, "Have a bath otherwise we'll make you." I would have had the bath.

'Grace'

Table 15.2 Relevance of The Human Rights Act to mental health law.

Article	Meaning	Application
2	*Right to Life*	Article 2 includes an obligation for authorities to prevent people in their care from committing suicide. This obligation is greater for detained patients but does apply to informal patients. Successful Article 2 cases have been brought by families of both detained and informal inpatients who committed suicide in hospital. It also imposes a duty to properly investigate any deaths or near-deaths in custody, which includes patients in hospital.
3	*Prohibition of torture and inhuman or degrading treatment or punishment*	Many cases have been brought under Article 3, arguing that various practices constitute inhuman or degrading treatment. These have typically failed, with the courts deciding that treatment like force-feeding and restraint don't constitute torture. The Court's view seems to be that the threshold to breach Article 3 is very high, and isn't reached when there's 'medical necessity'. However, there have been some cases where Article 3 breaches have been upheld, mainly involving lengthy segregation or lack of access to appropriate medical treatment whilst detained. The interpretation of Article 3 has been criticised by both professional and patient groups as holding the profession to a lower standard than should be expected.
5	*Right to liberty and security.* Article 5(4) states that anyone deprived of their liberty shall have the right to go before a court and have the court 'speedily' decide whether their detention is lawful – and order their release if not.	Article 5 is key to mental health legislation, and dictates the *criteria* for detention and evidence required to detain (or arrest) someone. Many Article 5 cases relate to Tribunals, and have resulted in changes to mental health legislation. A 2001 case showed that the wording of the MHA meant that patients had to prove the conditions of detention were no longer met. This was reversed to ensure the burden of proof was on the detaining authority, and the Tribunal *must* order release if not satisfied that the conditions for detention were *still* met. Tribunals must meet the *Winterwerp* criteria, i.e. must be of a 'judicial character', and allow the detainee to present their own case and challenge medical evidence. Article 5 is considered in cases pertaining to the MCA and DoLS and helps guide judgement. The 'Bournewood gap' resulted from a House of Lords judgement that non-objecting patients lacking capacity did not need to be detained under the MHA. This led to the question as to whether they were being deprived of their liberty. If so, Article 5 demands this is done under a clear legal framework, which resulted in the Deprivation of Liberty Safeguards (DoLS). This legislation has proven problematic, with an almost constant flow of case law altering the interpretation of statute. Following criticism from the House of Lords, it's expected to be substantially redrafted. Essentially Article 5 cases turn on closely following existing statute to deprive someone of their liberty – any deprivation outwith MHA/DoLS may constitute a breach.
8	*Right to respect for private and family life, including one's home and correspondence.* Includes the caveat that interference is lawful in some cases, e.g. to prevent crime, protect public health/ morals, and protect the rights and freedoms of others	Article 8 cases have been mainly brought from forensic hospitals, where telephone calls and correspondence, internet access and visits are subject to restrictions and monitoring based on risk assessment. These have generally failed due to the caveats in Article 8, and detaining authorities are only required to show that these restrictions are proportionate. Article 8 *did* change legislation by ruling it was an infringement of a detainee's rights to have their nearest relative informed, and resulted in the change to the MHA, allowing the detainee to apply to the courts to change their NR where there is a 'reasonable objection'. Article 8 includes an obligation on authorities to involve family and carers. There have been successful cases of Article 8 breaches where this has not happened adequately under both MHA and MCA.

Reference

Department of Health (2015) Mental Health Act 1983: Code of Practice. The Stationery Office, Norwich.

Further reading

Department for Constitutional Affairs (2007). Mental Capacity Act 2005 Code of Practice. The Stationery Office, Norwich.

Francis, R., Higgins, J. and Cassam, E. (2006) Report of the Independent Inquiry into the Care and Treatment of Michael Stone. South East Coast Strategic Health Authority, Kent County Council and Kent Probation Area.

Mental Health Law Online: a useful website explaining statute and particularly good for brief summaries of the cases which led to changes in the law: www.mentalhealthlaw.co.uk

Ministry of Justice (2008) Mental Capacity Act 2005: Deprivation of Liberty Safeguards: Code of Practice to Supplement the Main Mental Capacity Act 2005 Code of Practice. The Stationery Office, Norwich.

Ritchie J., Dick, D. and Lingham, R. (2004) The Report of the Inquiry Into the Care and Treatment of Christopher Clunis. HMSO, Norwich.

South London and Maudsley NHS Foundation Trust (2013). The Maze: A Practical Guide to the Mental Health Act 1983 (Amended 2007) 3rd edn. South London and Maudsley NHS Foundation Trust, London.

CHAPTER 16

Compliments, complaints and serious incidents

Anna M Burnside[1] and Sarah Stringer[2]

[1] *East London NHS Foundation Trust, London, England*
[2] *King's College London, London, England*

> **TIP:** Learn to be comfortable with your weaknesses, rather than showing off your strengths. For your team to recognise your limitations is a way to make you a better doctor.
>
> **Piers Newman, Family Therapist**

Hopefully, you'll mostly receive compliments for your hard work – especially after reading this book and fervently implementing its advice … However, complaints and Serious Incidents (SIs) happen to everyone at some time, and even experienced consultants find them upsetting and stressful.

Compliments

When people thank or compliment you, it's usually important to *them* to recognise something you've done. Don't undermine this by minimising your work (e.g. *It was nothing!*) – learn to accept praise, and thank people. Don't brag about compliments. Remember:
- Keep evidence (obscuring patient details) for your portfolio and 'bad' days …
  - E.g. cards, letters; store emails in an 'evidence' folder for easy access
- Include your team in thanks, when it's *not* all about you. Tell grateful relatives (etc) who else helped, then feedback praise to involved colleagues.
- Be wary if told you're the 'best'/'only' doctor to ever help or understand someone (Table 12.5, p80).

Never encourage or request gifts. Consider whether any gift could affect or *appear* to affect your practice/relationship with the patient (including in the eyes of other patients). Say thank you for cheap and ordinary presents; share food with your team. Politely decline, then discuss in supervision:
- Expensive gifts, money, cheques, gift vouchers
- Recurrent gifts – suggest the giver misunderstands/wants more from the relationship
- Anything the giver/their family may want back, e.g. once MSE settles
- Anything you'd feel awkward discussing in a team meeting
- Tickets to events – these erode your personal/professional boundaries (expect to 'bump into' the giver at that *One Direction* concert …)
- Suggestive gifts, e.g. the last Rolo™.

Psychiatry: Breaking the ICE – Introductions, Common Tasks and Emergencies for Trainees, First Edition.
Edited by Sarah Stringer, Juliet Hurn and Anna M Burnside.
© 2016 John Wiley & Sons, Ltd. Published 2016 by John Wiley & Sons, Ltd.
Companion Website: www.psychiatryice.com

If unsure, check:
- Trust guidance, e.g. nothing >£20; formally disclosing gifts
- GMC guidance: www.gmc-uk.org/guidance/ethical_guidance/21161.asp

Complaints

It's unlikely you'll receive a complaint directly, but if you do, discuss it with your consultant. Go through the notes and think honestly about:
- Things you may have done badly
- Things you could do differently next time
- Communication with the patient or team member – this often causes complaints.
  - Did you miss or misunderstand dynamics?
  - Could your language or body language have been misunderstood?
  - Are cultural or personality issues relevant?

Your consultant will help you decide how best to respond, depending on the nature and seriousness of the complaint. A written and/or face-to-face apology may help. If arranging a meeting:
- It's daunting, but often much easier than you'd imagine.
- Let the complainant bring a supporter, e.g. friend, carer, advocate; union representative for colleagues
- You must also have someone with you, e.g. your team manager
- Thank them for coming in – it takes courage for people to raise complaints
- Let them fully explain their grievance. Make notes and prompt until they've nothing more to add.
- Apologise for your mistakes and anything you've done to upset or offend them
- Address their points in turn
- Before the end of the meeting, check whether they have any other issues.
- Tell them what will happen next, e.g. you can write a letter to summarise the meeting
- Give details of the Trust's complaints procedure, if they wish to take it further.

More serious complaints (e.g. of sexual assault) require formal investigation, either by your consultant or an external investigator. Contact your medical indemnity provider immediately for advice. Your consultant should support you through the process, however hard it may be.

Serious incidents

An SI is an incident occurring within NHS care, resulting in:
- Unexpected or avoidable death
- Serious harm
- Allegations of abuse
- A threat to a service's ability to deliver healthcare
- Adverse media coverage or public concern.

Your Trust's Risk Management Department (or similar) will deal with SIs. They'll inform you of an SI if you didn't already know, and guide you through the internal enquiry process. A panel will be formed which usually includes a Risk Management Department representative, an independent Trust consultant, and a non-medical health professional. An external investigation may take place if the incident's very serious (e.g. homicide), or the Trust's investigation is considered unsatisfactory.

If you had contact with the patient, you may be asked to submit a report or attend an interview. This is a fact-finding exercise, and nobody is *blaming* you.
- Discuss the incident with your consultant and seek their support throughout
- If the incident was traumatic, you can access counselling through your Trust or GP
- Respond to SI emails swiftly and courteously
- Read the patient's notes and reflect on your role
  - Could you have done anything better?

- It's unlikely you'll have contact with the patient or relatives during this process, as the panel usually handles this
- If asked to attend an interview, dress smartly and arrive promptly
  - You can refer to the patient record and any notes you've made
  - Answer questions factually, politely and openly
  - If you don't know something, say so
- The investigation's outcome will be reported to your team. If you've moved on by then, return for this meeting if possible.
  - It aims to disseminate learning points to change practice.

If your Trust offers Root Cause Analysis training, undertake it and apply the learning to minor incidents you spot in everyday practice. Remember, one day you may be the SI's investigating consultant, so this is all useful practice.

TIP: People respect you more when you can honestly say:
- *I made a mistake there – I'm sorry*
- *I don't know*
- *What do you think about this?*
- *How do you think I could have done it differently?*
- *I'm not sure, but I'll find out.*

Research clearly shows that being aware of – and able to tolerate – the reality of yourself as a fallible clinician, will make you safer, more effective and more popular with patients and colleagues.

Nicola Gawn, Clinical Psychologist

Further reading

National framework for reporting and learning from serious incidents requiring investigation, NPSA, March 2010, available at: www.nrls.npsa.nhs.uk/resources/?entryid45=75173

The National Patient Safety Agency *Medical Error, a Guide for Junior Doctors*, available at: www.nrls.npsa.nhs.uk/juniordoctors/

CHAPTER 17

Training in psychiatry

Mujtaba Husain[1], Juliet Hurn[1], Rachel Thomasson[2], Christina Barras[3], Rory Conn[4], Laurine Hanna[1], and Sarah Stringer[5]

[1] South London & Maudsley NHS Foundation Trust, London, England
[2] Manchester Royal Infirmary, Manchester, Lancashire, England
[3] South West London & St George's Mental Health NHS Trust, London, England
[4] Tavistock and Portman NHS Foundation Trust, London, England
[5] King's College London, London, England

PATIENT VIEW:

There's two ways of looking at doctors in training. You lose the good ones, but you're not stuck with the bad ones for too long. The problem is though, either way, you have to reboot that rapport and it takes you a good few sessions before you're likely to.

'Beth'

Training Basics

This is a brief guide to get the most out of your placement, whatever your intended career. The Further Reading section points you to more detailed, specific and up-to-date resources.

TIP: Psychiatry may be a step along a career path elsewhere, and a psychiatry rotation is a goldmine for learning skills you won't encounter elsewhere, but will need in your day-to-day work.

Jocelyn Cherry, Academic Paediatric Ophthalmology SHO

---

1. Supervision

TIP: When the going gets tough, the tough get supervised.

Gwen Adshead, Forensic Consultant

All trainees receive weekly, hour-long supervision with their consultant (Clinical Supervisor). This should be marked as a regular, protected time-slot on your timetable – if you can't see it, ask. Good supervision is useful and enjoyable; bad supervision is a terrible waste of time. You and your supervisor are jointly responsible for ensuring the time's well spent.

A good supervisor sets the agenda with you at the start of a session, encouraging you to suggest topics, then adding things they think are important for your development. Think about what you'd like to cover *before* attending each week, e.g.

- Specific topics, e.g. early sessions might include history-taking/MSE advice, prescribing, or writing discharge summaries
- Personal Development Plan (PDP) and Workplace-based assessments (WPBAs) – see below
- Detailed discussion of complex or challenging patients
- Issues related to your team, service or difficulties while on-call
- Personal and professional issues affecting your ability to work, e.g. conflicts, stress, time management.
- Careers advice/planning.

There are common pitfalls. Supervision is *not* meant for:

- A general chat, e.g. the weather, football results, office gossip
- Updating your consultant on every patient on your list – this should be done in ward rounds/team meetings
- *Only* discussing clinical cases *or* non-clinical work *or* doing WPBAs
- Your supervisor dumping a list of jobs on you
- Free psychotherapy.

Different supervisors have different styles; offer gentle steering if your needs aren't being met.

2. PDPs

In the first or second week, set placement goals, and make a plan for achieving these with your supervisor. Each item on your PDP should relate to competencies in your curriculum (UK Foundation Programme or your Royal College's website).

> **TIP:** I ask myself three questions when mapping the PDP:
> - *1. What are my specific training needs?*
>   - I use the 18 Intended Learning Outcomes from the RCPsych curriculum, available via:
>   - www.rcpsych.ac.uk
>   - I write these in my own words as personal objectives for the year
> - *2. How will I tackle these objectives?*
>   - I write a short plan for each objective, e.g. assessing patients under senior supervision and proactively gaining feedback on technique
> - *3. How will I show I've met the learning objective?*
>   - WPBAs in a range of settings
>   - Written reflections on what went well/could improve
>   - Further reading on specific areas, e.g. transcultural psychiatry.
>
> Together, my objectives cover clinical skills, teaching, leadership, clinical governance, research, and personal qualities, e.g. team working, self-reflection. This prevents gaps and shows how different pieces of evidence map to different learning outcomes.
>
> **Manchester Trainee**

Your plan might include spending time with another team, getting feedback from a range of seniors, or attending a conference or teaching event. You're more likely to meet goals you agree at the start and review regularly.

3. WPBAs

It's easy to see WPBAs as a tick-box exercise, and if you treat them like that, that's all they'll ever be. The word *assessment* is a bit of a red herring: whilst they've assessment elements, WPBAs are most important as *feedback* tools. Good feedback is the most effective way to develop your knowledge, skills and attitude as a doctor. To make the most of WPBAs:

- Don't just use colleagues who only give 'nice' feedback
- Get WPBAs from different doctors and senior colleagues, e.g. nurses, social workers and psychologists. Non-medic feedback is just as valuable, and often picks up different issues.
- Spread WPBAs across your placement. It's stressful chasing people for WPBAs at the end of your job, and they're too late to improve anything.
- Get face-to-face feedback immediately after assessing or presenting a patient. Requesting an online WPBA a week later may irritate seniors and teaches very little.
- If you feel feedback isn't detailed enough or doesn't address what you could do differently, say so.

TIP: Whether or not your Trust offers a formal mentoring scheme, find a CT2 or CT3 to mentor you. They'll provide more than a friendly face over a cup of coffee – helping you navigate the practical and emotional challenges of your clinical work, as well as all the additional tasks which make up training, e.g. how to set up your psychotherapy patient, apply for exams, choose exam revision courses, keep on top of Journal Club presentations...

Lizzie Hunt, ST4

4. Psychiatrists in training

If you're a psychiatry CT1, there are a few extra things:
- Read the curriculum in your first fortnight
- Record your learning in the e-portfolio from day one. It'll give you a better training experience and prevent meltdown before your Annual Review of Competence Progression (ARCP).
- Attend the local MRCPsych course. This covers skills and knowledge for clinical practice and exams
- You'll sit the MRCPsych exams over the next three years. There are currently:
  - Two written papers
    - Paper A = scientific and theoretical basis of psychiatry
    - Paper B = critical review and clinical topics
  - A practical exam, the Clinical Assessment of Skills and Competencies (CASC)
- You'll hopefully belong to a Case Based Discussion ('Balint') group, where you'll discuss clinical experiences with other trainees and a senior practitioner. It's a useful introduction to psychotherapy *and* a space to think about the doctor-patient relationship.
- You'll complete two psychotherapy cases, usually in your second or third year.

Check www.rcpsych.ac.uk for current information, including your MRCPsych exam dates and training requirements.

TIP: MRCPsych Exams – I can't emphasise enough the importance of doing questions. And once you've done all the questions – do them again! As for the CASC, it's more important to be relaxed, and deal with the entire exam experience, than learning more lists of things the night before the exam.

Thom Proven, ST4

TIP: Psychiatric training has unique challenges that are quite difficult to share with people who aren't doing it. What I found most useful was the people I was training with – some of whom are still my best friends today. Having a group of people with whom you can talk, drink, rant about the difficulties of the training and the injustice of the universe, is essential to survive this quite complicated period and deal with the steep learning curve ahead.

Anastasia Apostolou, Psychotherapy ST5

Training – next steps

Being a good doctor is more than just face-to-face patient care. Once you've settled into the clinical work, it's time to think about your wider expertise:
- Teaching
- Leadership and management
- Research.

By the time you're a consultant, you'll feel clinically confident, but *won't* magically know how to do this other work – so start developing skills as a trainee.

> **TIP:** Find a mentor or two or three to guide you: one clinical, one academic and one to whom it appears work is a hobby. Balance of approach to your career is important.
>
> **Angus Brown, Consultant Liaison Psychiatrist**

> **TIP:** Something happens when doctors move into the senior ranks and particularly when they become consultants and sometimes a new arrogance can get in the way of communication with people they previously had good working relations with. So, when you reach the lofty heights of consultant, please don't change.
>
> **Cathi Francis, Business Manager**

1. Teaching

All doctors are teachers, though none are born excellent – it takes effort, training, feedback and reflection. You may feel you know too little to teach anyone *anything*, but you've actually got a lot to offer, whether it's explaining psychotherapy to patients, presenting at a grand round, providing medical student bedside teaching or feedback to a colleague. The first step is offering to teach. Your consultant should know about:
- Medical students' timetables
- Team teaching needs/opportunities
- Formal teaching programmes you might join
- Opportunities to observe experienced teachers in action.

Teaching Tips

Teaching is more complex than simply transmitting information from a teacher to a learner. Table 17.1's tips may help, whoever your audience.

Feedback and reflection

Use feedback to check what students thought of your teaching: do more of what worked and less of what didn't.
- *1-minute paper*
  - Give everyone a small piece of paper and 1 minute to write the best thing about your teaching on one side, and something for you to improve on the other
  - Likely to get responses from all learners, but lacks detail
- *Core Trainees' Guide to Clinical Teaching with Medical Students in Psychiatry*
  - See Resources
  - More detailed feedback form; takes longer

Table 17.1 Teaching basics.

Do	• Check what learners already know and what they want to know
	• Start by explaining what you want them to understand or be able to do by the end (set 'learning objectives')
	• End by checking they've met objectives and get them to summarise key points
	• Emulate your favourite teachers, adding your own personality
	• Change the stimulus every 10–15 minutes to keep attention high, e.g.
	  ◦ Role-plays, diagrams, pair/group work, debates, case studies, clinical anecdotes, videos …
	• Remember that less is often more
	• Respect and be interested in your learners. Be clear that there are no 'stupid' questions
	• Interact: ask questions, encourage questions and discussion
	• Be creative and remember people may need information presented in multiple ways
	• Role model acceptable behaviour
	• Use enthusiasm, humour, praise and encouragement
	• Deal with trouble-makers:
	  ◦ Make eye contact
	  ◦ Move closer
	  ◦ Direct questions their way
	  ◦ Politely ask them to stop whatever's annoying you
	  ◦ If needed, keep them behind to discuss the problem afterwards.
	• Know your subject – prepare beforehand, but don't be afraid to say when you don't know
	  ◦ You/learners can research the answer for the next session
	• Chunk information and check everyone's understood before moving on to the next point

Don't	• Emulate teachers you hated
	• Teach people what they already know
	• Patronise, humiliate or make fun of learners
	• Bore people: hour-long monologues or Powerpoint presentations are sedative
	• Overlook quiet or shy students. Gently involve them:
	  ◦ Make eye contact and smile
	  ◦ Use their names
	  ◦ Offer them easy questions or small group work
	• Let a single, keen student dominate a group session
	  ◦ Try, *That's brilliant [Name]. Now I want to find out what everyone else thinks …*
	• Run over time.
	  ◦ Learners won't retain the extra material
	  ◦ Students may be in trouble if late for their next clinic

- *Peer observation*
  - Ask another trainee to observe your teaching and give feedback
- *Assessment of Teaching (AoT)*
  - WPBA for seniors to formally assess your teaching
  - Helps you demonstrate teaching competencies and improves your teaching through constructive feedback, reflection and goal-setting
  - Try to find an assessor with medical education expertise.

Remember, there's no point getting feedback unless you reflect and act on it. All feedback and reflection can pad out your portfolio.

Further development

If you want to develop your teaching further, see your Deanery's website for options, or:

* *Teaching The Teachers* courses
  * Offered by many universities and Trusts
  * Provide education theory and practical advice to improve teaching
* *Medical education organisations*
  * Provide training, resources, courses and conferences
  * E.g. The Association For The Study of Medical Education (ASME), The Association for Medical Education in Europe (AMEE).

2. Leadership and management

Leadership and management can seem intimidating. You might worry you could never be a leader; that it would be arrogant to try; or that management suggests a 'dark side'. In reality, leadership is about values, attitudes and being the kind of doctor you'd want on your team or treating your family. All doctors are managers: we manage teams and services and are responsible for the quality of care our patients receive.

The NHS and psychiatric services: key themes

The political and financial context of psychiatry can seem overwhelming, so we'll start with a bite-size overview of the key themes. By understanding what's going on, you may feel more confident to change things *through* leadership and management.

Resource allocation

We're currently in a period of cuts rather than expansion. Many argue that psychiatric cuts highlight chronic underfunding, relative to physical health (lack of "parity") – due to stigma. You'll find under-resourcing everywhere, and the arrival of new referrals and pressures to discharge can seem relentless. You may want to understand how to best use resources (e.g. by learning about 'lean' service development), or get involved in addressing stigma (e.g. via the Time to Change campaign).

Commissioning

This is the planning and purchasing of NHS services from providers (e.g. NHS Trusts) to meet the local population's needs. It is currently done by Clinical Commissioning Groups (CCGs), giving commissioning power to clinicians, particularly GPs. This offers the opportunity to strengthen links between psychiatry and primary care, e.g. by developing psychiatric clinics embedded in GP practices. A current commissioning trend is the increased provision by non-NHS providers, whether *independent* (private) or *third sector* (voluntary).

Payment systems

Traditionally, commissioners paid providers a fixed amount for services, whatever the amount of work done (*block contracting*). *Payment by results (PbR)* aims to increase service efficiency by rewarding activity. Debate continues about the feasibility of PbR in psychiatry, but you'll notice increasing emphasis on:

* Outcome measures, e.g. Health of the Nation Outcome Scales (HONOS) – rates symptoms and problems, often linked to PbR. HONOS is usually completed at initial assessment, transfer between services, and discharge.
* Clustering – grouping patients according to resource needs. *Tariffs* are the set prices paid for each unit of healthcare; units are known as *currencies.*

Quality of care

The Francis report highlighted the failings of care in Mid Staffordshire NHS Foundation Trust. In psychiatric services, further reports (e.g. Schizophrenia Commission, National Audit of Schizophrenia) have pointed to shortcomings, for example, in service user involvement and standards of physical healthcare. Your Trust will be under pressure to meet targets, and will be reviewed by the quality regulator, the Care Quality Commission (CQC). You can directly contribute to quality of care through audits and Quality Improvement Projects – endearing yourself to your seniors.

Location of services

Recent trends have seen physical healthcare move from secondary to primary care, and from general hospitals to specialist centres. Mental health has had its own parallels, moving care from asylums to the community in the late 20th century, and more recently emphasising GP-led care of manageable mental illnesses. You may play a part in this, e.g. by visiting GP practices to offer education or advice on patients.

Getting involved

You've many options for building leadership and management experience.
- *Audits and Quality Improvement Projects:* aim to complete an audit per job (Box 17.1)
- *Trainee representation:* most Trusts have trainees' committees, which are a great introduction and can provide opportunities for Deanery, Local Education, Training Board or national representation
- *Management roles in your team*, e.g. arrange learning events, update local guidance policies or trial new initiatives
- *College resources*, e.g. the RCPsych has a Leadership and Management Study Guide on its website and runs an excellent Leadership and Management Conference
- *Connect with clinical managers and leaders*, e.g. follow them on Twitter; ask to shadow them to learn about their role and make new contacts
- *Check out the Leader Academy* (the Edward Jenner Programme is a good trainee-level course)
  ○ www.leadershipacademy.nhs.uk/grow/professional-leadership-programmes/
- *Use the Medical Leadership Competency Framework* (MLCF). This describes:
  ○ Competences needed to become more actively involved in planning, delivering and improving services
  ○ How to attain these
  ○ How to assess yourself in these areas.
- *Join the Faculty of Medical Leadership and Management.* This has a thriving trainee membership and provides resources, conferences and events.
- *The King's Fund* and *Nuffield Trust* provide events and resources, e.g. research, news and reports
- *The Health Service Journal* covers current NHS management issues.

Box 17.1 Audits

- Choose topics which matter, but are small enough to complete within your post:
  ○ Risk, patient satisfaction or outcomes – most likely to lead to satisfying changes
  ○ Documentation quality – straightforward and quick
- Make sure your audit leads to change by completing the audit cycle
- For ideas:
  ○ Ask your consultant, team manager, and other colleagues for areas needing improvement
  ○ Read national guidelines/publications, e.g. NICE, National Schizophrenia Audit
  ○ *Recipes for Audit in Psychiatry* – Oakley et al, 2011
- Most Trusts have a quality improvement group where you can get advice on registering audits and getting them off the ground. They'll tell you if similar audits have been done, and how to access reports.
- Use a team meeting slot to present your audit and findings
- If you can't complete the audit cycle in the post, think about coming back to do it (your successor may be keen to assist).
- Find other forums to present your findings, e.g. Trust audit meeting, RCPsych International Congress poster presentation.

TIP: Never expect your organisation to care for you. The *people* around you will care (especially if you care for them), but the organisation only sees you as something that does or doesn't work.

Phil Timms, Consultant

3. Research

As a CT, you probably won't run a double-blind, multi-centre randomized control trial, but there are always opportunities to undertake research.

Why?

There are many benefits to getting involved with research:
- In-depth knowledge in your field of study
- Understanding the research process
- Skills: data collection/handling, team-working, problem-solving, formal writing
- Critical appraisal skills (currently tested in the MRCPsych Paper B exam)
- Improved clinical use of evidence-based medicine.

It's never a bad thing to have a publication on your CV, and improves your chances of gaining ST and consultant posts.

How?

If your consultant or academic department undertake research, simply ask how you can help. Alternatively, every training programme has a Research Tutor who can:
- Discuss your research idea, e.g. whether practical, useful, or already being done by another team
- Suggest a supervisor
- Suggest relevant courses (Trust, affiliated university or academic department), e.g.
  - Quantitative/qualitative research methodology
  - Computer literacy, e.g. the European Computer Driving Licence
  - Data handling
  - Ethics, e.g. www.crn.nihr.ac.uk/learning-development/good-clinical-practice/
- Connect you with people for data handling help, e.g. statisticians.

Whether you're developing a new idea or joining an existing team, check you have everything listed in Table 17.2.

The final steps are the write-up and publication. Your supervisor should guide you towards the most appropriate peer-reviewed journal for publication. Think about the *impact factor* (measure of the number of citations to recent articles) as a proxy marker of the journal's importance, but be realistic: the Lancet probably won't give you a 10-page spread on spider naevi in people with OCD.
- Stick to the journal's submission criteria exactly when writing up your research, or you'll be rejected, no matter how fabulous your work
- Run drafts past your supervisor and trusted colleagues. Ask them to be as critical as possible, since this saves embarrassing critiques from the journal.
- Once submitted, your paper will be reviewed by two to three experts, and returned after a few *months*, hopefully recommending changes for publication
- If rejected, choose another journal and submit from scratch.

Once accepted, you may wait 6–12 months before publication, leaving plenty of time to remind yourself how it feels to have a life.

Taking it further

If you've enjoyed the research process, you may want to consider further opportunities.
- *Wellcome Trust Clinical Research Fellowship*
  - Funding for two to three years for clinicians entering the early stages of research
  - Research may lead to a diploma, MSc or PhD (only covers research expenses)

Table 17.2 Research essentials.

You need …	Reason and comments
An interesting question	Research drags if not clinically, educationally or ethically interesting
A good supervisor	• Choose an expert in your area of research and methodology • Beware the hands-off, name-on supervisor who wants you to produce papers *for* them – this is unfair and unethical. • Although you *can't* guarantee how the project will evolve, try to agree goal(s) in advance, e.g. gaining skills; poster presentation; journal publication; pilot data for future research
To have performed or read the literature review	• What's already known? • What requires confirmation? • Which questions still need answering? • Embrace research addressing controversial findings or new questions • Avoid replicating well-established results. A good literature review stops you reinventing the wheel
A clear research question/hypothesis	• Make sure you understand this if joining a team • If writing your own, your supervisor should help ensure it's simple and manageable for your timeframe. • Check it's a *SMART goal* (p72)
A clear role	• In joint ventures, clarify your role, and whether this will meet your goals. • Don't join projects where months of toil become a footnote in the acknowledgements
Ethics approval	• If joining an existing project, read the approved ethics application to understand this process and how successive revisions passed panel. • If leading your own project, ask your Trust's Research and Development Department for advice on the relevant forms and deadlines for panel reviews. Your supervisor should help you complete the forms and ensure you're not missing anything obvious, e.g. confidentiality/anonymity, consent, data storage
Funding	• If joining a team, check that you're comfortable with the source(s) of funding, e.g. are drug companies involved? • Your own research is likely to be self-funded, so think about costs of travel, interview venues, equipment or incentives for participation. • Your supervisor or Research Tutor may know of funds in the Trust, affiliated university or local charities
Realism	• Conducting research can be grueling, frustrating and repetitive • Set time aside, whilst maintaining your social life for a sense of balance • It's likely to take at least a year to complete even a simple project, though writing systematic reviews or analysing an existing dataset are quicker

- *Academic Clinical Fellowship (ACF) post*
  - Scheme run by the NHS Institute for Health Research
  - 25% of your training is spent in protected research time; the rest is clinical
  - Entry is usually during core training or the early part of higher training
  - Competition is fierce. Most deaneries offer one to two slots, per specialty, per year.
  - Deaneries organize the research time in different ways, e.g. three to six month blocks/1 day a week throughout a three-year fellowship
  - The scheme includes a research training programme, e.g. workshops around project design, statistical analysis, grant applications and scientific writing
  - There's a general expectation that the project you undertake will lead to a PhD application, but this isn't mandatory.

As a higher trainee, you might use your Special Interest sessions for medical education, leadership or research, e.g. undertaking a certificate, diploma, masters. There are also opportunities to take Out Of Programme Experience (OOPEs), e.g. a Fellowship in medical education or leadership, or a full-time research post.

TIP: Medical training doesn't have to be a conveyor belt, with your life neatly planned out. Take time out, develop yourself personally. Find out what your deanery offers in terms of OOPEs, etc. Although MBBS, then training, RCPsych Membership and even consultant status are fantastic achievements in their own right, it's about the journey, not the destination. Fulfilment and satisfaction aren't always the same as clinical and academic accolades.

Robin Wilson, ST6

TIP: I think enjoyment of autobiographies/biographies is a good proxy marker for being suited to a career in psychiatry. If you can't enjoy an autobiography, it's probably not for you.

Sharon Brown, Consultant

Further reading

The Mid Staffordshire NHS Foundation Trust Public Inquiry (2013) The report of the Mid Staffordshire NHS Foundation Trust Public Inquiry. The Stationery Office, Norwich.

Curriculum, training, exams information and more:

http://www.rcpsych.ac.uk/specialtytraining.aspx
Dearman, S.P., Joiner, A.B., Abbott, S. and Longson, D. (2014) *Passing the ARCP: Successful Portfolio-Based Learning*, RCPsych Publications, London.

Teaching information:

McKimm, J. and Swanwick, T. (2010) *Clinical Teaching Made Easy: A Practical Guide to Teaching and Learning in Clinical Settings*. Quay Books, London.
Impey, M., Bennett D., Casanova Dias, M., Lydall, G., McKinnon, I., Masson, N. and Simmons, M. (2009) *Core Trainees' Guide to Clinical Teaching with Medical Students in Psychiatry*. Royal College of Psychiatrists, London.

Management:

Brittlebank, A., Briel, R., Richardson, J., Swann, A., Thakur, A. and Whaley, J. (2012). *Leadership and Management Study Guide: for Higher Trainees in Psychiatry*. Occasional paper OP80. Royal College of Psychiatrists, London.
NHS England (2014) Understanding the New NHS. NHS England, London
Davies P. *The Concise NHS Handbook 2013/14*. NHS Confederation. 2014.
Whistleblowing Hotline for NHS staff 0800 0724725

Research:

The International Committee of Medical Journal Editors – useful information on authorship and preparing manuscripts: http://www.icmje.org/
Wellcome fellowships:
www.wellcome.ac.uk/Funding/Biomedical-science/Funding-schemes/Fellowships/Clinical-fellowships/
   wtd004435.htm
ACF posts:
www.nihrtcc.nhs.uk/intetacatrain/rtp
http://careers.bmj.com/careers/advice/view-article.html?doi=10.1136/bmj.g4415

PART II
Common tasks

CHAPTER 18

Outpatient clinics

Christina Barras[1], Rory Conn[2], and Laurine Hanna[3]

[1] South West London & St George's Mental Health NHS Trust, London, England
[2] Tavistock and Portman NHS Foundation Trust, London, England
[3] South London & Maudsley NHS Foundation Trust, London, England

---

RELATED CHAPTERS: Care Programme Approach (CPAs) (19), home visits (20)

Your consultant hands you a dictaphone and tapes: you have an outpatient clinic tomorrow morning.

Reviews happen in various settings: patients' homes, the team base, and even GP surgeries. You may have a traditional *outpatient clinic*, where you regularly see a list of patients, with or without their Care Coordinators (CCs).

Preparation

1. Consultant
- Consider shadowing them or asking them to sit in on your first clinic
- How involved do they want to be?
  - E.g. discuss every patient/only those you're unsure about
- Typical follow-up timeframes
- Can you discharge people? (Ch.33)
- Documentation, e.g. *immediate* event, GP letter, medication record, risk assessment, outcome scores
- Policy on latecomers (to include in appointment letters), e.g. if >15 minutes late, should you ask patients to rebook or wait until the next gap/end of clinic, rather than making *everyone* wait?

2. Administrator
- Can you dictate letters? (Box 18.1)
  - How long does typing take? (Urgent letters need special arrangements)
  - How will you make amendments? (Paper or email drafts)
- How do colleagues access your diary?
- How do you arrange follow-ups?

Psychiatry: Breaking the ICE – Introductions, Common Tasks and Emergencies for Trainees, First Edition.
Edited by Sarah Stringer, Juliet Hurn and Anna M Burnside.
© 2016 John Wiley & Sons, Ltd. Published 2016 by John Wiley & Sons, Ltd.
Companion Website: www.psychiatryice.com

3. Your team
If the CCs or administrator enter appointments on your online diary, discuss the time needed for appointments, e.g.
- Reviews: 0.5h
- CPAs: 1h
- New assessments: 1–1.5h
- *Double* times when using interpreters

4. Prepare your clinic
Find out where your clinic is, and block out time in your diary:
- Leave and teaching
- Admin time, e.g.
  - 0.5–1h before a clinic (read background notes)
  - 1h after/admin morning or afternoon (letters and related tasks).

Collect resources in a folder, locked drawer ± hard drive:
- Referral forms, useful phone numbers (Appendix F)
- Patient information leaflets (PILs)
- Prescription pad ± charts
- British National Formulary (BNF) ± *Maudsley Prescribing Guidelines*
- Investigation request forms, phlebotomy service details
- ±Dictaphone, tapes.

PATIENT VIEW:

If it's a first meeting with a new psychiatrist, probably best to spend at least an hour to get to know you. After that, half an hour each time. I know resources are tight but this is people's lives. They *don't* make you all better, but having a psychiatrist who listens, helps and supports you in keeping stable, that would be a good start.

'Wendy'

During

1. Time management
Set the agenda. Ask how the *patient* wants to use the time, then say what you'd like to cover.
- Explain time constraints and negotiate how the session should run, e.g. 10 minutes on medications, 15 minutes on housing
- Be realistic: you can't solve everything at once
- Start wrapping up five to ten minutes before the end: summarise and outline the plan
- Book a speedy follow-up appointment if you haven't covered key issues, or need to seek advice
- If certain people always take more time, consider lengthening their appointments

2. Make notes
No matter how brilliant your memory, you'll struggle to write accurate letters without keeping notes, especially when dictation or typing are delayed.

3. Be useful
Make every review useful. Patients can obediently languish in clinics for years without clear reason, so avoid 'junior doctor inertia' – don't automatically review people every 3–6 months without specific needs. Clarify why they're attending:
- Period of assessment/MSE review, e.g. spotting early relapse
- Active management e.g. medication change; social intervention
- Patient issues, e.g. *My care coordinator doesn't understand me/I'm lonely …*
- Your issues, e.g. anxiety; seeing 'favourite' patients; needing to be needed …

If assessment/management are the focus, explain and document a reasonable timescale (SMART goals, p72). Review this frequently ± handover to your successor to keep plans active. Address other reasons for appointments with your team, and consider non-medical ways to meet needs, e.g. help lonely people find a social network. If somebody needs frequent appointments, they may require a CC (if they have one, check what's happening in *their* contacts).

Book timely follow-ups. Six-monthly appointments suggest you're doing little to help, but should address team/patient fears around discharge.

PATIENT VIEW:

The junior doctor was very good, she helped me a lot: wrote letters for me and really seemed to go the extra mile ... Very good at explaining the medication. I was really, really frightened they were going to drug me senseless, so I was really glad of that explanation and she gave me leaflets and things.

'Stacey'

After

- Organise your notes
- Deal with immediate tasks, e.g. referrals, telephone calls
- Dictate (Box 18.1)/type letters as soon as possible.

Box 18.1 Dictation etiquette

Dictation is harder than typing initially, but worth learning if you have access to it.
- Find a quiet room
- Speak clearly and slightly slower than usual
- Don't eat, drink or chew gum (they add unpleasant and distracting sound effects!)
- Say hello and thank the typist at the start. Rewind the tape and check you can clearly hear this, before continuing.
- State clinic date
- For each patient, state:
  - The recipient (add address if not easily accessed)
  - Patient's full name, date of birth, address
- Pause the tape when thinking, yawning, coughing, sneezing ...
- If you make a mistake, rewind and tape over it
- State punctuation or style, e.g. *Full stop. New paragraph. New heading in bold: Plan.*
- Pin a phonetic alphabet on your wall and 'spell' medications and medical words, e.g. ABC = Alpha, Bravo, Charlie.
- Enunciate easily confused words extra clearly, e.g. Hypo/hyper; sixteen/sixty
- Letter endings:
  - Add a closing remark, e.g. *Please do not hesitate to contact me, should you require further information.*
  - *Yours faithfully* – if you started *Dear Sir/Madam*
  - *Yours sincerely* – if you started with a formal name, e.g. *Dear Dr Hurn*
  - *Kind regards* or *Best wishes* – if writing less formally, e.g. Dear Juliet
  - State if it should be copied to anyone (include names and addresses)
  - State any enclosures, e.g. reports/results you'd like included
- Thank the typist at the end of the tape.

The administrator should send you drafts to check before posting letters – these often include '_____' for words they couldn't make out. Keep your notes until then, in case you can't remember what you said. Ask the typist for feedback on your dictation, and give feedback (sensitively) on recurrent problems.

What If ... ?

... They do not attend (DNA)?

Don't just send another wasted appointment slot. Consider *why* someone isn't attending, e.g. they're angry with you/relapsing/moved house so didn't get the appointment letter. Check your local DNA policy, but think flexibly, e.g. *three DNAs = discharge* isn't safe or useful if disengagement signals relapse.

- Get information: notes; contact patient, relatives, GP
  ◦ New or longstanding DNA?
  ◦ Risks
  ◦ Barriers to attendance
  ◦ Recent concerns/contact with GP?
- If they don't *want* to come anymore, consider discharge *or* need for assertive follow-up
- Address reasons for non-attendance and consider offering a *better* appointment, e.g. early morning if drinking alcohol; afternoon if sedative medications; home visit if housebound
- If you're worried/can't contact them, discuss with your team and consider an urgent home visit (Ch.20)
- Don't get frustrated – use the time for admin, audits or seeing the next patient early.

Take-home Message

Organisation makes the difference between an efficient, useful clinic, and a weekly nightmare.

CHAPTER 19

Care programme approach (CPA) meetings

Abigail G Crutchlow[1], Christina Barras[2], Rory Conn[3], and Laurine Hanna[1]

[1] South London & Maudsley NHS Foundation Trust, London, England
[2] South West London & St George's Mental Health NHS Trust, London, England
[3] Tavistock and Portman NHS Foundation Trust, London, England

RELATED CHAPTERS: Outpatient clinics (18), home visits (20); watch Video 6 to see a discharge CPA in action

Femi is 48 and has schizoaffective disorder. His CC requests a CPA meeting.

Some of your patients will be under the CPA (Box 19.1). You'll support CCs in reviews and management; they may ask you to attend, minute or lead CPA reviews. "Non-CPA" patients are more common in teams providing brief assessment and treatment, or may be maintained with only outpatient clinic contact.

Box 19.1 The CPA

Eligible patients:
- Severe/complex mental illness
- Co-morbid complexity, e.g. substance misuse, housing issues, physical illness
- Ongoing risks
- Historic disengagement
- Recent/current detention under MHA

Essential CPA elements:
- Allocated CC
- Regular CPA reviews (6–12 monthly)
- Assessment of needs
- Holistic care planning
- Emphasis on patient and family involvement
- Written care plan for all involved, including patient and GP

CARER VIEW:

The CPA is very difficult. If you have a voice, you can speak up for [your relative], but then [staff] don't ask to hear from you, and that just really annoys me. Too much of the time they don't even invite you … sometimes, only last minute.

Psychiatry: Breaking the ICE – Introductions, Common Tasks and Emergencies for Trainees, First Edition.
Edited by Sarah Stringer, Juliet Hurn and Anna M Burnside.
© 2016 John Wiley & Sons, Ltd. Published 2016 by John Wiley & Sons, Ltd.
Companion Website: www.psychiatryice.com

Preparation

Femi's CC will set the date, and make invitations, asking Femi who to invite (e.g. relatives, advocate, GP, housing officer). You can help by:
- Suggesting possible attendees
- Contacting the GP for a physical health update, including the annual physical health check results/current medications. Your team may have a standard letter for this.
- Reading Femi's notes thoroughly
- Checking your Trust's policy on CPA paperwork: who completes what?
- Printing off the last CPA plan, new CPA forms ± drug chart.

CCs are encouraged to lead, but may prefer you to chair, or co-chair with them. If they lead, offer to take minutes.

TIP: Your patients are often right. Your boss is often wrong (but be gentle if pointing this out!)

Chris Douglas, Consultant Psychiatrist and Psychotherapist

During

1. Approach

Allow time for introductions. Don't plough through a full psychiatric assessment: the meeting should focus on positive care planning.
- Give Femi space to talk and respond to comments
- Ensure *all* attendees have their say.

2. Coverage

Use the CPA forms to guide structure:
- Progress since last CPA
- Current symptoms or problems
- MSE
- Social issues, e.g. housing, finances, activities, education, social network
- Medication: adherence, views, side-effects
- Physical healthcare
  - If Femi hasn't seen his GP, discuss this and consider offering simple investigations, e.g. bloods, Body Mass Index (BMI)
- Goals and aspirations (use recovery principles, p45)
- Risks/safeguarding
- Relapse signature: what are the usual signs when he becomes unwell?
  - Encourage *Femi* to identify these if possible

3. Discuss the care plan

- For each area of need – decide clear actions and who will be responsible
- Risk management plan
- Crisis plan (p315) – steps to take if relapse/crisis.

After

The CC will type and circulate the CPA plan within 14 days; Femi and his GP must receive copies. You may be asked to:
- Write a GP letter
- Update diagnosis/outcome measures
- Advise on risk assessment/management.

What if ... ?

... Femi's an inpatient?
The same applies, but the CC (±CMHT doctor) attend the ward for the meeting. CPA meetings should be held:
- When care plans or circumstances significantly change, e.g. admission, discharge
- Every 6–12 months in long admissions.

... You're the CC?
Doctors sometimes act as CCs for less complex CPA patients. If so, go through your responsibilities with an experienced CC, and don't be afraid to refer to teammates for help.

Take-home message

Use your medical expertise in CPA meetings, and support CCs to lead.

Further reading

Rethink Mental Illness (2013) *Rethink Factsheet: Care Programme Approach (CPA)*, Rethink, London. Available at: www.rethink.org/resources/c/care-programme-approach-cpafactsheet
Department of Health (2008) *Refocusing the Care Programme Approach: Policy and Positive Practice Guidance*. COI, London.
Watch Video 6 on this book's companion website to see a ward discharge CPA in action.

CHAPTER 20

Home visits

Laurine Hanna

South London & Maudsley NHS Foundation Trust, London, England

RELATED CHAPTERS: non-engagement (27), acute relapse (62)

Stephanie is 32 and has depression. She hasn't attended her last 5 appointments. You decide to organise a home visit.

Home visits are revealing, fascinating, and a welcome break from the office. They're also time-consuming, so plan them well to avoid wasted journeys, and be clear about *why* you're visiting, e.g.

- The person *won't* come to you (unwell/relapsing) or *can't* come to you (e.g. poor mobility, severe agoraphobia, negative symptoms)
- To encourage engagement
- To assess the home environment/family/risks.

Preparation

1. With the CC/team
- Decide whether the visit will be:
  - *Planned* – tell Stephanie you're coming (obvious, but often overlooked!)
  - *Unannounced* – useful if she's chaotic/avoiding you, but can feel intrusive
- Access – do you need help, e.g. housing officer/relative?

2. Safety
- Read your Trust's home visit policy
- Check risks, especially aggression
  - Environmental, e.g. dangerous pets, infestations, electrical hazards
  - If high risk, you may need police present (which will usually require a formal MHA assessment)
- Always visit in pairs (with the CC)
- Travel together/arrange to meet CC outside the house
- Tell someone at the team base *where* you are and *when* you'll be back.

3. Practicalities
- *Travel*
  - Print a map of your catchment area $\pm$ download public transport apps, e.g. Traveline, Citymapper

Psychiatry: Breaking the ICE – Introductions, Common Tasks and Emergencies for Trainees, First Edition.
Edited by Sarah Stringer, Juliet Hurn and Anna M Burnside.
© 2016 John Wiley & Sons, Ltd. Published 2016 by John Wiley & Sons, Ltd.
Companion Website: www.psychiatryice.com

- ○ Check if you should claim for travel costs, or whether your Trust has a scheme to help you buy a bicycle
- ○ If cycling, plan how you'll look professional, despite sweat, rain or snow
- ○ If driving, check parking regulations ± ask if your team has a parking permit
- *Carry*
  - ○ Stephanie's address and phone number; relatives' numbers.
  - ○ Colleagues' phone numbers
  - ○ ID
  - ○ Mobile phone/personal alarm
  - ○ Team details/compliment slip
  - ○ Necessary equipment, e.g. blank prescription, stethoscope
- Calling Stephanie beforehand may save a wasted journey.

During

1. Approach
Remember your manners: you're a *guest,* and must respect Stephanie's home. Aim to engage – not upset or annoy – her.
- Introduce yourself clearly, showing your ID
- If she declines your visit, try polite persuasion but don't be pushy: you're not selling double-glazing. Explain how you could help, and offer a CMHT appointment.
- Without a warrant, you can't legally enter or stop her shutting the door in your face
- If she's watching TV or listening to music, ask – don't *tell* – her to switch it off.

2. Manage the setting
- Do what you can to relax Stephanie
- Never assess in a kitchen (knife risk)
- Scan the area for potential weapons
- Stay near an exit
- If feeling uneasy, trust your instincts and leave quickly
- Ask if pets can stay in another room (plead dog phobia or allergies!)
- If relatives or older children are present, request time together and separately.

3. Spot environmental clues
- *Neighbourhood,* e.g. deprivation, antisocial behaviour, thin walls, noisy neighbours
- *Neglect*: ask for a guided tour – which Activities of Daily Living (ADLs) are affected?
  - ○ Self/home: hoarding, dirt, disrepair, insects, empty/mouldy fridge
  - ○ Others, e.g. children, pets
- *Substance misuse*, e.g. cigarette butts, empty alcohol bottles, drug paraphernalia
- *Psychosis*, e.g. unusual writing on walls/paper, blocked vents, covered windows, excessive security, signs of barricading, damage to property
- *Medications* – can she locate them?
  - ○ Note the prescription date and how many she's taken
- *Mobility* – can she safely get around/out?

After

1. Wrap up
- Thank her and try to book a follow-up appointment
- Call the CMHT to say you're safe (if this was agreed beforehand)
- Document clearly and decide on next steps, e.g. in the team meeting.

2. Address problems

- *Mental illness/relapse:* offer treatment $\pm$ HTT/admission
- *Unsafe home*: discuss with the housing officer (if available)
- *Unsanitary* (e.g. infestation) contact social services about re-housing.
  - ○ The National Assistance Act 1948 allows an infirm/physically or mentally ill person living in unsanitary conditions, and unable to self-care, to be removed without consent to a suitable place for care/assessment
  - ○ In practice, gentle persuasion, or the MHA/MCA are more often appropriate
- *Neglect:*
  - ○ Children: contact social services (Ch.64)
  - ○ Pets: contact the Royal Society for Prevention of Cruelty to Animals (RPSCA)
- *Bullying* by neighbours: consider adult safeguarding (Ch.63)
- *Not managing at home*: consider OT assessment (via the GP/team OT).
  - ○ Aids, alterations, home support, or relocation to supported accommodation
  - ○ You may be asked to assess capacity around these decisions (p102).

What if...?

... She doesn't answer?

Search for clues. Peep in through her windows or (*cautiously*) via her letterbox (never poke fingers through):

- Uncollected post
- Unattended pets
- Smell of decay

Call through the letterbox and ring her mobile. *Consider* asking neighbours if they've seen Stephanie lately, but avoid breaching confidentiality or stigmatising her by revealing your professional role.

Leave a note with your team details, when you called, and how she can contact you. Discuss in the team meeting and see Ch.62 (acute relapse).

Take-home message

Home visits are extremely useful, but require planning and manners.

CHAPTER 21

Depression

Rory Conn[1] and Rachel Thomasson[2]

[1] Tavistock and Portman NHS Foundation Trust, London, England
[2] Manchester Royal Infirmary, Manchester, Lancashire, England

RELATED CHAPTERS: electroconvulsive therapy (47), self-harm (51)

Denise is a 36-year old, single mother. First diagnosed with depression at 17, she's had 4 hospital admissions and attempted suicide once. Her GP writes: "She's had every antidepressant in the BNF but is still depressed. I'm running out of ideas ... "

As the letter hints, depression can be a draining illness for clinicians and sufferers. GPs expertly manage mild to moderate depression and refer:
• Moderate depression with complex problems
• Severe depression
• Significant risk
• Treatment-resistant depression
• Complex presentations
This referral could mean many things: persistent unhappiness, heavy social burdens, personality difficulties, medication non-adherence or severe, treatment-resistant depression. Start from scratch and try to bring fresh eyes to the problem.

Preparation

1. Gather information – GP, old notes, previous CC/psychiatrist
• Reason for referral *now*
• Immediate risks (including child welfare)
• Current medication: does Denise always collect it?
• Previous treatments: efficacy and reasons for stopping
  ◦ Antidepressants: duration, adherence, side effects
  ◦ Antipsychotics, mood stabilisers, electroconvulsive therapy (ECT)
  ◦ Psychological therapies. Psychologists' closing summaries can highlight key issues and 'psychological-mindedness'.
• Physical illness; latest blood results
• Personality difficulties.

2. Family (with permission)
• Key concerns
• Premorbid personality
• Support available at home.

Psychiatry: Breaking the ICE – Introductions, Common Tasks and Emergencies for Trainees, First Edition.
Edited by Sarah Stringer, Juliet Hurn and Anna M Burnside.
© 2016 John Wiley & Sons, Ltd. Published 2016 by John Wiley & Sons, Ltd.
Companion Website: www.psychiatryice.com

If Denise needs to bring her children, ask if a relative can attend, so you can see her alone for at least part of the assessment.

Assessment

1. Approach

Don't rush the interview and leave space for silences: psychomotor retardation, poor concentration, shame or guilt may slow Denise's responses.

- Use reflection if she trails off, e.g.
  - Denise: *It's all gone wrong since January…*
  - You: *January…?*
- Don't jump to mop up tears – allowing crying shows *you* can cope and contain her distress. Offer tissues if tears or a runny nose are distracting or upsetting *her*.
- Arguing with negative cognitions can feel dismissive, e.g. *You're not fat and stupid!* Instead, empathise, e.g. *It must be horrible feeling like that.*

> **TIP:** If people struggle to describe their mood, ask them to rate how they feel out of ten (ten is the best day ever and zero the worst). Their answer can guide you towards stressors *and* protective factors, e.g.
>
> Denise: *Three.*
> You: *What stops it being a four or five?*
> D: *Work … and back pain.*
> Y: (After exploring these) *What stops it from being a two or one?*
> D: *My kids.*
>
> **Dr David Okai, Consultant**

2. Full history, remembering…

Some factors may masquerade as depression, be co-morbid, or make depression harder to treat.

- *HPC:*
  - Triggers – particularly loss, shame, stress.
  - Impact – on work, relationships
  - Symptoms
    - Core: ↓mood, energy, enjoyment
    - Biological: changed sleep, appetite, ↓libido
    - Cognitive: helpless, hopeless, worthless, guilty; ↓concentration, memory; thoughts of suicide/self-harm
    - Psychotic: *typically* nihilistic/persecutory delusions; unpleasant auditory hallucinations
  - Co-morbid anxiety
- *PPHx* (draw a timeline, p31)
  - Pattern and episodes of illness (Table 21.1)
  - *Bipolar affective disorder (BPAD)*
    - Past hypomanic/manic/mixed affective episodes
    - Antidepressant 'switching' to agitation/irritability/elation?
  - What helped most? E.g. medication, therapy, admissions
- *PMHx*
  - Painful, chronic or neurological illnesses are linked with depression

○ Mimic depression: *anaemia, hypothyroidism, hypocalcaemia, SOL, hypoactive delirium, diabetes, chronic fatigue syndrome, coeliac disease …*
- *DHx*
  ○ All current, including OTC, e.g. St John's Wort
  ○ Depressogenic, e.g. steroids, antihypertensives, antiretrovirals, antipsychotics
  ○ Psychotropics
    - Past and present
    - Which helped most?
    - Side effects (NB: sexual side-effects are rarely volunteered)
    - Adherence – if poor, why?
- *FHx*
  ○ Depression/suicidality
  ○ BPAD – may suggest undiagnosed BPAD
- *Personal history* – childhood abuse, losses
- *Substance misuse* – cause or effect of low mood
- *Personality difficulties* – particularly affecting relationships
- *SHx* – supports, stressors, carer responsibilities.

TIP: *Is there secondary gain,* i.e. a conscious/unconscious reason to stay ill? Broaching this directly will lose rapport: Denise may feel disbelieved or accused of malingering. But these issues are important to *your* formulation, so ask …
- *What does your depression stop you doing?*
- *What would you do if you were well that you can't do now?*
- *What do your family think about your depression?*

3. MSE, remembering …
- Self-neglect, weight loss
- Affect: flat/reactive
- Incongruent mood (personality factors, psychosis?)
- Prominent anxiety
- Depressive cognitions
- Thoughts of self-harm/suicide
- Psychotic symptoms, including commands to self-harm.

4. Physical assessment (you/GP)
- *Examination*
  ○ General health check, e.g. BMI, BP
  ○ Exclude organic causes, e.g. thyroid, diabetes
- *Investigations – consider*
  ○ FBC, glucose/HbA1c, TFT, B_{12}, folate, ESR/CRP (exclude organic)
  ○ Drug levels if relevant, e.g. mood stabilisers.

5. Risk assessment, remembering …
- Self-harm/suicide (Ch.51)
- Self-neglect, social vulnerability, isolation
- Children.

Table 21.1 Depression differential diagnoses.

Differential	Subtype	Presentation
Depression	Depressive episode	≥2 weeks' symptoms *Mild:* few/mild symptoms; still functioning socially *Moderate:* increased severity and number of symptoms; considerable problems with social functioning *Severe:* all core symptoms, plus many/very severe other symptoms. Loss of social function. *Psychotic:* severe depression + delusions/hallucinations
	Recurrent depressive disorder	>1 depressive episode, separated by at least 2 symptom-free months Focus on relapse indicators and early intervention
	Chronic depression	Depression ≥ 2 years Distinguish from • *Dysthymia* = milder low mood and anhedonia, of such chronicity it's almost seen as someone's personality • Inadequate treatment • Treatment-resistance
	Treatment-resistant depression	Fails to respond to ≥2 sequential antidepressants, at adequate doses for an adequate time (p138)
	Atypical depression	↑appetite/weight, sleep; leaden sensation in limbs. Mood may remain reactive.
	Seasonal affective disorder (SAD)	Recurrent seasonal depression (usually autumn/winter) Often atypical features Light therapy may help Relapse prevention focuses on high-risk seasons
	Agitated depression	Depression + motor agitation, inner tension, racing thoughts (exclude mixed affective episode or antidepressant side effects)
	'Double depression'	Depression superimposed on *dysthymia*
Adjustment disorder		Low-level depressive +/or anxiety symptoms within a month of a clear stressor Usually remits spontaneously, within 6 months (may need support + risk monitoring)
Grief	*Normal*	Gradual shift *towards* recovery over weeks/months Normalise, signpost to GP/bereavement counselling, e.g. Cruse Psychiatric involvement only if high risks
	Pathological	Unusually intense/prolonged/'stuck' Hallmarked by severe depressive symptoms May need secondary care psychology
Bipolar affective disorder (Ch.25)		2 or more affective episodes, at least one of which is hypomanic/manic, or mixed affective (p344)
Schizoaffective disorder		Psychotic and depressive symptoms are equally weighted, and arise together (rather than mood worsening and becoming psychotic) May suffer schizomanic episodes

Management

1. Approach and psychoeducation
Acknowledge Denise's probable weariness and frustration with her depression – this may be compounded by barely-disguised exasperation from her friends, relatives and GP. Don't replicate that exasperation!
- Explain the biopsychosocial model of depression, and explore Denise's explanatory preferences. This helps treatment-planning, as different models may make more sense to her, e.g. learning how to stop criticising herself; understanding how her upbringing affected her; changing brain chemicals.
- Gently move the focus from current disability to Denise's wishes for the future. Show her you're hopeful things can improve, even if she can't see this at present.
- A clear treatment plan is essential: consider SMART goals (p72) ± rating scales to measure response to treatment (p57).
- Treatment might range from advising the GP on next steps, to a period of care co-ordination in the CMHT. If unsure, explain that you'll discuss with your team and feedback to her via a letter ± telephone ± follow-up appointment.

Extend psychoeducation to Denise's family and friends. If they understand depression as a real illness, legitimately needing support and treatment, they'll be more likely to support her. Mind have useful resources:

www.mind.org.uk/media/42904/understanding_depression_2012.pdf

2. Risk management
Address immediate risks.
- Consider HTT or admission if:
  - Risk of self-harm/suicide
  - Severe self-neglect. e.g. not eating or drinking
  - Marked retardation/poor insight means she'll struggle to follow the plan
  - Psychotic depression
- Discuss a crisis plan if her mood/risks worsen, e.g. call CMHT/attend ED.

Refer to Children's Social Services if concerned about risks to her children, including the need for childcare support if admitting Denise (Ch.64).

3. Practical advice
Focus on *relevant* things she can *do* to start feeling better and address triggers:
- Behavioural activation (p73)
- Sleep hygiene (p72)
- Exercise (shown to reduce depressive symptoms)
- Reducing or stopping alcohol or drugs
- Problem-solving
- Help with carer responsibilities
- Time off work (p87).

Don't overload her with ideas. Keep it simple, and recruit carers to ensure things happen.

4. Medication

> **TIP:** The sixth antidepressant is unlikely to do the trick.
>
> Chris Douglas, Psychiatrist and Psychotherapist

Your judgement in choosing antidepressants will only come with experience. Use the BNF/Maudsley Prescribing Guidelines (MPG) and call your pharmacist or consultant for advice. People often request anxiolytics, but these should be avoided where possible; anxiety usually improves as the depression lifts, and may improve with sleep hygiene or relaxation techniques. If there's prominent anxiety or insomnia – whether primary or due to medication side effects – you might consider a *short-term* benzodiazepine or sedative antihistamine.

If Denise hasn't received adequate trials of antidepressants:

- Offer medication choices, and information on side effects (p57–62); PILs help
- Address previous reasons for non-adherence, e.g. suggest slower titration to decrease side effects
- Ensure adequate trials (4–6 weeks) of at least two antidepressants, from different classes.
  - Start with an SSRI or the antidepressant which helped most before
  - After four weeks increase the dose if needed
  - If tolerated, try to increase to the maximum dose before swapping
  - Monitor for early agitation and suicidality, reviewing Denise within two weeks (1 week if higher suicide risk)
  - Thereafter, review monthly if possible.
  - MPG – useful guidance on swapping and stopping antidepressants.

Advise shorter prescriptions if there's a risk of overdose, and discuss this with her GP. In psychotic depression, an antidepressant and antipsychotic should be combined (Box 21.1).

TIP: St John's wort may help in mild/moderate depression, but advise caution: preparations often have unclear 'doses' and can interact with other drugs, e.g. oral contraceptives, anticoagulants, anticonvulsants.

Box 21.1 The antidepressant debate

There are fierce arguments about antidepressants, including how much of their effect is placebo-driven, and whether they are over-prescribed. Be pragmatic rather than dogmatic, giving accurate information on risks and benefits, and offering choice whenever possible.
- Use other treatments when people decline antidepressants – don't just discharge them!
- If patients want antidepressants when you *don't* think they're indicated, discuss with your consultant.

If treatment-resistant (Table 21.1):

- Discuss with your consultant
- Extra care is needed to exclude/treat differentials and offer psychosocial treatments
- Options include *augmentation* with lithium, antipsychotics, or another antidepressant e.g. mirtazapine
  - Remember any routine monitoring needed with these additions
  - Side effect load may worsen
- Electroconvulsive therapy is an effective last-line treatment in resistant depression (Ch.47)

Medication is recommended for:

- 6–9 months after a single depressive episode resolves
- ≥2 years if recurrent depression, perpetuating factors or significant risk

5. Psychological interventions (p66–70)

Local Improving Access to Psychological Therapies (IAPT) services may suffice, but Denise may need secondary care input – discuss with the team psychologist. Evidence-based treatments include:

- Cognitive Behaviour Therapy (CBT)
- Mindfulness-based therapy
- Interpersonal therapy.

Consider couples therapy if problems with her partner are key. Counselling/psychodynamic psychotherapy have a weaker evidence base, but may be offered if Denise prefers them.

6. Other interventions
- Optimise physical health (via GP)
- Offer social interventions (Ch.13)
  - Even without acute risks, Denise's depression may impact on her children; the family could benefit from parenting support groups, babysitting services, etc.
  - Carer's assessment/support groups. Don't forget young carers (children)
- Frustration and therapeutic nihilism are not uncommon when working with chronic depression. Express these feelings in supervision or team case discussions, rather than taking them out on Denise. Clear, focused plans will also help keep a sense of direction and purpose.
- If it's unrealistic for Denise to be completely depression-free at the point of discharge, focus on *recovery principles* (p45).

> **TIP:** If they're not getting better, you may have the diagnosis/treatment wrong, or they may not *want* to get better.
>
> **Chris Douglas, Psychiatrist and Psychotherapist**

7. Documentation
It's particularly important to write down simple plans in depression, due to concentration and memory problems, e.g. Denise's initial plan might read:
- Do one 'pampering' activity a day
- Take citalopram 20 mg each morning
- Book GP appointment for blood tests this week
- If in crisis, e.g. suicidal
  - Office hours: contact CMHT (telephone …)
  - Out-of-hours: attend casualty.

If discharging Denise back her GP, ensure she and her GP have a clear discharge letter and plan, with guidance on re-referral.

What If … ?

… You're seeing her in ED?
Ensure she's been screened by the ED doctors for overt organic causes and undisclosed self-harm. Focus on assessment and *initial* management, containing risks and alleviating distress (Table 21.2).

Table 21.2 ED depression management.

Risk	Severity/complexity	Willing to engage	Usual next step
Non significant	Low–moderate	Yes	GP within one week
Significant *but* protective factors/ able to seek help	Moderate – severe	Yes	CMHT $\pm$ HTT
Significant	Moderate – severe	Yes/no	Admit (if unwilling, consider MHA assessment)

It's rarely helpful to start antidepressants in ED – the immediate impact is side effects, rather than mood improvement. Medications are usually best started and monitored by the GP/CMHT, or the ward team if admitted. Any suspicion of BPAD should prompt CMHT referral, since antidepressants may trigger a manic episode.

If sleep's a big problem, consider *short-term* night sedation, e.g. 3 days' zopiclone 3.75–7.5 mg *or* promethazine 25 mg.

Always fax a copy of your assessment with a cover letter to the GP, clearly stating any recommendations, (e.g. CBT +SSRI). Refer as necessary to the CMHT/HTT and provide Denise with a written plan.

Take-home message

Depression is a challenge, and your patient *and* team may feel jaded. Take time to re-examine the problem and think broadly: holism becomes *more* – not less – important in complex case management.

Reference

Mind:
  ○ www.mind.org.uk/media/42904/understanding_depression_2012.pdf

Further reading

Depression Alliance: patient information; online and face-to-face support groups
  ○ http://www.depressionalliance.org
Depression UK: National Self-help organisation
  ○ www.depressionuk.org
NICE Guideline CG90 Depression in Adults: the treatment and management of depression in adults
NICE Guideline CG91 Depression in adults with a chronic physical health problem: treatment and management.
RCPsych patient information leaflets:
  ○ www.rcpsych.ac.uk/healthadvice.aspx
Timonen, M, and Liukkonen, T. (2008) Management of depression in adults. *British Medical Journal* **336**, 435–439.

CHAPTER 22

Generalised anxiety disorder (GAD)

Laurine Hanna

South London & Maudsley NHS Foundation Trust, London, England

> **RELATED CHAPTERS:** Post-traumatic stress disorder (PTSD, 31), Obsessive Compulsive Disorder (OCD, 56), panic attacks (57), somatisation (61)

The GP refers Craig, 26, for repeatedly presenting in high distress, begging for diazepam to 'stop him going mad'. Craig's on sick leave from work as a chef in a Michelin-starred restaurant, where he was terrified of causing food poisoning.

Most anxiety disorders are managed in primary care. Stepped care advises secondary referral for:
- **Inadequate treatment response** *or*
- **Significant risk/functional impairment/co-morbidity.**

A thorough assessment is essential: Craig's food-poisoning worries may indicate GAD, vomiting phobia, OCD … or psychosis! Revise your differentials with Table 22.1.

Preparation

1. Gather information – GP ± old psychiatric notes
- Content of worries
- Organic causes excluded?
- Treatments offered/accepted
- Clarify risks and urgency
- Will anxiety prevent attendance at your clinic?

2. Flexibility
- Encourage Craig to bring a friend to the appointment, or offer a home visit if he's too anxious to attend the CMHT.

Assessment

1. Approach
Don't mirror Craig's anxiety! If pressured and over-inclusive, let him talk for a few minutes, rather than interject. Then try:
- *"You've got lots to tell me, and might worry we'll miss something important. Could you trust me to ask some very specific questions to ensure we get to the bottom of this? I may need to interrupt or redirect you if you're going off track."*

Psychiatry: Breaking the ICE – Introductions, Common Tasks and Emergencies for Trainees, First Edition.
Edited by Sarah Stringer, Juliet Hurn and Anna M Burnside.

Table 22.1 Anxiety disorders: differential diagnoses.

Disorder	Continuous or episodic anxiety? C E	Anxiety focus/worry	Check for...
GAD	C ✓	Just about everything, e.g. work, health, family, money, future...	Apprehension Chronic physical anxiety symptoms, e.g. tension headaches, shakiness, dry mouth, palpitations...
Panic disorder (Ch.57)	E ✓	No clear trigger – panic seems *out of the blue*	Recurrent panic *attacks* (Ch.57) within a month
Specific phobia	E ✓	Particular feared thing, e.g. spiders	
Agoraphobia	E ✓	Inability to escape to a safe place, thus: open spaces, enclosed spaces (lifts, public transport), crowds	Panic attacks
Social phobia	E ✓	Scrutiny or judgement, e.g. public speaking, eating, intimate groups	Symptoms which draw attention, e.g. blushing, tremor, sweating Self-scrutiny, e.g. *I'm being boring, I'm embarrassing myself*
PTSD (Ch.31)	C ✓* E ✓	Severe trauma, then reminders of this	Re-experiencing: flashbacks, nightmares, intrusive memories Emotional changes, e.g. numbness, irritability, depression
OCD (Ch.56)	C ✓	Obsessions and their triggers	Obsessions, e.g. contamination, morality, violence, sex, religion Compulsions, e.g. clean, count, check, order

*Hyperarousal – feeling constantly on edge/alert.

Letting anxious patients ramble seems kind, but generally fuels – rather than resolves – anxiety.

TIP: There's a danger in believing that reflective thinking is the *only* thing. You still need to prioritise and act – navel-gazing is not psychiatry! You need an objective, which is to find a solution, which is an action, *even if only verbal*.

Duncan McLean, Consultant Psychiatrist and Psychotherapist

2. Full history, remembering...
- *HPC:* pattern, triggers, physical anxiety symptoms
  - Avoidance/escape
  - Safety-seeking behaviours (coping mechanisms which make him feel safer, but don't address the problem, e.g. seeking reassurance from relatives)
  - Distress and effect on life
  - Triggers, especially threat events/ongoing stressors
- *Comorbidity*
  - Depression, other anxiety disorders, substance misuse
  - Identify the *primary* problem (first/most prominent)
    - *Would you still be depressed if your anxiety improved?*

- *PPHx* – including treatments – what's helped?
- *PMHx*
  - Causative: hyperthyroidism, arrhythmias, phaeochromocytoma
  - Exacerbating, e.g. arthritis, gastrointestinal/respiratory disorders, pain
  - Health *worries* suggesting somatisation (Ch.61)?
- *DHx*
  - Benzodiazepines
  - Exacerbating, e.g. steroids, oral contraceptives, decongestants, thyroxine, SSRIs, methylphenidate
- *Substance misuse:*
  - Caffeine, nicotine, alcohol, drugs
  - Relationship to anxiety (self-medication, triggering anxiety)
- *Premorbid personality,* e.g. avoidant traits
- *SHx* – coping, carers; work situation.

3. MSE, remembering …
- Agitation, reassurance-seeking, panic attacks, compulsions
- Worries, feared outcomes, obsessions, covert compulsions
- Suicidal ideation
- Depersonalisation/derealisation
- Symptom interpretation; psychological mindedness.

TIP: Rating scales can help when unclear/measuring response to treatments (p146).

4. Risk assessment, remembering …
- Self-harm/suicide (anxiety *isn't* protective)
- Self-neglect
- Social, e.g. losing job
- Risk to children/dependents.

5. Physical assessment
- Basic examination, observations
- Appropriate investigations, e.g. ECG, TFTs.

Management (for GAD)

Simple plans can be organised via the GP; more complex or risky presentations may need regular clinic appointments or care coordination. With very mixed pictures, consider defining the primary diagnosis, then making a functional problem list, rather than giving 5 or 6 diagnoses!

1. Deal with immediate risk
Craig's desperation may be alarming, and he might want admission to 'stay safe'. This is unlikely to help unless significant risks, e.g. suicide. If so, discuss with your consultant, and consider HTT.

2. Treat 'red herrings'
- Treat comorbid/primary psychiatric conditions
- Ensure GP addresses physical conditions

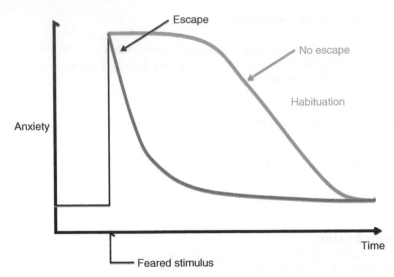

Figure 22.1 Anxiety exposure graph.

3. Psychoeducation

Craig may be desperate for a quick fix, but you'll help him most by *teaching* him about anxiety and how to manage it. Carers are often drawn into safety-seeking behaviours, especially reassurance, so extend psychoeducation to them. Explain:

- Anxiety is unpleasant, but normal. It's the primitive 'fight or flight' response to life-threatening situations.
- These days, there's less to fight or flee, but anxiety can kick in unhelpfully, due to stress, genetics and thinking habits.
- Anxious people tend to worsen their anxiety by:
  - *Avoiding* and *escaping* anxiety-provoking situations (Figure 22.1), so they never learn:
    - Anxiety passes if they stay with it (habituation)
    - They *can* cope without safety-seeking behaviours
  - Looking for danger in everyday situations
  - Worrying about worrying, e.g. *I'm going mad! Why's my heart pounding?*
  - Needing to be certain, e.g. about the future.

4. Self-help

Craig can reduce anxiety himself:

- Relaxation exercises (p71)
- Mindfulness (p68)
- Sleep hygiene (p72)
- Reduce/stop caffeine; address alcohol, drugs ($\pm$ substance misuse service)
- Problem-solving, SMART goals (p72), time-management
- Behavioural changes:
  - Schedule relaxing activities e.g. seeing friends, hot bath
  - Physical exercise
  - Set aside daily limited 'worry time' – *just* to worry (e.g. 10 minutes)
- Contact self-help organisations (Resources, p146).

TIP: Valerian, chamomile, ginkgo biloba? There's no conclusive evidence for these, but they're harmless, and placebo's a powerful thing ... If Craig's keen, don't waste time dissuading him.

5. Psychology
Anxiety management includes learning how to:
- Accept and 'stay with' anxiety
- Face anxiety-provoking situations
- Think about situations more realistically or helpfully
- Tolerate uncertainty.

Self-help works, but encourage formal support – it's hard to fight anxiety alone.
- CBT (p67–68) – three to four month course
- Applied relaxation: using relaxation techniques during exposure to anxiety-provoking situations
- Lower intensity options, e.g. psycho-education/anxiety groups, computerised CBT.

Discuss options with a psychologist: primary care (via IAPT) or secondary care.

6. Medication
Discuss options with your consultant or pharmacist.
SSRIs (p59–61) are first line, preferably combined with psychology:
- Start at half the usual dose, warning that anxiety/insomnia may briefly increase
- Regularly review response and risk
- Continue for a minimum of six months after remission
- If ineffective, alternatives include:
  - Different SSRI
  - Different antidepressant class, e.g. SNRI see Appendix B5
  - Buspirone
  - Pregabalin
  - Propranolol – useful for somatic symptoms, but can be depressogenic

Avoid benzodiazepines:
- Effects quickly wear off (tolerance)
- Addictive
- Counter-productive, e.g. prevent habituation or naturally learning to relax.

You may occasionally use them low dose and briefly in highly distressing or disabling anxiety, e.g. diazepam 2 mg BD, maximum two to four weeks. If Craig's *using* regular diazepam, implement psychological approaches and negotiate a gradual reduction via his GP.

Sedating antihistamines and antipsychotics aren't addictive, but again prevent habituation, so can prolong problems or obstruct CBT.

7. Tertiary referral
If Craig's anxiety is intractable or particularly complex, consider tertiary service review.

What if ...

... Craig has a different anxiety disorder?
Most of the above guidelines apply to the other anxiety disorders, but also remember:
- *PTSD* – Ch.31
- *OCD* – Ch.56
- *Panic disorder* – Ch.57
- *Agoraphobia* – treatment as for panic disorder
  - Prepare for more home visits initially, reducing these with time
- *Social phobia*
  - Consider differentials/co-morbidities: autism, avoidant PD, negative symptoms of schizophrenia.
  - Craig may find appointments daunting, so make them easier, e.g. initial home visit, off-peak appointment times
  - CBT and antidepressants are evidence-based.

Take-home message

Psychoeducation is central.

Further reading

NICE (2011) CG 113 Generalised anxiety disorder and panic disorder (with or without agoraphobia) in adults: Management in primary, secondary and community care. NICE, Manchester.

Hoge, E., Ivkovic, A. and Fricchione, G. (2012) Clinical review. Generalised anxiety disorder: diagnosis and treatment. *British Medical Journal* **345**, e7500.

Patient resources:

PIL: www.nhs.uk/Conditions/Panic-disorder/Pages/self%20help.aspx

Anxiety UK: www.anxietyuk.org.uk
Phobics Society: www.phobics-society.org.uk
No More Panic: www.nomorepanic.co.uk

Moodjuice (self-help guide): www.moodjuice.scot.nhs.uk/anxiety.asp

Meares, K. and Freeston, M. (2008) *Overcoming Worry*. Constable and Robinson, London.

Shafran, R., Brosan, L. and Cooper, P. (2013) *The Complete CBT Guide for Anxiety*. Constable and Robinson, London.

Anxiety rating scales

Generalised Anxiety disorder-7 (GAD-7): self-rating. Public domain.
  ◦ http://www.phqscreeners.com/pdfs/03_GAD-7/English.pdf

Hamilton Anxiety Rating Scale (HAM-A): clinician-rating. Public domain.
  ◦ www.outcometracker.org/library/HAM-A.pdf

CHAPTER 23

First episode psychosis (FEP)

Christina Barras[1] and Juliet Hurn[2]

[1] South West London & St George's Mental Health NHS Trust, London, England
[2] South London & Maudsley NHS Foundation Trust, London, England

RELATED CHAPTERS: psychosis in ED (53), longer-term management (24), side effect management (36); Videos 1–6 (see companion website)

Alex is 20 and recently dropped out of university. His mother lives with him and told the GP that Alex mutters to himself, and became very frightened last week, dismantling the electric sockets in the lounge. He was angry when she suggested seeing a doctor. The GP requests your assessment.

Developing a psychotic illness – or witnessing psychosis in a relative – can be bewildering and desperately upsetting. The first experience of care can affect someone's view of services forever, so try to make your contact as positive as possible. Apply Early Intervention (EI) principles (Box 23.1) to Alex's management, whether you are working in an EI service (p6), or a generic CMHT.

Box 23.1 EI Principles

- The shorter the Duration of Untreated Psychosis (DUP), the better the prognosis
- Diagnose and treat early (keep DUP < 3 months)
- Optimise early years of treatment
  - Use evidence-based interventions; medication doses should start low and increase slowly
  - Work closely with GPs, Child and Adolescent Mental Health Services (CAMHS), schools, employer, etc.
  - Emphasise psychoeducation and patient/family involvement
  - Promote recovery (return to social/vocational activity)
  - Increase public awareness; reduce stigma.

PATIENT VIEW:

To be honest, I don't really believe I get unwell. I believe I lose control and The Controller comes in and takes over … I actually like having him around because sometimes I can't know what to do and he tells me what to do … There's something scary about it at the same time, because you have to trust him, and I don't really trust him, not completely … I'm scared a little bit about what he can make me do. On the whole, it's a comfort … When I was jogging, I sometimes got into trouble with men in the dark park and he made me go *whoosh*! Really fast. Yeah, seriously. Sometimes I drop something and he tells me I've dropped it. I don't know I've dropped it, but he's seen from somewhere, satellite probably.

'Sarah'

Psychiatry: Breaking the ICE – Introductions, Common Tasks and Emergencies for Trainees, First Edition.
Edited by Sarah Stringer, Juliet Hurn and Anna M Burnside.
© 2016 John Wiley & Sons, Ltd. Published 2016 by John Wiley & Sons, Ltd.
Companion Website: www.psychiatryice.com

Preparation

1. Gather information – GP, mother
- Details about presentation, risks, PMHx, medications, substance misuse
- Does Alex know about the referral?
- Is his mother happy for you to disclose her worries?
  ◦ If not, discuss how you'll negotiate this with her, the GP and your team.
- If you decide on a home visit (Ch.20), consider safety and take:
  ◦ A colleague ± GP
  ◦ Relevant PILs
  ◦ UDS kit
  ◦ ± Blank prescription, blood test forms

2. Discussion
- Check your consultant's preferences for antipsychotics: types, doses, etc.

Assessment

1. Approach
Your key task is *engaging* Alex and those close to him – without this bedrock, all your excellent knowledge and skills will be for nothing. This may mean some flexibility, i.e. not always pushing your management plan if temporarily sacrificing it builds a relationship with Alex.

Your empathy is essential: try to understand Alex's agenda (e.g. why he's terrified of electric sockets) before addressing your own (i.e. psychosis) – see p32.

Be as honest as possible: if Alex decides you (and therefore other professionals) aren't to be trusted, it'll be a hard view to shift. At the same time, use your judgement in deciding how 'medical' to be about his problems. He may not be ready to hear that you believe this is psychosis, and may respond better to initial discussions about 'stressful experiences' and offering support.

2. Full history, remembering…
- *Prodrome:* low-level symptoms predating more overt psychosis, e.g. withdrawal, poor self-care, mood/personality changes, loss of function, blunting
  ◦ Estimate the DUP
- *Triggers:* stressors, substance misuse
- *Psychotic symptoms:* understanding his 'story' of these will help your empathy and engagement
- *Impact:* on function/relationships
- *Comorbidity:*
  ◦ Depression, anxiety
  ◦ Premorbid personality traits, e.g. paranoid, schizotypal
  ◦ Substance misuse.

3. MSE, remembering…
- Self-care
- Positive and negative psychotic symptoms
- Insight into need for help. What help?

4. Risk assessment, remembering…
- Self-harm/suicide (desperation/command hallucinations?)
- Environmental risk, e.g. tampering with electrics

- Risk to others, especially anyone involved in paranoid delusions
- Contact with children?
- Risk *from* others due to his behaviour (e.g. by drawing attention to himself/being provocative)
- Longer-term social disability, e.g. isolation, impact on education.

5. Physical health (you/GP)

He may be young, but Alex's mental illness already increases his future physical health risk – start taking this seriously *now* (p49–51; Appendix A1 + A3).

- Physical exam
- Baseline investigations (ideally *before* starting antipsychotics):
  - Weight (+ BMI/waist circumference if possible), BP
  - FBC, U&Es, LFTs, glucose, lipids, prolactin, CK
  - ECG
- UDS
- ± Brain scan: *if* you suspect an organic cause (Box 23.2)
  - CT is quicker and shows gross pathology
  - MRI required for more subtle changes.

Alex may refuse investigations or it may be more important to start treatment immediately. If you haven't investigated, document reasons, including capacity status – and keep trying.

Box 23.2 Organic cause!

> The likelihood of FEP being organic in this age group is low. Suspect if
> - Established medical condition which could feasibly account for it, e.g. SLE
> - Marked personality or cognitive change (including confusion)
> - Physical symptoms/signs, e.g. localising neurological signs, fever, headache, confusion, weakness
> - Older, e.g. >40 y.
> NB: Visual hallucinations *may* suggest an organic cause, but are by no means uncommon in functional psychosis.

6. Collateral

Ask Alex's permission to talk to his family. Stress that you'll *ask* about their worries, not disclose his information without his consent. If he declines, consider risk and confidentiality (p37–38).

PATIENT VIEW:

At night I feel him taking over my breathing. Sometimes my saliva changes, and I know he's done something to make it a bit more poisonous, so I feel like spitting. Sometimes he won't let me spit, he makes me swallow, so, you know, he can control me from the inside. Sometimes I want to turn left, he says, "No". So I think, *Right* – I *think* it – I don't *say* it. But he knows I've thought that, so he won't let me turn right. Sometimes I'll just pop out and leave the door on the latch because I think I'll just be a second, and I'm not a second at all – I'll be gone for hours because I've stood in the bloody alleyway like that. Waiting for him to tell me I can go.

'Sarah'

Management

Alex will probably benefit from being placed on CPA and having a CC allocated. Organise proactive and regular meetings with him.

1. Deal with immediate risk

Consider HTT/hospital admission if worried about severe symptoms, an unmanageable home situation, high risks, chaotic presentation, or need for help initiating/monitoring medication. You'll usually have time to discuss this in the next team meeting, but contact your consultant or team leader if urgent.

2. Psychoeducation

Try to understand Alex's explanatory model for his experiences. *Then* suggest your model: you can emphasise different angles, depending on what makes most sense to him, e.g.

- *An illness called psychosis can cause experiences like this*
- *Changes in a brain chemical called dopamine can make you more sensitive to everything going on around you*
- *Stress can cause unusual experiences, or can make you feel less able to cope with things*
- *Cannabis is often used to cope with stress, but can also make you worry a lot about people around you ...*

Mind your language: even if absolutely sure about the ICD diagnosis, *psychosis* may be a more helpful word than *schizophrenia* at this stage. If asked about schizophrenia, explain that it's very difficult to diagnose the type of psychosis so early.

Remember that psychosis may make information processing that much harder:

- Keep things simple
- Check frequently for questions or worries
- Offer a leaflet.

People often ask if psychosis gets better. Explain that a psychotic episode may occur just once in a lifetime, but further episodes *can* happen. Emphasise that support and treatment now offers the best chance of getting and staying well.

Don't forget Alex's family: their explanatory model is also important, and they may greatly influence his engagement. Discuss their worries, recognising they may be experiencing grief, as they seem to be 'losing' the man they know and love.

3. Initial plan

In the community, you usually have time to discuss management at team meetings, so don't feel you have to come up with a comprehensive care plan after a first assessment. Think which colleagues could help Alex the most through further assessment and management, e.g. assessing accommodation, occupation/education/activities, social networks, benefits (Ch.13). The more useful your team is to him, the greater your chances of longer-term engagement.

Alex's explanatory model may guide your initial emphasis, e.g.

- *How about meeting with us regularly to talk about how to cope with these worries ... ?*
- *Medication to lower dopamine/help you cope with feeling monitored*
- *Psychology to help deal with stress ...*
- *Our football group might take your mind off things and help you connect with people again*

4. Medication

Alex may consider an antipsychotic if you explain it well (p57–9) and offer choice (Appendix B1.1; B2 includes doses). Start dose low and increase slowly. Monitor response for 4–6 weeks.

Consider short-term symptomatic relief for agitation or insomnia, particularly if using a non-sedative antipsychotic (aripiprazole/amisulpride) e.g.

- Zopiclone 7.5 mg/promethazine 25 mg nocte for a week.

Take side effects seriously. They're a major barrier to effective treatment – ask about and manage them proactively (Ch.36).

If Alex doesn't respond to the first antipsychotic at adequate dose:

- Check adherence
  - Would he agree to drug levels/temporary HTT input?
- If you're pretty sure he's concordant, check alternatives with pharmacist/consultant, then discuss with Alex.

5. Physical health

Encourage good physical healthcare early and organise monitoring for:
- SMI (Appendix A1)
- Antipsychotics (Appendix A4 and 5).

6. Substance misuse

See *What if…?*

7. Psychotherapies

Discuss options with the team psychologist.
- *Family intervention*: may reduce risk of relapse by improving communication in families
  - You can offer this to other members of the household/family, even if Alex doesn't want to be involved
  - *High expressed emotion (EE)* refers to family attitudes/communication styles which can worsen prognosis and trigger relapse, i.e.
    - *Emotional over-involvement*, e.g. over-protectiveness, taking over tasks from the patient
    - *Hostility*, including blaming the patient
    - *Critical comments*
  - Low EE families show great *warmth* and *positive remarks* (e.g. supportive comments, appreciation) towards the patient
- *CBT for psychosis*: may reduce symptom severity, readmission rates, admission duration
  - Ask Alex how he thinks this could help, e.g. dealing with voices/anxiety; helping him understand the illness
- *Arts therapy*: reduces negative symptoms
  - Can be offered early in the illness. Often very popular.

Counselling and supportive psychotherapy aren't evidence-based, but worth considering if they'd help Alex, e.g. for engagement or feeling supported. Psychodynamic therapy *isn't* recommended.

8. Longer-term (+Ch.24)

- Provide access to information and mental health support groups
- Support the team in helping Alex pursue interests, social opportunities, education, and employment (Ch.13)
- Support carers. Check *they're* OK, and invite questions – they may otherwise hold back. Tell them about carers' support groups and ensure the CC offers a carer's assessment.

EI services increasingly recommend continuing antipsychotics for anywhere between 18 months and 3 years after a first episode of psychosis, to minimise the risk of relapse.
- Acknowledge this is *hard* and explain that people often don't manage this
- Offer to keep discussing it with him, or review it, e.g. every 3–6 months
- Consider explaining things in terms of risk. Risk-averse people ('I'll do *anything* not to relapse') might be happier with longer-term medication than risk-takers.
- If Alex might benefit from a depot, don't see this as a sign of failure – discuss sooner, rather than later (p58; Appendix B1.2)
- Consider clozapine if two trials of antipsychotics don't work (Ch.37)
- Monitor side-effects closely
- Encourage adherence (p177–8)
- Involve HTT swiftly if relapsing: getting the medication back on track *early* might prevent an admission.

Ask Alex to be honest with you and the team if he's stopped or considering stopping medication.
- Explain that you'll still support him if he *does*
- He and the team should discuss relapse indicators and have a crisis plan
- Keep him engaged with the team in all other ways, if he stops medication.

For discharge back to GP, see Ch.33.

PATIENT VIEW:

I've sometimes felt very distressed and wanted to get rid of The Controller, but the trouble is he knows what I'm thinking – there's no escape. I'll think *I'll go there and ask for a scan and ask them to take out these fucking things that are in my brain*, but he knows what I'm going to ask. Even when you start the thought, he's got the thought, the beginning of it, so he probably knows the rest. Totally distressing sometimes, really. Nothing you can do about it because he's got access to all your thoughts.

'Sarah'

What if ... ?

... He's also using drugs?

You'll see a spectrum of 'dual diagnosis' in the community: from people with severe mental illness intertwined with substance misuse, to those who function well, but use substances 'behind the scenes' to cope with depression or anxiety. In a general CMHT, your roles are to help Alex think about his drug use, manage co-morbid conditions, and liaise with addictions services (Ch.41).

General points
- Whether or not his psychosis is 'drug-induced', it's still a psychosis, and he still needs help
- When he's intoxicated/high, you can make a limited assessment but not hold a useful meeting. Unless immediate risks, re-arrange the meeting for a time when he can more easily attend sober.
- Immediately focusing on drug use may be counter-productive. Successfully tackling Alex's most pressing problems first can build trust and may allow substance misuse work.
- Psychology for psychosis may not be useful until substance use is controlled – discuss with the team psychologist
- Consider risks, e.g. targeted by drug dealers, contact with children?
- Physical health may be poor: can you or the GP offer screening or interventions?

Medication
Take extra care when prescribing psychotropics alongside substance misuse.
- Adherence may be chaotic: avoid long prescriptions
- Antipsychotics may increase sedation from depressant substances, e.g. opiates
- Avoid anticholinergics, benzodiazepines and opioid analgesics – all have a street value and misuse potential
- Liver impairment (e.g. from Hepatitis B/C) may impair drug metabolism
- Check interactions if prescribed antiretrovirals
- Seek advice from addictions services if unsure about doses/safety.

Psychoeducation
Use a motivational interviewing approach (p74). Try to understand Alex's reasons for substance misuse. This may help you to explore the relationship between psychiatric symptoms and substance use:
- "Self-medication"? (Drug used to suppress distressing feelings/symptoms)
- Increased use triggers relapse?

If Alex is receptive, offer information on substance misuse and mental health. You can explain:
- Many people use drugs to cope with their symptoms (e.g. voices, depression, paranoia) or medication side-effects

- This feels helpful, short term, but causes longer term problems:
  - Worsens symptoms e.g. cannabis – paranoia; alcohol – depression;
  - Increases likelihood of relapse and readmission
  - Makes symptoms harder to treat
  - Can cause a vicious cycle of illness/drug use.
- Drugs/alcohol can also interact with medication, increasing side effects, e.g. drowsiness, arrhythmia.

Addictions services
- Check local services, referral methods and what they offer
- Get leaflets/contact details for Alex if interested
- If Alex engages with them, find out:
  - Keyworker's details – invite them to CPAs and reviews
  - Prescriber's details – which medications and doses? E.g. benzodiazepines, methadone
- Avoid duplication between you, addictions and the GP. Document and communicate well, e.g. include keyworker and GP in all correspondence; add a prescribing alert to his notes.

> **TIP:** If you don't do an Addictions job, consider some training or special interest sessions to increase your confidence.

Take-home message

If 'all' you manage at a first appointment is an agreement to meet again, consider your assessment a success: engagement is the best first step.

Further reading

Stefan, H., Bracha, M.D. and Wolkowitz, O.M. (1989) High prevalence of visual hallucinations in research subjects with chronic schizophrenia. *American Journal of Psychiatry*, **146**, 526–528.

Singh, S. and Fisher, H. (2005) Early interventions in psychosis: obstacles and opportunities. *Advances in Psychiatric Treatment*, **11**, 71–78.

NICE (2014) Psychosis and schizophrenia in adults: treatment and management (CG178). NICE, Manchester. Available at: http://www.nice.org.uk/Guidance/CG178.

NICE (2011) Psychosis with coexisting substance misuse: Assessment and management in adults and young people. NICE, Manchester. Available at: http://publications.nice.org.uk/psychosis-with-coexisting-substance-misuse-cg120.

Resources for patients and carers:

Psychotic Experiences:
  - www.mind.org.uk/information-support/types-of-mental-health-problems/psychosis/what-is-psychosis/#.VCaOqxY1DXMtal_health_a-z/8043_understanding_psychotic_experiences

Schizophrenia:
  - www.rcpsych.ac.uk/healthadvice/problemsdisorders/schizophrenia.aspx

Cannabis and Mental Health:
  - www.rcpsych.ac.uk/expertadvice/problems/alcoholanddrugs/cannabis.aspx

CHAPTER 24

Psychosis – longer term

Stephanie Young

South London & Maudsley NHS Foundation Trust, London, England

RELATED CHAPTERS: first episode psychosis (23), disengagement (27), discharge (33), common side effect management (36)

Jenny, 52, lives alone in a housing association flat. She has schizophrenia, attends the CMHT for her monthly depot (if reminded), and hasn't been admitted for 6 years. She goes out twice a week, to the corner shop. At the CPA review, Jenny's dishevelled and quiet. Her CC seems frustrated, and suggests discharging Jenny to the depot clinic.

Patients with dramatic or worrying presentations can take up most of your time and energy, whilst people like Jenny – who are highly disabled but don't cause any 'trouble' – can slip under your radar. Negative symptoms are challenging, and need a thorough reassessment and recovery-oriented approach (p45). Try to help Jenny find goals and meaning in life, even if you can't 'cure' all her symptoms.

> **PATIENT VIEW:**
>
> I said to my nurse, "I think I'm going mad," and she said, 'No, you're not going mad." It was helpful, because I get so scared I'm going in hospital and going mad again, and because I don't know when I am – that's the trouble... I don't want to go mad. My dog needs me. My dad needs me, he's had a stroke. My mum needs me – she's elderly and dependent on me because she loves me so much. So I can't afford to get ill, so I'm taking the risperidone every day. It's very rare I don't.
>
> 'Sarah'

Preparation

1. Gather information – CC, GP, notes
- PPHx: previous relapses/admissions; relapse signature
  - Has she received OT or psychology input before?
- Risks including self-neglect
- DHx, including adherence.
  - Ever offered clozapine?
- PMHx: does she see the GP for annual health checks?
- Premorbid personality
  - Previous occupations, interests, social networks

Psychiatry: Breaking the ICE – Introductions, Common Tasks and Emergencies for Trainees, First Edition.
Edited by Sarah Stringer, Juliet Hurn and Anna M Burnside.
© 2016 John Wiley & Sons, Ltd. Published 2016 by John Wiley & Sons, Ltd.
Companion Website: www.psychiatryice.com

- CC's relationship with Jenny: duration, problems and frustrations?
  - Jenny's strengths.

2. Arrange a home visit (Ch.20)
- If Jenny agrees, this is far more useful than a CMHT appointment.

3. Check local resources
- Your service may have written 'Recovery' tools and plans for use with patients; take a look at these.

> **TIP:** Don't take diagnoses made by previous doctors for granted. Question, analyse, read up and ask your supervisor if you think someone's got the diagnosis or treatment wrong. There are hundreds of people out there with 'schizophrenia' who actually have nothing of the sort. We all find it easier to go along with what others have said – but learning to think for yourself will stand you in excellent stead for your future career.
>
> Daniel Harwood, Old Age Consultant

Assessment

1. Approach
You're not the CC who's met Jenny for years, and may be exhausted or bored. Acknowledge these feelings, and offer your support. Occasionally, words like 'lazy' creep into the language, even of professionals. Without being 'holier-than-thou', try to combat this, if it's an issue.

2. Full history, remembering ...
- *Negative symptoms and effect on life*
  - Poor motivation
  - Social withdrawal/no desire to form relationships
- *Residual/overlooked positive psychotic symptoms*
  - Paranoia may cause withdrawal
- *Medication*
  - Side-effects, especially mimicking/exacerbating negative symptoms, e.g. sedation making activity difficult; cognitive blunting; EPSEs
  - Adherence and smoking status (smoking lowers some antipsychotic levels)
- *Screen for psychiatric co-morbidity/differentials:*
  - Dementia – new memory problems or marked recent decline
  - Depression – cognitive and biological symptoms help distinguish depression from the negative syndrome's anhedonia. Remember Jenny may have *both*.
  - Social anxiety/loss of social confidence
- *Drugs/alcohol:*
  - Does she self-medicate for psychosis, insomnia or boredom?
  - Fatigue and low motivation are common with chronic alcohol/cannabis use
- *SHx:*
  - Home environment (NB: institutionalisation can worsen negative symptoms, e.g. in high-support placements)
  - ADLs
  - Social networks.

3. MSE, remembering ...

- Negative symptoms:
  - Poor self-care
  - Poverty of speech
  - Flat affect/anhedonia
- Hallucinations, delusions; formal thought disorder
- Cognition: formal testing (Appendix D).

PATIENT VIEW:

There's people who talk to themselves ... Now, is that some sort of psychotic reaction, or is that a natural thing that we do, to think over things?

'Ben'

---

4. Physical assessment

- Remember higher risks of co-morbidity due to schizophrenia (Ch.10)
- Exclude or treat conditions that mimic negative symptoms or limit activity, e.g. hypothyroidism, anaemia, shortness of breath.

Management

1. Manage immediate risks

If the home visit revealed unpleasant surprises (e.g. infestation, severe neglect), consider admission/HTT.

2. Treat comorbid conditions

- Consider SSRI for depression or anxiety
- Ask GP to address physical conditions/refer possible dementia to Memory Clinic
- Encourage Jenny to attend substance misuse services if appropriate.

3. Psychoeducation

Jenny may not realise that poor motivation is part of schizophrenia and hard to battle. Explain this, ensuring she understands she isn't being 'lazy' or 'stupid'. Also acknowledge if she *isn't* battling it, because she's 'content' with life as it is.

Carer psychoeducation is as important. Frustration levels can be high, due to, e.g.

- Jenny's 'laziness' or 'tiredness'
- The CC's failure to 'give her things to do'.

Acknowledge the frustration and sadness of 'losing' a relative to schizophrenia. Explain how they might support Jenny, e.g. by avoiding criticism and encouraging even small successes. Consider a carer's assessment ± family intervention.

TIP: With relatives, anger is often driven by guilt. Saying, "It must be really difficult for you looking after your husband," (or similar) can help conversations move on from complaining and defensive responses to thinking about what the problems are and what can be done to help.

Daniel Harwood, Old Age Consultant

4. Medication

- Blood levels if relevant and possible
- Optimise current medication
  - Manage side-effects (Ch.36)
  - Enhance adherence (p177–8)
  - Jenny's probably tried a number of different antipsychotics, but if not, consider switching (avoid FGAs due to EPSEs)
  - Aripiprazole *may* help with motivation, and can be added to an existing antipsychotic; discuss with your consultant
  - Proactively discuss clozapine if Jenny qualifies for this (Ch.37)
  - If clozapine isn't feasible, consider other treatment-resistant options with your consultant.

TIP: The French psychiatry professor, Marc Bourgeois said, "Le troisieme psychotrope est toujours de trop" – it means something like, "the third psychotropic drug is always excessive". I find it useful to remember when adding an extra drug. Ask yourself, *what am I actually treating? Is it psychosis, depression? What's the evidence for this combination?*

Dr Anna Lasis, LD Consultant

---

5. Recovery approach (p45)

Encourage autonomy by actively involving Jenny in her management and crisis plans:
- Ask how she already copes with symptoms; encourage this
- Ask what she enjoyed previously
  - Can she identify activities or goals she'd like to re-instate?

6. Psychosocial interventions

Help the CC brainstorm possibilities, e.g.
- OT referral if available and not recently done. An assessment can guide interventions or lead to specialist OT input.
- Discuss possibilities with a psychologist:
  - Cognitive remediation therapy/arts therapy (evidence-based for improving negative symptoms)
  - CBT for social anxiety
  - Behavioural therapy for goal-setting
  - Social skills training
  - Family interventions
- Check Jenny is receiving her full benefits entitlement (p89). Lack of money may make her reluctant to enrol in courses or activities.
- Support any application for transport passes if needed, e.g. Freedom pass. The case is usually strengthened when people use public transport to treatment-related activities.
- Brainstorm social opportunities and support, e.g.
  - Befriending, peer support
  - Volunteering opportunities
  - Day centres
  - Vocational training, college courses
- A support worker may be available to help her attend/try new activities.

TIP: Throughout your post, gather information on local services/resources (consider handing this on to the next trainee). Don't assume that every CC has considered all available resources – *you* might come up with the bright idea.

7. Longer-term plans

- Treat negative symptoms as you would any symptoms, i.e. review regularly and monitor the effect of interventions. Rating scales may help, e.g. PANSS
- Consider floating support or a move to higher-support accommodation
- Your team may have policies on the duration of input for people like Jenny, but think carefully before moving her to the depot clinic, since this may end active interventions
- Consider referral to a specialist rehabilitation service
  - www.rcpsych.ac.uk/pdf/fr_rs_1_forwebsite.pdf

> **TIP:** If your team has a regular case discussion, ask to present people like Jenny, not just your more dramatic or worrying patients.

Take-home message

Don't let patients with negative symptoms 'drift'. Actively think about management and assess their response to interventions.

Further reading

Shepherd, G., Boardman, J. and Slade, M. (2008) Making Recovery a Reality, *The Sainsbury Centre for Mental Health*, London.

Roberts, G., Davenport, S., Holloway, F. and Tattan, T. (eds) (2006) *Enabling Recovery: Principles and Practice of Psychiatric Rehabilitation*, Gaskell, London.

CHAPTER 25

Bipolar affective disorder (BPAD)

Rory Conn[1] and Juliet Hurn[2]

[1] Tavistock and Portman NHS Foundation Trust, London, England
[2] South London & Maudsley NHS Foundation Trust, London, England

RELATED CHAPTERS: mania (54), pregnancy (29, 43), lithium toxicity (69)

Josie Soler, 24, has just been discharged from hospital following a second lengthy admission for mania. She's an architecture student, repeating her third year. Her CC arranges a review, explaining that Josie's unsure about her diagnosis, and wants to stop lithium.

Developing a serious mental illness is often devastating, particularly when someone's focusing on career goals and the excitement of university. Possible problems are:
- Stigma
- Ambivalence about manic symptoms, e.g. highs may feel exciting/creative, or a welcome relief from depression
- Medication side effects
- Long-term adherence is difficult.

The 'kindling' theory (e.g. Bender, 2011) suggests that repeated relapses worsen prognosis in BPAD, so the earlier you address Josie's concerns and support her to manage her illness, the better.

Preparation

1. Gather information – GP, notes (including latest discharge summary), CC, family
- Previous episodes, triggers, engagement
- Medication history and adherence
- Blood results: lithium levels, renal function, TFTs
  - Frequency
  - Who's responsible? (You/GP)
- Risk history
- Social situation and relationships.

2. Encourage Josie to bring a relative/friend

Psychiatry: Breaking the ICE – Introductions, Common Tasks and Emergencies for Trainees, First Edition.
Edited by Sarah Stringer, Juliet Hurn and Anna M Burnside.
© 2016 John Wiley & Sons, Ltd. Published 2016 by John Wiley & Sons, Ltd.
Companion Website: www.psychiatryice.com

Assessment

1. Approach

Don't assume anyone's actually discussed BPAD properly with Josie when well enough to take on the information. Go back to basics where needed.

Acknowledge losses and readjustment difficulties. Answer Josie's questions and explore her worries about lithium. She may be feeling quite helpless, so you don't want to *impose* management, if at all possible. Focus on empowerment: give choices and encourage her to take control through self-management.

> **TIP:** Consider drawing Josie's illness with her, as a timeline (p31)

2. Focused history, remembering ...

- *Symptoms when unwell* – noticed by her and others
  - Hypomanic/manic
  - ± Depressive
  - ± Psychotic
- *Triggers*, e.g.
  - Stress, insomnia, international air-travel
  - Antidepressants, non-adherence
  - Substance misuse
- *Effect on life:*
  - Family, relationships.
  - University: impact on studies. Does her tutor know about her illness? Is the university supportive?
- *Medication:*
  - Lithium – reasons for stopping (Box 25.1)
  - Side-effects
  - Adherence with medication *and* monitoring
- *Comorbidities:*
  - Substance misuse – self-medication/trigger?
  - Anxiety disorder
  - Personality disorder.

Box 25.1 Common reasons for stopping lithium

- Side-effects (p61–3) including feeling blunted
- Loss of highs
- Blood tests
- Fear of damaging the brain/body
- Reminder of illness
- Planning pregnancy
- Poor insight

3. MSE, remembering ...

- Signs of manic relapse, depression or residual illness

4. Physical assessment (interventions via GP, if preferred)

- PMHx, smoking status
- Contraception/pregnancy plans
- Examination, including BP, BMI, thyroid disease
- Investigations, including:
  - Yearly BPAD checks (Appendix A1 and 4)
  - Medication monitoring (Appendix A6)
- Pregnancy test/GUM referral if appropriate.

5. Risk assessment

Current *and* relapse risks, e.g.
- Self-harm
- Self-neglect
- Deterioration of mental ± physical health
- Sexual, financial, social vulnerability (e.g. relationship breakdown)
- Driving
- Aggression.

Management

Some Early Intervention services include BPAD – check local protocols.

1. Manage acute relapse

Acute mania often needs admission; hypomania *can* often be managed in the community – see Ch.54 (mania) and Ch.62 (relapse). For depressive relapse, see *What if … ?*

2. Talking about the illness

Josie may be bewildered, scared or angry about recent events. Answer questions and discuss:
- Why she 'qualifies' for the diagnosis of BPAD (Table 54.1, p342)
- Genetic contribution and importance of triggers (stress vulnerability model)
- Natural illness course (relapsing-remitting)
- Prognosis – usually well between episodes
  - Good management can decrease episode frequency and severity.

Offer a leaflet, and links to support groups (see resources on p164).

3. Self-management

This work may be offered more formally with a psychologist, but you can start the conversation, involving Josie's carers wherever possible.

Use her timeline, or suggest a symptom/mood diary (Bipolar UK link, p164) to help her identify:
- Triggers
- Early warning signs, e.g. insomnia, irritability, concerned friends
- Relapse signature
- Impact of relapse on her life.

Encourage Josie to take control of triggers:
- Establish a routine, increasing relaxation, decreasing 'busy-ness'
- Sleep hygiene (p72); avoid pulling 'all-nighters'
- Care if flying across time zones

- Stress-management and problem solving
- Seek help from carers when stressed
- Medication – stopping or omitting medication increase her relapse risk

Agree a crisis plan for early warning signs, e.g.

- Get advice quickly from GP/CMHT; attend ED
- ± Swift access to night sedation, benzodiazepines or an antipsychotic in early relapse or high-risk periods, e.g. travelling abroad
  - ○ Discuss doses and indications
  - ○ Some people hold a small 'emergency' supply themselves.

4. Medication

Go back to basics, explaining the rationale for long-term BPAD medication, and encourage Josie to consider lithium's costs/benefits (p61–63, Appendix B6). If she doesn't want lithium, discuss options with your consultant ± offer a meeting with a pharmacist. Explain alternatives, giving full and written information on *effects*, *side-effects*, and *monitoring*. Decisions should recognise her preferences and past response to treatment.

- *Lithium*: tried and tested; significant side effects, monitoring and toxicity risks
- *Sodium valproate* (Appendix B6): common alternative to lithium – less monitoring/toxicity, though slightly less effective
- *Olanzapine, aripiprazole, risperidone, quetiapine* (p57–9, Appendices B1&2) – effective mood stabilisers, but carry antipsychotic risks and monitoring needs
- *Carbamazepine* – if poor response to above options (Appendix B6).

All mood stabilisers are teratogenic (Table 29.1, p186), so discuss reliable contraception with all women of child-bearing age. Avoid using valproate or carbamazepine, but prescribe folate if unavoidable. Document your information-giving and consent.

> **TIP:** If you see women of child-bearing age prescribed valproate/carbamazepine, raise this with your consultant and consider safer alternatives.

5. Physical health

Josie should be on her GP's SMI register and receive annual monitoring (Appendix A1) in addition to medication monitoring. Decide whether the GP or CMHT will take responsibility, and ensure results are shared between primary and secondary care.

Provide simple, non-judgemental information about the possible impact of substance misuse on symptoms, offering information on substance misuse services if needed.

6. Psychotherapies

Discuss options with your psychologist:

- Psychoeducation
- Relapse prevention work/coping strategies
- CBT
- Family intervention if there are particular issues to address.

7. Longer-term

- Student issues:
  - ○ Would Josie like you/CC/vocational worker to liaise with her tutor or university health service about her illness?
  - ○ Could you advocate for extra support, e.g. a study mentor?

- ○ Plan for care during term-time *and* holidays. You may share care with a CMHT local to her studies, or offer more flexible appointments to enable attendance during term-time.
- Keep carers involved. Tell them about carers' support groups and ensure they've had a carers' assessment via the CC.

Although some people need to take medication long-term, this is *difficult.* Review medication regularly and tackle side effects or worries proactively. Ask Josie to be honest with you and her CC if she wants to stop or has *stopped* medication.

- Explain you'll still support her if she decides to go medication-free, but it's generally safer to withdraw mood stabilisers (especially lithium) slowly, to reduce the relapse risk
- She and her CC should discuss relapse indicators and the crisis plan
- If she stops medication, keep her engaged with the team in all other ways.

For discharge back to GP, see Ch.33.

What if ... ?

... Josie's renal function deteriorates?

Abnormal renal function is *commonly* found in people using lithium, but may relate to other factors, e.g. vascular disease:
- ↑ urea, creatinine, ↓ eGFR – may be reversible *or* irreversible
- Lithium levels can rise and therefore cause toxicity (Ch.69).

Discuss with nephrology before making the cost/benefit decision with Josie to continue or stop lithium. (See also the patient management problem on the Breaking the ICE website.)
- GFR <50 ml/min: discontinue *or* reduce dose and increase monitoring frequency
- If GFR <10 ml/min and lithium *must* be continued, reduce dose to 50% or less of normal dose.

... Josie's develops hypothyroidism?

You don't usually need to stop lithium. Discuss with Josie's GP ± endocrinology.
- Abnormal TFTs but asymptomatic: continue monitoring
- Symptomatic hypothyroidism or ongoing mood problems (e.g. rapid cycling): prescribe thyroxine.

... Josie's depressed?

Depression's often severe and risky in BPAD: take it seriously and monitor closely for suicide risk. Treatment is generally as for unipolar depression (Ch.21), but recognises that antidepressants can trigger mania/hypomania ('switching'). Prioritise non-medical treatments, e.g. CBT.

Antidepressants should *not* be prescribed:
- Without mood stabiliser 'cover'
- Without close mood monitoring, e.g. via a mood diary
- For long periods once depression's resolved.

... Josie has bipolar II? (Table 54.1, p342)

Bipolar II may not require admission, but often evolves into recurrent depression with more occasional hypomanic episodes, and may include high suicidality. It's *frequently* misdiagnosed as recurrent depression.
- Treat as for bipolar I, though lamotrigine or quetiapine may be particularly helpful for depression
- Take extra care with antidepressant switching.

Cyclothymia may be treated similarly, though self-management/psychology intervention alone are often preferred to medication.

...Josie has rapid cycling disorder? (Table 54.1, p342)

Like bipolar II, this has a high depressive morbidity and suicide risk.
* Withdraw antidepressants
* Discuss options with your consultant, e.g. combining lithium and valproate; lamotrigine; SGAs
* Focus on mood diary and triggers.

TIP: Audit ideas include:
* **Valproate in women of reproductive age: documented informed consent about risk/prophylactic folate**
* **Lithium monitoring adherence**
* **Patient knowledge of lithium management**

Take-Home Message

Help Josie prevent relapse by managing her triggers and providing bio-psycho-social interventions.

Reference

Bender, R.E. and Alloy, L.B. (2011) Life Stress and kindling in bipolar disorder: Review of the evidence and integration with emerging biopsychosocial theories. *Clinical Psychology Review*, **31**(3), 383–398.

Further reading

Jamieson, K.R. (1995) *An Unquiet Mind: A Memoir of Moods and Madness.* Vintage Books, London.
Psychologist's account of her own bipolar illness – useful for doctors and patients.
NICE (2014) CG185 Bipolar disorder: the assessment and management of bipolar disorder in adults, children and young people in primary and secondary care. NICE. Available at: http://www.nice.org.uk/Guidance/CG185.
Patients, carers ± clinicians:
  ○ www.bipolaruk.org.uk (includes downloadable mood diaries)
  ○ www.bipolar-foundation.org
  ○ www.mind.org.uk/information-support/types-of-mental-health-problems/bipolar-disorder/
  ○ http://www.rcpsych.ac.uk/healthadvice/problemsdisorders/bipolardisorder.aspx
  ○ www.beatingbipolar.org/ (interactive site for patients and clinicians including psychoeducation modules)

CHAPTER 26

Emotionally unstable personality disorder (EUPD)

Jane Bunclark and Juliet Hurn

South London & Maudsley NHS Foundation Trust, London, England

RELATED CHAPTERS: ward EUPD (45), self-harm (51)

Karen, 35, has EUPD and has needed numerous admissions for self-harm. She frequently texts her CC, saying she's suicidal and that her CC 'doesn't care'. You're asked to review.

Personality disorder (PD) is as much a mental disorder as psychosis, dementia or mania, but *by definition*, these patients have problems managing relationships, including those with psychiatric services and professionals. This can make it hard for them to seek or accept help, and hard for services to provide help. They're often mistreated, not least because the 'PD label' dredges up memories of particularly difficult patients, which staff may link unfairly with anyone given this diagnosis.

EUPD (sometimes called "borderline" PD) patients can provoke strong reactions; you may find that staff are reluctant to work with them, or believe these patients are 'untreatable' or 'undeserving' (Table 26.1, Box 26.1). A more useful view is that EUPD *can* be helped, but management is more a marathon than a sprint: you can't treat a lifetime of difficulties with a couple of outpatient appointments and a swift prescription. Relationships with Karen may be the source of difficulties, but they're also the key to recovery.

> **TIP:** One way of seeing it is that personality disordered patients can be very controlling in relationships because they're very anxious about them. It's a mistake to be endlessly empathic, just listening – you can become the dustbin to the patient's distress. Therefore, an empathic relationship involves staying in touch with their distress, limit-setting and thinking about how to help them manage it better.
>
> **Duncan McLean, Consultant Psychiatrist and Psychotherapist**

Psychiatry: Breaking the ICE – Introductions, Common Tasks and Emergencies for Trainees, First Edition.
Edited by Sarah Stringer, Juliet Hurn and Anna M Burnside.
© 2016 John Wiley & Sons, Ltd. Published 2016 by John Wiley & Sons, Ltd.
Companion Website: www.psychiatryice.com

Table 26.1 EUPD psychological mechanisms.

Mechanism/ pattern	Karen …	You/team …	Management tips
Poor anxiety containment	Passes anxiety onto you, e.g. hints mysteriously at suicide, but won't elaborate	Feel anxious ± over-react to manage own anxiety, e.g. detain	• Acknowledge anxiety • Discuss with senior/team • Make decisions based on calm risk assessment, rather than anxiety. Explain that this may take time, so Karen doesn't interpret this as procrastinating/being dismissive
Black and white (polarised/ dichotomous) thinking	Idealises some staff (e.g. helpful, caring) and denigrates others (e.g. cold, stupid). Dynamics can change: Karen may praise you today and 'sack' you tomorrow.	Emotional roller-coaster, e.g. *I'm so caring … I'm incompetent!*	• Remember it's not about *you* • Reinforce the idea for Karen that you're part of a team, which has strengths, weaknesses and limitations
Splitting	Plays team members off against each other; may refuse to work with some.	Team division/conflict. Spend disproportionate time discussing Karen.	• Recognise and discuss splitting • Regular but boundaried staff meetings/case discussion slots to discuss and resolve splitting • Involve psychologists/ psychotherapists
Idealised attachments/ boundary breaking	Seeks more than patient–professional relationships, e.g. offers 'secrets'/ opportunities to be 'the only one who understands'. Asks disingenuously about your personal life.	Over-involvement/ unease. Feel flattered or drawn into 'becoming a friend'.	• Explain and hold professional boundaries • Be reliable and consistent • Don't disclose personal information
Abuse	Re-enacts previous abusive experiences in your relationship	Feel 'abused' yourself, e.g. by Karen's criticism. Become drawn into 'abuser' role, e.g. harsh tone; 'teaching her a lesson'; sub-standard treatment.	• Monitor your reactions • Discuss decisions with the team if you're acting out-of-character • Consider discussing the dynamic with Karen (often best with senior colleague present)
Testing behaviour	Tries to elicit a response, e.g. harms herself in clinic when you decline a prescription	Feel personally attacked; react disapprovingly or over-protectively.	• Don't condemn or condone • Take a balanced stance: the behaviour is understandable but not acceptable.
Catastrophising	Experiences general life events/problems/ relationships as overwhelming, leading to crisis.	Need to 'rescue'/go into crisis mode	• Discuss crisis plans in advance • Give Karen warning if usual staff taking leave, arranging alternative (experienced and well-briefed) staff cover

Table 26.1 (*continued*)

Mechanism/ pattern	Karen …	You/team …	Management tips
Ambivalence towards services	Oscillates between unrealistically high expectations ('insatiability') and disappointment	Offering too much (e.g. over-run meetings because disclosures are made at the end). Feel you've failed.	• Manage expectations, e.g. reasonable frequency and duration of appointments • Don't offer what you can't guarantee • Explain your limitations and acknowledge she may feel disappointed • Check you're offering only what you'd reasonably offer *any* patient • Significant crises should be managed more flexibly, rather than enforcing 'treatment as usual'
Difficulty in thinking/ feeling	Uses mind-numbing behaviours to avoid/evacuate emotions, thoughts or memories, e.g. self-harm	Find yourself struggling to think clearly; feel pushed into action yourself.	• Model listening/thoughtfulness, rather than rushing to suggest solutions • Encourage Karen to mentalise (p69)

Box 26.1 Difficulties in EUPD (borderline/impulsive subtypes conflated)

- *Emotion/behaviour:*
  - Unstable mood, difficulty regulating/expressing emotions
  - Uncertain self-image/desires; feeling 'empty'
  - Impulsivity, poor planning; angry outbursts
- *Relationships*: conflicted, intense/unstable
  - Efforts to avoid abandonment/rejection
- *Recurrent self-harm/suicidal thoughts*
- *Transient psychotic symptoms*, e.g. hearing voices when stressed
- *Harmful coping mechanisms*, e.g. substance misuse, 'comfort' eating

Preparation

1. Gather information – notes, CC, GP

- Previous engagement/relationships with staff and services
  - Strengths and positive experiences
  - Difficulties, including complaints
- Self-harm: triggers, pattern, function (Table 51.1, p321)
- Past management, including boundary-setting, crisis plans, admissions
  - What did/didn't help?
- Personal history (helps understand personality development and therefore current patterns of behaviour)
  - Childhood; relationships, employment, life events.

2. Plan joint review *with* CC

- Take a team approach to minimise misunderstandings/splitting (Table 26.1)
- If Karen refuses, explain that you'll discuss with your team (including the CC)
- Aim *not* to change CC (problems are likely to recur with *anyone*). Instead, try to help Karen manage the difficulties of working closely with one person.
- See Table 26.1 for practical tips, should the meeting become tricky.

> **TIP:** Speak to clinicians who've met Karen before – they may have useful insights, not elaborated in the notes. Expressions of frustration are *information*, not a cause for despair!

Assessment

1. Approach

- Agree an agenda and explain time constraints
- Be calm, open, curious and empathic
- Let Karen voice distress/frustration, rather than bracing yourself for conflict
- Showing frustration yourself won't make this interview go faster or smoother
- Notice Karen's interactions with you and colleagues. Don't label her as 'dramatic'/'fake'/ 'manipulative' – store observations as information about how she experiences others, and discuss this with your team, afterwards.
- Be aware of your *counter-transference* (p78) to Karen, e.g. irritation, helplessness. Notice whether you're 'taking up a role', e.g. disapproving parent.
- Think *why* she's reacting this way, e.g. childhood trauma, adult experiences of frustration and disappointment in others.

> **PATIENT VIEW:**
>
> They just talked to me like a normal, intelligent human being that also had a mental health diagnosis. It felt quite equal. Once it starts feeling unequal, you start regressing to a childlike state when the teacher's telling you what to do, and you get into this weird dynamic.
>
> **'Adele'**

2. Full history, remembering ...

- *HPC: What do you find most difficult now?*
  - Let her express problems that others are causing her, then try ...
    - *What's caused you to feel/behave in this way?*
    - *Why did X (events/feelings) cause you to do Y (e.g. text messages/suicide threats)*
    - *Did Y help you? (How?/Why not?)*
    - *What else have you tried to manage X?*
  - Explore coping mechanisms and strengths
- *Experience of care:*
  - *How have you got on with staff before?*
  - *What's made relationships difficult?*
  - *What's been helpful/unhelpful?* (Including admissions)
- *Comorbidity:* especially other personality disorders/strong traits
  - Mood, anxiety (especially PTSD), eating, psychotic disorders
  - Exclude differentials, e.g. BPAD II (discrete, *sustained* periods of hypomania); ADHD
  - NB Personality disorder worsens the prognosis of other disorders
- *DHx:* perceived usefulness, adherence
  - Dependence on prescribed medications, e.g. benzodiazepines

- *Substance misuse*: role in self-medication/coping/triggering conflict or self-harm
- *Relationships*:
  - Early family: abuse, neglect, inconsistency (rejection/abandonment) – causing disordered attachments
  - Previous patterns/conflicts with friends, family, partners
  - Current social networks: quality (supportive or dysfunctional)
  - Own children: relationships, perception of *their* personalities, behaviours and interactions with her and others
  - Views on carer involvement
- *Sexual history*: childhood sexual abuse; rape; abusive partners; sex-working
- *Forensic*: crime and antisocial behaviour.

3. MSE, remembering ...

- Rapport; intense emotional responses; outbursts
- Observed dissociation, other psychological mechanisms (Table 26.1)
- Depression, elation, lability
- Current thoughts or plans for self-harm/suicide
- Pseudohallucinations/hallucinations
- Flashbacks.

> **TIP:** It's debatable whether the experience of pseudohallucinations in EUPD is different from hallucinations in psychosis. Don't argue or imply that an experience of voices 'isn't real'. Instead, ensure you're not missing a first episode of psychosis and explore, e.g.
> - *Do the voices feel like something alien, a part of yourself, or a memory of someone from the past?*
> - *How do they make you feel?*
> - *How do you cope?*
> - *Have your experiences changed recently?*

4. Risk assessment

- *Previous self-harm/suicide attempts* (Ch.51 for details)
  - Explore methods and function (Table 51.1, p321)
  - Triggers (check significant anniversaries, e.g. birthdays, bereavements)
  - Warning signs
  - Does she 'own' her risk and seek help *or* await 'rescue' by others?
  - Which behaviours does she think place her at most risk?
  - Protective factors
  - Coping skills; obstacles to using these
  - Previous helpful care/crisis plans
- *Other risks to self*:
  - Vulnerability, e.g. sexual abuse, domestic violence
  - Substance misuse.
  - Accidents/retributive violence (excess mortality in PD)
- *Risks to others*:
  - Children, e.g. neglect, witnessing self-harm; abuse
  - Violence.

5. Physical health, especially

- Self-harm injuries, e.g. scars, burns, liver damage
- Misuse of alcohol/drugs/prescribed medications
- Sexual health: contraception, GUM

6. Collateral

Although carers' views may be coloured by their own frustration or distress, they'll give insights into how people perceive Karen, and the dynamics of her wider relationships. It's essential to get carers 'on board' with the treatment plan – and asking their views can be the first step.

Management

For immediate risk of self-harm, see Ch.51.

1. Psychoeducation

Check whether Karen knows/agrees with her diagnosis. Develop your own ways of explaining this, e.g.

- Summarise her main problems, and relate these to diagnostic criteria, e.g.
  - *You've explained how your emotions change quickly, and sometimes feel overwhelming. They make it hard for you to plan your days, or have long-lasting relationships, as you never know how you'll feel next. This* emotional instability *is really common in people who've been through extremely difficult experiences, especially in childhood.*
- Link life experiences to difficulties coping with emotions and relationships
  - *After a lifetime of being let down or hurt by people, it's really hard to trust or believe people can be kind or reliable.*
  - *It sounds like you weren't given the space or support to cope with difficult emotions when you were younger – and the ways you developed [e.g. self-harm] were the best you had at the time. Some coping strategies cause you more harm than good, but are hard to change after years of use.*
- Recognise that you can't change the past, but it's possible to understand it and learn ways to cope, which don't cause Karen such harm.

2. Planning treatment

Management plans should be:

- *Collaborative* – encourage Karen to see herself as a partner, working *with* you
- *Consistent* – plans may evolve, but try to maintain an agreed direction/goal
- *Contracted* – as far as possible:
  - Be realistic about the team's resources, e.g. agree frequency/duration of contacts, including telephone calls; content/focus of conversations
  - Agree acceptable behaviours e.g. *If I feel suicidal, instead of texting my CC, I'll [follow crisis plan]*
  - Agree acceptable team responses, e.g. *My CC won't immediately respond to a text, but will remind me (maximum once a day) to follow my crisis plan.*

Agree treatment goals

Encourage Karen to focus on realistic goals, e.g.

- Learn more about coping with emotions
- Develop plans for when she wants to self-harm
- Learn to work with her CC
- Tackle substance misuse
- Cope with work stress; find voluntary or paid work if unemployed.

If you can't cover this today, arrange a further planning meeting.

Crisis plans

A 'crisis' often means escalating self-harm, but may also present as unbearable anger, anxiety, or worsening psychotic symptoms. Adapt the plan accordingly, taking these problems into account. Remember, you can mitigate – but not eliminate – risk.

Construct the crisis plan together, including:
- Triggers and early warning signs, e.g. arguments; loneliness, tension
- Coping strategies/alternatives to self-harm (Table 51.4, p325)
- Proactively seek help if suicidal or worried she'll seriously self-harm, e.g. attend ED/call Samaritans
- *Harm minimisation*: if unrealistic to stop self-harm, consider harm minimisation (p325)
  - Discuss with your team/senior before discussing with Karen as part of a longer-term plan to reduce self-harm
  - Advise her there's no safe way to self-poison
- If Karen presents in crisis, try to *contain* her emotions, rather than jumping in to react (either with exasperation or piling on safety measures). Options include:
  - Help her express her feelings. Be calm, reassuring and empathic.
  - Review her crisis plan with her and encourage her to use it
  - Increase support, e.g. CC contact/enlist carer support
  - *HTT*: agree indications with HTT beforehand, e.g. increased risks, reduced support
  - Consider admission (Box 26.2)

Box 26.2 Admissions and EUPD.

- Don't make admissions a battleground
- Early on, discuss indications with your consultant and Karen
  - Karen might consider a goal, e.g. maximum number of admissions/year
- *Remember it's difficult for colleagues who don't know Karen to 'fend off' an admission*
  - Clarify admission criteria and any plans for out-of-hours presentations
  - Add an alert to her record, drawing attention to this plan
  - Any admission should be on the understanding that your team will review her and the plan, the next working day
- Ideally, admissions should:
  - Be to a ward where staff know her and won't overreact. Better an acute ward (e.g. Triage), rather than a long-stay ward.
  - Have clear goals, e.g. contain a crisis, review medication, treat depression
  - Be brief, with agreed time-frames
  - Be informal. Detention removes *Karen's* responsibility and may reinforce views of herself as helpless, or others as controlling/abusive
- Clarify plans with ward staff
- Ensure her team/CC are involved throughout admission and at discharge

(*Source*: Adapted from Bateman and Tyrer 2004.)

3. Medication

Polypharmacy is common in EUPD – often due to misdiagnosis or therapeutic desperation. Avoid futile arguments about whether Karen 'needs' existing medication; it's likely to be an important coping mechanism, even if placebo-based. Explore why she finds it helpful.
- There are no evidence-based medications for EUPD. The following are sometimes tried and may modestly help some people:
  - Antidepressants – low mood, anxiety, impulsivity
  - Antipsychotics – voices
  - Mood stabilisers – affective instability
- Medication may be used for *comorbid conditions*, e.g. depression
- If considering medication:
  - Discuss with your senior first (they may have strong views)
  - Discuss NICE recommendations and risks/benefits with Karen
  - Monitor effect, e.g. symptom diary, rating scale, number of ED presentations

- ∘ Consider risks in OD (including cumulative effect if taken with existing medications). Limit scripts *with* Karen, e.g. don't give a 3–month supply of amitriptyline.
- ∘ Discuss safety at risky times, e.g. Karen could agree to hand supplies to carers
- Medication in crises:
  - ∘ Avoid initiating if possible; discuss benzodiazepines/antipsychotics with seniors
  - ∘ Choose time-limited, safer sedatives (e.g. 1 week of promethazine 25 mg)
  - ∘ Review frequently with a view to stopping (e.g. planned, gradual reduction for benzodiazapines)
- Withdrawing medication
  - ∘ Withdrawal will be *far* more successful if Karen agrees
  - ∘ Explain reasons for stopping
  - ∘ Consolidate other coping strategies and reduce gradually
  - ∘ Discuss conflicts with seniors.

4. Psychological treatments (p66–70)

Karen may have had numerous psychotherapies before. Summarise these (including benefits) and discuss with your psychologist.

- Karen needs good overall engagement and motivation
- The evidence base is limited, but options include:
  - ∘ Dialectical Behavioural Therapy (Linehan, 1993) and Mentalisation Based Therapy (Allen and Fonagy, 2006) – both usually as part of a treatment programme. May reduce self-harm (in women), anger, aggression and depression.
  - ∘ CBT/CAT – may help specific problems (e.g. self-harm, anger management) and comorbid symptoms (e.g. depression, anxiety)
  - ∘ Local specialist services, e.g. therapeutic communities.

5. Other considerations

- Remember to discuss Karen's strengths and positive qualities (recovery, p45)
- Don't let the PD label blind you to comorbid psychiatric/physical problems
- Offer help with substance misuse (p152–3)
- Involve, educate and support carers
- Address practical problems, e.g. housing, finances, domestic violence
- Rather than always focusing on how to change Karen, think about whether you can help her change her *environment* to make life easier (Tyrer 2009).
- Document and communicate carefully. This helps ensure management is consistent and all staff use the same approach, boundaries and plans (including GP, wards).

6. Support yourself and the team

- Suggest team discussion slots to plan Karen's care
  - ∘ An external facilitator may help if particularly fraught
- Be aware of her taking up too much time at the expense of other patients
- Avoid pejorative terms, e.g. *attention-seeking, manipulative, time-waster*
- Discuss your own reactions in supervision Balint/psychotherapy group.

7. Discharge

This can be problematic, so discuss with your team. The usual principles apply (Ch.33) but remember:

- Karen may interpret discharge/transfers as rejection
  - ∘ Acknowledge this, discuss fully and never discharge suddenly
- Give extra care to crisis planning and good communication with the GP.

Take-home message

Working with people with EUPD can be challenging, but a compassionate, boundaried and reflective stance is most helpful.

References

Allen, G. and Fonagy, P. (2006) *The Handbook of Mentalization-Based Treatment*. John Wiley and Sons, Chichester.
Bateman, A.W. and Tyrer, P. (2004) Services for personality disorder: organisation for inclusion. *Advances in Psychiatric Treatment*, **10**, 425–433.
Linehan, M. (1993) *Cognitive-behavioural Treatment of Borderline Personality Disorder*, Guildford Press, New York.
Tyrer, P. (2009) *Nidotherapy: Harmonising the Environment with the Patient*. RCPsych, London.

Further reading

Adshead, G. and Jacob, C. (2012) Personality disorder, in Core Psychiatry, 3rd edn, (eds P. Wright, J. Stern and M. Phelan), Saunders, Elsevier, London, pp. 193–206.
Davison, S.E. (2002) Principles of managing patients with personality disorder. *Advances in Psychiatric Treatment* **8**, 1–16.
NICE (2009) CG 78 Borderline Personality Disorder, *NICE*.
NICE (2011) CG 133 Self-harm: Long Term Management, *NICE*.
Norton, K. (1996) Management of difficult personality disorder patients. *Advances in Psychiatric Treatment*, **2**, 202–210.

Patient/Carer resources:

BPD world: www.bpdworld.org (US website: patient and professional resources)
Emergence: www.emergenceplus.co.uk (for patients)
RCPsych leaflet: www.rcpsych.ac.uk/healthadvice/problemsdisorders/personalitydisorder.aspx
Mason, P.T. and Kreger, R. (2010) *Stop Walking on Eggshells: Taking Your Life Back When Someone You Care About has Borderline Personality Disorder*, New Harbinger, Oakland CA.

CHAPTER 27

Non-engagement or disengagement

Rory Conn

Tavistock and Portman NHS Foundation Trust, London, England

RELATED CHAPTERS: home visits (20), psychosis – longer-term (24), discharge (33), relapse (62)

Mick Styles, 58, has schizoaffective disorder and self-neglects when relapsing. He engages erratically, sometimes leaving home for several weeks and missing his depot, before suddenly reappearing. His CC raises him at the team meeting: Mick hasn't been opening his door.

Every team has patients who are hard to work with, for various reasons (Table 27.1). For some, non-engagement is a sign that they're well, getting on with life, and don't need you. For others, it's a red flag of relapse, heralding risk events or the need for admission. Non-engagement usually means there are barriers, needing more flexible, creative or intensive interventions.

Preparation

1. Gather information – CC, notes, GP, family
- Does Mick have a pattern of poor/intermittent engagement or is this unusual?
  - Don't be complacent – there may be new reasons for non-engagement
- How does he usually get on with his CC?
- Usual relapse signature
  - What's helped re-engage him before?
- Historic risks
- Recent concerns:
  - Signs of relapse
  - Medication adherence
  - New psychiatric problems e.g. cognitive decline
  - Recent discharge from psychiatric/general hospital
  - Risks, e.g. expressions of hopelessness
  - Physical health (Is he seeing his GP/allowing investigations or treatment?)

2. Efforts to make contact
- Usual and recent: texts, calls, letters, home visits
- How many contacts has he missed/declined?
- Home visits: announced or unannounced?
  - Timings (likely to be in?)
  - Signs of life, e.g. post collected, curtains being opened/closed
  - Called through letterbox? Left a note?

Psychiatry: Breaking the ICE – Introductions, Common Tasks and Emergencies for Trainees, First Edition.
Edited by Sarah Stringer, Juliet Hurn and Anna M Burnside.
© 2016 John Wiley & Sons, Ltd. Published 2016 by John Wiley & Sons, Ltd.
Companion Website: www.psychiatryice.com

Table 27.1 Reasons for non-engagement.

Factor	Reasons for non-engagement
Psychiatric	Acute: relapse Chronic: • Negative symptoms, paranoia • Anxiety, agoraphobia, social phobia • Depression • Personality traits, e.g. dismissive or feels undeserving of help • Low energy, motivation, confidence Disorganisation/chaotic: • Cognitive problems, e.g. dementia, depression • Unstable illness, social situation, homelessness • Substance misuse
Practical/environmental	Away, e.g. holiday, visiting family Physical illness/poor mobility Medication side effects, e.g. over-sedation prevents morning appointments Forgetful, e.g. around medication/appointments Appointments, e.g. inconvenient, letters sent to wrong address/illiterate patients Cultural, e.g. correct interpreter not provided; overlooking religious festivals Team base: • Dislikes environment/sitting with unwell patients/stigma • Far from home/travel problems • Neighbourhood problems, e.g. victim of crime/gangs Home visits: • Feel intrusive • Embarrassment, e.g. because cluttered, dirty
Health beliefs/ experiences	Well or managing symptoms – wants to move on 'Benefits' of illness, e.g. if well, would miss voices/'creativity' Conflict with medical model, e.g. • Feels stigmatised (medication can add to stigma) • Doesn't want/like/believe in treatment • Poor insight • Influenced by sceptical others, e.g. family, GP Anxious about: • Seeing a doctor • Receiving a diagnosis/unwanted treatment • Being detained Relationship with team: • Mistrust of professionals • Past negative experience of care • Expecting a negative reaction, e.g. criticism for non-adherence • Perceived lack of: communication, warmth, helpfulness, thoroughness, competence, listening • Frequent changes in CC/doctor • Treatment decisions feel non-collaborative • Unclear goals
Serious event	Death/illness/accident

Initial Management

> **TIP:** Always assume the patient *doesn't* want to see you. Make it as easy as possible for them.
>
> **Phil Timms, Consultant**

1. Collateral history

Ensure all potential sources of information have been contacted: GP, relatives, housing officer, day centre staff, neighbours (discreetly)
- Is anyone else worried?
- When did they last see him?

PATIENT VIEW:

When I see a person I know, I think, *That's not X, she has a good sense of humour, she's a really lovely woman.* So, I wonder what upset her. But when *you* see someone and they're very upset, all you might think is, *that's part of an illness* – because you don't know the person. You don't know that this could be for a reason and you need to find out about that. Where is she coming from, why is she behaving like this?

'Alexia'

---

2. Immediately risky presentation (see also Ch.62)

You may need to act assertively and swiftly if:
- The team's exhausted ways of seeing him
- Other people are worried, e.g. family
- Relapse indicators have reappeared
- Risk, e.g. recent expressions of self-harm
- Recent discharge from hospital
- Worrying signs at property, e.g. post piling up, unusual smells, distressed pets
- Poorly managed medical problems.

Discuss options with your team, including consultant, e.g.
- Further home visit
- Police *welfare check* (p245), if extreme concerns about physical health/suicide
- MHA assessment if strong suspicions of relapse. The AMHP will probably need to apply for a warrant (s135), since Mick isn't opening his door.

3. Less worrying presentations

Make more efforts to communicate – discuss ideas with the team, e.g.
- Write: say you're worried and would really like to see him, at a clear time and place
- Offer a team-based group/activity (e.g. football), rather than a medical review
- Ask family or GP to facilitate contact, e.g. open the door/joint visit
- Opportunistic engagement, e.g. at day centre or favourite cafe
- If a colleague has a better relationship with Mick, could *they* try to see him?

Keep reviewing risk and the need for more assertive action.

Management

When you *do* see Mick, explain he's not in any trouble, but you've been worried. Find out why he hasn't been in touch (Table 27.1). Review his current circumstances, MSE, risk and physical health.

Table 27.2 Solutions to non-engagement.

Problem	Possible solution
Appointment practicalities	Liaise with team/administrator ...
	Reminders, e.g. CC calls/texts 24h beforehand
	Choose appointment times, e.g. flexible/open access booking
	Offer afternoon appointments (generally better attended)
	Avoid clashing with Mick's commitments, e.g. work, religious festivals
	Book correct interpreter
Problems attending	Liaise with GP – address physical/mobility problems
	Arrange benefits advice/free bus pass
	Suggest initial meeting at non-CMHT site, e.g. cafe local to home
	Help to access travel apps, maps
	CC to bus/walk the route to and from the team base *with* Mick at first
	Support worker/carer to accompany him to appointments
	Consider befriender referral
Experience of care	Apologise for problems
	Build therapeutic alliance: if Mick likes and trusts you, he's more likely to attend
	Clarify and agree: treatment plan, likely duration, and purpose of reviews
	Psychologist to work on insight/medication adherence
	Improve continuity, e.g. suggest Mick sees consultant rather than transient trainees
	Be as flexible as possible, e.g.
	• Ask *where* he'd like to be reviewed, at *what time*, and *by whom*
	• Offer treatment choice
	• Involve Mick ± carers in care planning
	• If patchy engagement with doctor/CC, he might prefer mainly seeing another colleague, e.g. psychologist, vocational worker
	• Increase relevance, e.g. football group rather than 1:1 psychology

1. Address psychiatric factors

Treat symptoms assertively, e.g. paranoia, agoraphobia.
• Your psychologist might do the initial psychology assessment at Mick's home
• For negative symptoms, see Ch.24 and Table 60.1 on p370.

2. Address barriers

Problem-solve around Mick's reasons for not meeting with the team, involving carers if possible (Table 27.2).

> **TIP:** If visiting someone a lot at home, question whether you're fostering dependence. You may help them more by supporting them to come to you or a middle point, e.g. cafe. Consider alternating home and team-base appointments, then gradually weaning this down.

3. Improve medication adherence

The recovery model can help, e.g. by discussing medication as a means to an end in achieving life goals, rather than 'treating symptoms'.
Go back to basics:
• Acknowledge it's not easy taking medication long-term
• Answer medication questions/worries and give information (Ch.11), including PILs
  ◦ Offer choice, including formulation, e.g. liquid rather than tablets
  ◦ Discuss risks/benefits

- Encourage honest discussion of adherence and side-effects, remembering Mick may use medication:
  - Sporadically
  - Excessively, e.g. doubling antidepressant on bad days
  - PRN, e.g. olanzapine only if sleep is poor
- Assertively address side-effects.

Make it easier to take, access and remember medication:

- Simplify regime, e.g. single long-acting doses, avoid polypharmacy
- Be flexible with timings, e.g. take earlier in the evening to avoid morning sedation
- Make prescriptions easier to collect, e.g. from GP, team base or pharmacy; organise repeat prescriptions
- Aids/reminders, e.g. dosette box, mobile phone alarm; keep medication prominent; keep spare tablets in wallet
- Diary/phone reminders for monitoring and repeat prescriptions
- Plan ahead for holidays
- Check medication packets/blood levels if he agrees.

Provide regular follow-up and extra support where complex monitoring is needed e.g. lithium.

What if ... ?

... Despite your best efforts, Mick's engagement remains poor?

If Mick is well enough, consider discharging him (Ch.33)! Otherwise, discuss whether to refer to an Assertive Outreach Team (if you have one – p6) and negotiate a realistic plan, e.g.

- Minimal engagement's better than nothing
- Contract, e.g. *We'll visit to check on you if you don't text to say you're OK*
- Involve others: can provide further safety net/link for contact. Ensure they have your team's contact details
  - Formal services, e.g. housing worker
  - Family
  - GP
- Community Treatment Orders (CTOs, p99): if admitted under s3 at some point, discuss whether a CTO might facilitate ongoing engagement.

> **TIP:** Some things can't be helped, our meddling will only make them worse.
>
> **Chris Douglas, Psychiatrist and Psychotherapist**

Take-home message

Engage imaginatively, collaborate effectively, communicate clearly, set shared goals.

Further reading

Mitchell, A.J. and Selmes, T. (2007) Why don't patients attend their appointments? Maintaining engagement with psychiatric services. *Advances in Psychiatric Treatment*, **13**, 423–434.

Mitchell, A.J. and Selmes, T. (2007) Why don't patients take their medicine? Reasons and solutions in psychiatry. *Advances in Psychiatric Treatment*, **13**, 336–346.

Moritz, S., Favrod, J., Andreou, C. *et al.* (2012) Beyond the usual suspects: positive attitudes towards positive symptoms is associated with medication noncompliance in psychosis, *Schizophrenia Bulletin*, **10**,1093.

CHAPTER 28

Patients with forensic histories

Penelope Brown

South London & Maudsley NHS Foundation Trust, London, England

RELATED CHAPTERS: ward forensics (43), aggression (74), violent threats (80)

James, 28, has paranoid schizophrenia. His last admission was under Section 37, after committing Grievous Bodily Harm (GBH) against his girlfriend. His CC reports he was arrested but released 2 days ago, for assaulting a member of the public. She's very worried, and asks for your review.

Though community forensic mental health teams exist, their extent and scope vary widely across the country. In practice, some of your general community patients could be defined as 'forensic' (histories of offending and/or significant risk) – and may cause high anxiety. Some key skills are needed:
- Attention to detail
- Confident risk assessment/management
- Supporting the team.
You'll also need some knowledge of the criminal justice system and other agencies who can help share the load.

Preparation

Gather information: notes, CC, police ± probation officer
- Current risk assessment (± forensic risk assessment, e.g. HCR-20?)
- Relapse indicators/evidence of relapse
- Circumstances of recent assault
  - Victim? Weapon? Similarities to previous GBH?
  - Charged? If so, with what?
  - Does he need to attend a police station/court?
- Police: consider requesting a record of previous convictions
- Pre-existing legal restrictions, e.g.
  - *Conditional discharge*? (Box 28.1)
  - CTO? What are the conditions? (p99)
  - Exclusion zones
  - Probation order (may include conditions of mental health treatment)
- Previously under other forensic sections? (Appendix E3)
- Is he known to the Multi-Agency Public Protection Arrangements (MAPPA)? (p42).

Psychiatry: Breaking the ICE – Introductions, Common Tasks and Emergencies for Trainees, First Edition.
Edited by Sarah Stringer, Juliet Hurn and Anna M Burnside.
© 2016 John Wiley & Sons, Ltd. Published 2016 by John Wiley & Sons, Ltd.
Companion Website: www.psychiatryice.com

Box 28.1 Conditional discharge

You'll sometimes work with patients previously on a restriction order (Sec 41/49) who are *conditionally discharged*. They are required to meet with their social and clinical supervisors (usually the CC and consultant) who provide regular reports to the Ministry of Justice (MOJ), and may arrange random UDS. Patients may apply, through a tribunal, for *absolute discharge* with no further restrictions.

Assessment

1. Approach
Before seeing James *with* a colleague (± his probation officer), review the safety tips (Ch.6).
   Explain that you'll document the assessment and share it with the team. You may need to break confidentiality if:
• You're worried about risks to James or others, *or*
• The courts later direct it.

2. Full history, remembering...
• James' account of the assault/arrest
  ◦ *Instrumental* motivation, i.e. external gain, such as theft
  ◦ Were psychiatric symptoms relevant? (E.g. "God told me to protect myself"/ "I was on a short fuse because the voices were bothering me")
  ◦ Was he intoxicated?
• Detailed forensic history:
  ◦ Criminal record, including reasons for past GBH; sentences; current conditions, e.g. bail
  ◦ Risk incidents, e.g. assaults whilst an inpatient
• Substance misuse
• Premorbid personality: especially antisocial/impulsive traits
• Current social situation
  ◦ Stability of accommodation/support networks
  ◦ Does he have contact with his (ex-)girlfriend? *Is she safe?*
• Recent adherence to care plan: engagement and medication.

3. MSE, remembering...
• Evidence of relapse
• Thoughts of harm to others.
Don't assume these would have been noticed at the arrest!

4. Risk assessment (p38–42)
Focus on violence, then other risks, e.g. sexual, fire-setting, self-harm, harm from others.
• Systematically note exacerbating and protective (Table 80.1, p478)
• Are risks low, moderate or high?
• Consider both immediate and longer-term risks.

5. Legal practicalities
• Note any bail restrictions and if/when James is due in court
• Does he understand the charges and court procedure?
  ◦ This is useful information if the team/consultant are asked to provide court reports.

Management

Seek senior advice: don't feel you need to handle this alone.
If aggressive see Ch.74; for threats of immediate violence, see Ch.80.

1. Deal with immediate risks
Discuss admission with your consultant if:
- James is relapsing
  - His forensic history lowers your threshold for admission
- He's breached CTO conditions (consultant may consider recall)
- You're worried about increased immediate risks (even without clear relapse).
Admission may require PICU (p7) if risky – discuss with the team and bed manager. Your consultant might arrange admission to a forensic unit if the recent offence was very serious (unlikely, given that James was released).

2. If managing him in the community
Consider how your risk management plan can address *dynamic* (modifiable) risk factors and enhance *protective* factors, e.g.
- Increase support: increase frequency of contact with CC ± HTT.
- Treat symptoms: check adherence; review/change medication if necessary
- Substance misuse: discuss links with violence; offer support to reduce/stop
- Psychology: discuss options with your team/psychologist
  - CBT, e.g. addressing command hallucinations, insight
  - Anger management (often provided by non-statutory agencies)
- Social situation: via CC, e.g. housing issues; increase daily activities.

3. Communicate with your team
Some patients *will* make you and your team anxious: accept this. You're not all-powerful and can't infallibly predict the future – but you can think calmly and systematically about risk and, reduce it where possible.
- Always share anxiety and risk management with your consultant and team
- Place James in the red zone to ensure he's seen and discussed at least weekly, keeping the whole team aware and involved in care planning.

4. Communicate outside your team
Inform relevant agencies about recent events, e.g. probation officer, local police, MAPPA co-ordinator (Box 8.1, p42), children's services (p398).
- Consider the need to breach confidentiality (p38, 481)
- *Forensic referral:* may be appropriate if James is particularly risky. Check local provision, referral criteria and discuss with your consultant, e.g. a community forensic team may also offer one-off risk assessment/advice.
- *MAPPA* – if not known to them, discuss James' eligibility for referral with your team.

5. Document
Update the risk assessment: latest incident and reformulation of risk/risk management. Involve James with his care plan as you would anyone else, e.g. giving him a written crisis plan (p315).

TIP: If you understand someone more you are likely to hate them less. There will still be people you hate, but it is safer to recognise this than pretend you don't.

Elizabeth Venables, Consultant

What if ... ?

... James is held in custody?

Check whether he's been charged/interviewed, and inform seniors. You're unlikely to be involved in his immediate assessment, but may be asked for information. Possible scenarios are:

• The police, custody nurse or forensic medical examiner (FME) request a MHA assessment at the police station
• Assessment by the court diversion scheme. If available, this nurse-led team can assess James ± arrange diversion to hospital.
• The custody sergeant may request an appropriate adult if James is being charged. This is an advocate for mentally vulnerable individuals; his CC may take the role.

If James is remanded to prison, ensure your team shares information with prison in-reach mental health services, e.g. PPHx, medication, depot due date.

... James shows no clear symptoms of mental illness, but seems at high risk of violence?

Always discuss with your consultant. Admission may sometimes be warranted, e.g. if his presentation is atypical, or for brief containment if he has a personality disorder. Inform the police if he has named a victim or is carrying a weapon.

... He walks out, but you think he needs admission?

You've no powers to stop James leaving the CMHT. Call the police (p386) if immediate concerns about his mental health/risk, and discuss with the team how you'll organise admission.

Take-home message

'Forensic' patients are common in general psychiatry, and will hone your risk assessment and management skills. Notice your anxiety levels: they may alert you to an impending risk event, or indicate you're holding too much responsibility yourself. If worrying a lot, take it to supervision.

CHAPTER 29

Pregnancy

Anna M Burnside[1] and Noreen Jakeman[2]

[1] East London NHS Foundation Trust, London, England
[2] Lewisham & Greenwich NHS Trust, London, England

> **RELATED CHAPTERS:** bipolar affective disorder (25), pregnant inpatients (42), child protection (64), puerperal psychosis (78)

Josie Soler, 25, has bipolar affective disorder (BPAD), and last relapsed a year ago. During a routine review, she tells her CC that she wants to become pregnant soon.

Women with mental illnesses at are higher risk of:
- Unplanned pregnancy
- Poor access to antenatal services
- Poor physical health
- Substance misuse
- Birth complications
- Social deprivation
- Single parenthood/domestic violence

This doesn't mean you should try to put Josie off having children! It *does* mean she'll need extra support to optimise mental health and the safety of any pregnancy, including safe prescribing and close liaison with obstetric and perinatal services.

> **TIP:** Routinely discuss sex and contraception with female patients of child-bearing age. Encourage them to tell you as soon as possible if planning pregnancy or they become pregnant.

Preparation

1. Gather information – GP, psychiatric notes, CC
- History and response to medications
- Other children? Any previous concerns/social services involvement?
- Linked in with GP surgery?

2. Research beforehand

- Local perinatal services – referral criteria, scope of case management
  - They may offer medication advice *before* you see Josie

- Medication safety
  - See Management section (p185) for a list of useful contacts/resources

3. Invite Josie to bring her partner

Assessment

1. Full history, remembering ...
- *Current mental health*
- *Medication*: adherence and effectiveness
- *Sexual history:*
  - Current partner
  - Contraception
  - Last menstrual period (LMP) ± pregnancy test (see *What if ... ?*)
  - Recent STI checks
- *PMHx:* problems that could affect pregnancy (e.g. hypertension, diabetes) or drug choice (e.g. renal/liver problems)
- *Substance misuse*, including smoking
- *SHx* – relationship stability, family support; sensitively check – any domestic violence?
- If she has children:
  - Past experience of pregnancy and labour
  - Were medications used? Did she relapse?
  - Contact with perinatal services/social services
  - Current childcare arrangements, difficulties.

2. MSE, remembering ...
- Low/elevated mood
- Psychotic symptoms
- Views on medication.

3. Risk assessment, remembering ...
- Relapse if medication changes/becomes pregnant
- Self-harm
- Neglect, including of antenatal care
- Child risks.

Management

1. Psychoeducation
Explain the importance of good mental health during and after pregnancy.
- Pregnancy itself can be stressful; relapses are common, post-delivery
- Untreated mental illness can harm an unborn baby, e.g. increased risk of preterm delivery/perinatal mortality
- Stopping medication suddenly is risky
- Medication risks to the foetus are often uncertain due to limited data
  - Many other factors are of greater overall importance, e.g. spontaneous malformation in 2–4% pregnancies; smoking, alcohol, diet.
If Josie wants to discuss the heritability of her illness, you may need to do some research! Be clear there's no way to test beforehand or be certain of outcomes. Her partner's psychiatric history is

obviously relevant. She may be able to decrease the risk of her child developing problems, e.g. by providing a supportive home environment, teaching her child to manage stress and avoid illicit drugs. This can be discussed further with perinatal services.

> **TIP:** You may feel strongly about Josie's intended pregnancy, e.g. if she has several children already in care. It's not your job to offer your moral view, but to provide factual information. If this is hard, discuss it in supervision.

2. Perinatal service referral

If your local perinatal team offers clinics to discuss pregnancy planning, refer on and advise Josie to continue her current medication and reliable contraception. If on carbamazepine or valproate, add folate 5 mg daily.

3. Seek medication advice

Ask Josie for time to seek up-to-date advice (e.g. rebook for a week's time), after checking with:
* Your consultant and a senior Trust pharmacist
* The perinatal team
* UK Teratology Information Service (UKTIS):
  ○ www.uktis.org
  ○ www.toxbase.org
  ○ 0844 892 0909
  ○ Free access (including Toxbase) through doctors.net website.
* British National Formulary
* Maudsley Prescribing guidelines
* NICE guidelines.

Urge Josie *not* to stop medication until you've clarified information. Box 29.1 and Table 29.1 provide basic guidance.

4. Feedback information and make a plan

The decision depends partly on the degree of risk associated with relapse and Josie's response to previous medications. Your consultant or registrar may wish to see Josie with you. In all cases, offer written information about risks (often available from perinatal teams) and note Josie's *capacity* to make a decision (p102–3). Weigh factors together, remembering that risks change in different stages of the pregnancy.

Box 29.1 Prescribing in pregnancy – general principles

Give choice where possible and document all decision-making clearly.
* Weigh medication risks against the risk of relapse, both to mum (e.g. suicide, chaotic accident) and foetus (e.g. neglect, infanticide)
* Psychological and social interventions can decrease medication needs
* *When medications are needed*:
  ○ Use the lowest effective dose of the safest drug
  ○ Avoid multiple agents, whether together or sequentially
  ○ Inform obstetrics, especially nearing delivery
* *Potential exposure risks*:
  ○ 1st trimester: major organ malformation
  ○ 3rd trimester: neonatal toxicity
  ○ Long-term neurobehavioral effects (risk across pregnancy)

Table 29.1 Medication in pregnancy.

Medication	Recommended	Avoid if possible
Antipsychotics	Most experience with FGAs: • Haloperidol • Chlorpromazine • Trifluoperazine SGAs: • Olanzapine and clozapine – relatively safe, though gestational diabetes risk • Risperidone and quetiapine – little evidence, but no clear harm	Depots Anticholinergics
Antidepressants	Use in moderate – severe depression Most experience with: • Amitriptyline • Imipramine • Nortriptyline • Fluoxetine Sertraline has least placental exposure and is safe in breast-feeding. SSRIs are not clearly teratogenic	Paroxetine – may be the least safe SSRI MAOIs NB: SSRIs in 3rd trimester are associated with neonatal withdrawal, toxicity or persistent pulmonary hypertension

Mood Stabilisers	Antipsychotics are generally preferred for BPAD	Mood stabilisers are teratogenic:
		• Lithium: Ebstein's anomaly (tricuspid defect)
		  ○ Risk increases from ~1 to ~10/20,000 pregnancies
		• Valproate – highest risk, including neural tube defects
		  ○ Risk increases from ~6 to ~150/10,000 pregnancies
		• Carbamazepine: high risk, including neural tube defects
		  ○ Risk increases from ~6 to ~40/10,000 pregnancies
		• Lamotrigine: lower risk; may increase cleft palate

Sedatives	Use psychological approaches instead Promethazine – widely used and probably safe, but limited information.	Avoid sedatives in late pregnancy due to neonatal problems, e.g. floppy baby syndrome. Benzodiazepines are probably not teratogenic. If *needed*, use low dose and short-acting, e.g. lorazepam.

If newly-diagnosed/on medication, with low risk of relapse:

- Try to avoid (or *consider discontinuing*) medication, particularly in first trimester
- Avoid stopping medication suddenly
- Offer alternative support, e.g. psychology
- If medication's necessary, use the lowest risk drug, at the lowest possible dose.

If high relapse risk:
* Consider switching to a lower-risk drug, e.g. from valproate/carbamazepine to SGA.

5. Other steps
* Liaise with Josie's GP and carers
* Agree a clear follow-up plan, monitoring closely for relapse
* Address substance misuse: use an MI approach (p74) and discuss risks
  * Opiate/alcohol detoxification is risky *once* pregnant; try to organise *beforehand*
  * Strongly encourage smoking cessation/NRT
  * ± Signpost to local services.

> **TIP:** The psychiatrist at the moment is good, she has a very respectful manner, and she's calm and she does things quickly. If a letter needs writing, she'll do it. You don't feel it's gone off into this strange doctorly world that you can't access.
>
> 'Donna'

6. Once pregnant
Perinatal psychiatry usually takes over.
* Liaise with Josie's GP; encourage attendance of antenatal appointments
* Place an alert on Josie's notes that she's pregnant
* Specialist advice is needed around medication dose adjustments, e.g. increase in third trimester; withdrawal towards delivery
* A care plan for the birth and perinatal period should be made by 32 weeks
* Your team should have the delivery centre and midwife's details; obstetrics need a summary of Josie's history and medication
* Pregnant women may be fast-tracked for some services e.g. psychology.
* Discuss with your team whether to refer to children's social services (Ch.64).

7. After delivery
* Ensure a thorough handover from perinatal services/Mother and Baby Unit
* If Josie's breast-feeding, seek advice on medication
* Keep reviewing the need for children's social services input
* Discuss contraception.

What if ... ?

... Josie's *already* pregnant?
Don't panic. Assess as above, include:
* *The pregnancy:*
  * LMP date (often unclear if hyperprolactinaemia from antipsychotics)
  * How has pregnancy been confirmed?
  * Is she comfortable disclosing the father? Has she told him, and does he want to stay involved?
  * Feelings about the pregnancy
  * Plans: go ahead versus termination of pregnancy (TOP)
  * Antenatal care plans
  * Social support: who's she told; who can help?

- *Medication exposure since conception (psychotropic, physical, OTC)*
  - Explain that many women stop their medication in case it harms the baby – this may encourage her to disclose if she's already stopped her tablets!
- *MSE:* negative thoughts; psychotic or grandiose beliefs regarding the baby.

Signpost Josie to GUM/emergency contraception services, if needed. If she's considering a TOP, offer to liaise with her GP or signpost to family planning clinics if preferred. Discuss any requests for reports with your consultant, e.g. capacity to consent/likely effect of a pregnancy on MSE. You *don't* have to write a recommendation for a TOP if your personal beliefs interfere with this, but must recommend another doctor willing to write one.

If going ahead with the pregnancy, contact perinatal psychiatry early for advice. They may take over Josie's care or offer co-working. Advise Josie *not* to stop medication until you've clarified the plan: stopping medication *she's already taking* may not reduce risks to the foetus, but risks relapse, which may be disastrous. Options are:

- Continue current medication if effective, rather than exposing the foetus to a new drug
  - Prescribe folate if valproate or carbamazepine
- Change to a safer drug, e.g. from valproate to SGA
- Stop medication and monitor closely for relapse.

The rest is as above.

... She's pregnant but alcohol or heroin-dependent?

Seek urgent advice from addictions services. Alcohol detox carries more risks in pregnancy, but is safer than sudden, unassisted withdrawal or continued heavy use. Addictions may recommend an inpatient detox for alcohol-dependency. For opiate misuse, they may aim for substitute prescribing during pregnancy, rather than total withdrawal.

... Josie stops medication against your advice?

Unless she's detainable (Table 15.1, p98) or lacks capacity to make medication decisions (p102–3), simply offer close follow-up and support. Document clearly, explore her willingness to engage with antenatal care, and liaise with perinatal psychiatry.

Take-home message

Seek the latest advice on medication safety and explain risks/benefits clearly. Remember physical and supportive aspects of care.

Reference

Taylor, D., Paton, C. & Kapur, S. (2015) *The Maudsley Prescribing Guidelines in Psychiatry*, 12th edn, Wiley-Blackwell, Chichester., pp. 92–93.

Further reading

NICE CG45: Antenatal and postnatal mental health: clinical management and service guidance (2014)
Family Planning Association: www.fpa.org.uk
Henshaw, C. and Protti, O. (2010) Addressing the sexual and reproductive health needs of women who use mental health services. *Advances in Psychiatric Treatment*, **16**, 272–278.

CHAPTER 30

Older adults

Vivienne Mak[1] and Sean Lubbe[2]

[1] South London & Maudsley NHS Foundation Trust, London, England
[2] UNSW Black Dog Institute, New South Wales, Australia

RELATED CHAPTERS: ward older adults (46), delirium (55)

The GP refers retired accountant, Brian, 64, due to concerns from his husband, Jeremy. Brian's become uncharacteristically 'snappy' over the last 6 months, and was recently fined for not submitting his tax returns. Brian thinks it's 'a fuss about nothing,' but reluctantly agrees to see you.

Newly referred older adults (>65/75, depending on local protocols) are usually seen by Mental Health of Older Adults (MHOA) services. Nevertheless, in general adult CMHTs, you'll see:
* New under-65s with cognitive impairment
* Existing patients who pass the 65y age bracket while under your team.

You'll manage most problems as usual, but should know when to refer on or seek MHOA advice.

In Mild Cognitive Impairment (MCI), there's greater cognitive decline than expected for age/educational level, but it doesn't yet interfere with ADLs; over half will develop dementia. See Table 30.1 for the three commonest types of dementia.

Consider rarer dementias if unusual (particularly neurological) symptoms: frontotemporal, dementia in Parkinson's disease, Huntingdon's disease (family history, chorea), Creutzfeldt Jakob Disease, AIDs-related encephalopathy, neurosyphilis, progressive supranuclear palsy.

Preparation

1. Contact GP
* PPHx, including depression
* PMHx, vascular risk factors
* DHx – especially changes in the past year
* Request a dementia screen (Box 30.1) – try to get results before meeting Brian.

2. Appointment
* Offer a home visit (Ch.20): it's more comfortable for Brian, and gives useful insights, e.g. hoarding, safety, empty/mouldy fridge

Psychiatry: Breaking the ICE – Introductions, Common Tasks and Emergencies for Trainees, First Edition.
Edited by Sarah Stringer, Juliet Hurn and Anna M Burnside.
© 2016 John Wiley & Sons, Ltd. Published 2016 by John Wiley & Sons, Ltd.
Companion Website: www.psychiatryice.com

Table 30.1 Differentiating the three main dementias.

Feature	Alzheimer's disease (AD)	Vascular dementia (VD)	Dementia with Lewy bodies (DLB)
Onset/ course	Gradual, progressive decline	Acute onset Stepwise progression Worse at night: 'sun-downing' NB: gradual progression if multiple small infarcts	Fluctuating confusion (symptoms more enduring than in delirium)
Prominent features	4A's: • Amnesia: memory loss initially short term > long term • Aphasia (e.g. word finding problems) • Apraxia • Agnosia Poor insight	Vascular risk factors Emotional incontinence/ lability/depression. Slowed thinking Personality and insight often initially preserved	Hallucinations – often visual. Repeated falls Mild parkinsonism Antipsychotic sensitivity

- Your letter should ask Brian to bring/have ready:
  - Relative(s)
  - All medication
  - Glasses, hearing aid, mobility aids as needed

Box 30.1 Dementia screen

This screens for reversible causes of cognitive impairment and vascular risk factors (Table 30.2).
- FBC, U&Es, eGFR, LFTs, glucose/HbA1c, lipids, TFTs, Vitamin B_{12} + D, folate, corrected calcium, CRP
- MSU
- Delirium screen (Appendix A2)

Assessment

1. Approach

Older people have longer histories and complex problems – be patient, and use more than one meeting if needed.

At the start, explain that you *routinely* see people together and separately. This will assure Jeremy that he'll be able to tell you things he can't say in front of Brian, and may temper Brian's anxiety/irritability when you speak to Jeremy alone.

Acknowledge Jeremy and Brian's emotions, e.g. denial, grief, embarrassment, irritation. Ask them what their *worst fear* is about the underlying problem – this will help you gauge your approach. Don't jump to diagnose: there are many possible reasons for memory problems. At the same time, don't talk about dementia as 'the worst case scenario' – in case this *is* the outcome. If it's dementia, there are lots of ways to help, and it's good they've sought early help.

PATIENT VIEW:

I said to the doctor, "Please don't say it's Alzheimer's!" I was so relieved when he said it was a form of dementia but there was a lot they could do.

'Betty'

Table 30.2 Reversible causes of cognitive decline.

Diagnosis	Clues
Delirium (Ch.55)	Sudden, acute onset; fluctuating course
	Clouded consciousness
	Physical illness
Depression (pseudodementia)	Depression *before* memory problems
	Gradual decline
	Triggers: life events, e.g. bereavement
	Other depressive symptoms
	May *complain* of poor memory / concentration (not hide/deny them)
	Cognitive testing: apathy / 'I don't know' answers
Medication	Common culprits: antidepressants, anti-Parkinson's, anticonvulsants, sedatives, steroids
B$_{12}$ deficiency	Insidious apathy, irritability, paraesthesia, jaundice, anaemia.
	Common causes: pernicious anaemia, dietary deficiency (e.g. vegans)
Endocrine	Hypothyroidism/hyperthyroidism
	Hypoparathyroidism (hypocalcaemia): paraesthesia, cramps, muscle twitches/spasms, depression, irritability, anxiety
Wernicke-Korsakoff syndrome (Table 40.1, p253)	Alcohol history
	Wernicke triad: ataxia, confusion, ophthalmoplegia
	Korsakoff: prominent chronological confusion, confabulation; intact working memory
Normal pressure hydrocephalus (NPH)	Hesitant gait, falls, urinary incontinence
Space occupying lesion (SOL)	Personality change
	Headaches, vomiting, seizure
Subdural haematoma (SDH)	Previous head injury (often minor; may have been forgotten)

2. Full history, remembering ...

- *HPC:*
  Onset; triggers, especially life events, physical illness, head injury
  - Preceding mood changes, especially depression, anxiety
  - *Sudden, recent onset – always think delirium!*
  Course:
  - Gradual decline (AD/pseudodementia)
  - Stepwise (vascular)
  - Fluctuating (DLB/delirium)
  Memory problems and effect on life:
  - ADLs/*Take me through a typical day ...*
  - Also: problems in planning, judgement, adapting to change
  - Brian's an ex-accountant: small financial mistakes may indicate severe problems
  Behavioural and psychological symptoms of dementia (BPSD):
  - Mood/personality changes, e.g. apathy, anxiety, irritability, depression
  - Sleep disturbance, restlessness, shouting, hoarding, wandering
  - Aggression, sexual disinhibition
  - Psychotic symptoms
- *PMHx*: vascular risk factors, parkinsonism, head injury, falls; alcohol-related illnesses

- *DHx:* prescribed and OTC
- *Social history:* housing, social supports, carer stress
  - Educational level/occupation
- *Substance misuse:* especially alcohol and smoking
- *FHx:* memory problems, especially early onset (<65y).

3. Collateral history

Carers' views are essential and often more accurate for onset, course and extent of problems. Check specifically for:

- Worries
- Risks
- Carer stress.

4. MSE, remembering…

- Self-neglect, dressing dyspraxia (e.g. when removing coat)
  - Agitation, apathy, distractibility, disinhibition
  - Sensory impairments
- Dysarthria/dysphasia
- Depression, lability, irritability/frustration
- Psychotic symptoms
- Assess baseline cognition using a standardised test (ACE-III is the gold standard)
  - You can find the following in Appendix D (scores shown indicate impairment):
    - Montreal Cognitive Assessment (MOCA) ≤25/30
    - Addenbrooke's Cognitive Examination-III (ACE-III) <82/100
    - Mini-Addenbrooke's Cognitive Examination (M-ACE) ≤25/30
  - ± Frontal lobe testing
  - Note repetitions in the interview, poor understanding/judgement
- Insight: particularly any mismatch between subjective/objective accounts.

5. Physical health assessment, remembering:

- *Examination:*
  - Dentition, weight loss, pain, sensory impairment, incontinence, constipation, poor mobility/falls
  - Parkinsonism, including problems walking, turning
  - Safeguarding 'alarm bells', e.g. injuries, malnutrition, bruising, pressure sores (Ch.63)
- *Investigations:*
  - Dementia screen (Box 30.1) – if outstanding
  - Brain scan:
    - CT excludes gross problems, e.g. tumour, subdural haematoma, normal pressure hydrocephalus. Request specific features, e.g. atrophy: excessive/regional/hippocampal; small vessel disease and extent of this
    - MRI – more sensitive to early atrophy/subcortical or vascular changes. Request if CT unusual/shows nothing or the patient is young
- ECG – before starting "anti-dementia" medication
- MSU ± full septic screen.

6. Risk assessment, remembering

- Vulnerability, e.g. self-neglect, malnutrition, wandering, falls, fires, accidents
- Self-harm/suicide
- Safeguarding
- Risk to others, e.g. sexual disinhibition, aggression, driving (Ch.32), contact with children (e.g. babysitting).

7. Legal practicalities
* Check for Lasting Power of Attorney (LPA)
* Advance directives.

Management

1. Immediate risk issues
Discuss with your consultant and consider psychiatric admission, if high risks to self or others. If you suspect delirium, liaise with the GP to review urgently and consider a medical admission (Ch.55).

2. Treat differentials/reversible causes of impairment
Depression and anxiety may *accompany* early dementia. Treat these or any physical comorbidity before reviewing cognition. Avoid antidepressants with anticholinergic side effects.

3. Refer?
If you suspect dementia, you'll usually refer to specialists. Check local referral criteria for:
* MHOA team (p290) – may accept younger adults with cognitive problems
* Memory clinic – for mild and uncomplicated presentations, including MCI
* Neuropsychiatry – especially uncommon dementias.
Include your full assessment, cognitive score, and tests (results/awaited). If Brian's cognitive impairment is below the threshold for these services, ask his GP to address risk factors and monitor e.g. 6–12 monthly cognitive testing; MCI may progress to dementia.

4. Psychoeducation and advice
If relevant, offer Brian and Jeremy written information about MCI/dementia and signpost to:
* Local/national support services (see Resources p195)
* Carers' groups; ensure Jeremy is offered a carer's assessment.
Suggest practical steps
* To help with forgetfulness, e.g.
  ○ Diary, calendar, mobile phone alarms
  ○ Carry a notepad/make lists
  ○ Start and embed routines *now* – will help if memory problems worsen, e.g. keep keys somewhere specific
* Protect against memory loss:
  ○ Mental exercise, e.g. Sudoku, crosswords, reading
  ○ Physical exercise
  ○ Healthy lifestyle: stop smoking, limit alcohol, improve diet.

5. Optimise physical health (via GP)
* Assertively manage vascular risk factors (whatever the underlying dementia)
* Refer for exacerbating problems, e.g. pain, hearing, vision, mobility, nutrition
* Medication: advise if current drugs affect cognition, function or physical risk.

6. 'Anti-dementia' medications
In most areas, specialists initiate these, but Brian may have heard of them and want to know more. There are two main types:
* *Acetylcholinesterase inhibitors (AChEIs)*, e.g. donepezil, galantamine, rivastigmine
  ○ For mild and moderate AD, mixed type Alzheimer's
  ○ Rivastigmine used for DLB

◦ They slow dementia's progression, and may modestly and temporarily improve function and behavioural and psychological symptoms of dementia
◦ Effectiveness is measured by the prescribing team, patient and family. Medication is only continued if clearly helpful.
◦ Side-effects: nausea, vomiting, diarrhoea, dizziness, insomnia
◦ Cautions: bradycardia, asthma, gastrointestinal bleeding
• *Memantine* (NMDA receptor antagonist)
◦ Works differently to AChEIs, but similar effect
◦ Lacks the side effects of AChEIs
◦ For *moderate* AD when AChEIs are contraindicated/not tolerated
◦ For *severe* AD.

7. Psychology
Consider:
• Neuropsychological/psychometric testing if the diagnosis is unclear
• CBT for low mood, anxiety.
• Behavioural/family interventions to help carers manage symptoms
• Cognitive stimulation, reminiscence therapy (usually via MHOA).

8. Other interventions
Ask your team whether other input would help at this stage, e.g.
• OT: assess/address home environment and activities
• Social services: needs assessment, care package
• Benefits assessment/advice.

9. Document
Write to the GP, offering Brian a follow-up appointment if the referral to another team will take time.

What if ... ?

... Brian is a long-term CMHT patient and turns 65?
'Graduate patients' (who pass across usual service age limits) usually stay under your care, unless they have specific MHOA *needs* (p290). Check local referral criteria, and discuss with your team and Brian before making any referrals; if he's attached to his CC, any transfer will be disruptive.

Monitor if unsure, ensuring he receives at least yearly physical and social needs reviews. If you *do* refer, clearly state:
• Reasons – related to MHOA criteria (usually frailty)
• Relevant investigations, e.g. cognitive scores, scans, OT assessments
• Your team's care plan, should Brian not be accepted; highlight any limitations.
It may help to offer a joint review with the MHOA or a period of co-working.

Take-home message

Be alert to changes in function or symptoms in aging patients, which might point to cognitive decline. Equally, don't let a dementia diagnosis distract you from addressing psychiatric co-morbidities such as depression and anxiety.

Further reading

Sternberg, S.A., Wershof Schwartz, A., Karunananthan, S., Bergman, H. and Clarfield, A.M. (2011) The identification of frailty: A systematic literature review. *Journal of the American Geriatric Society*, **59** (11), 2129–2138.

NICE (2006) CG 42 Dementia: Supporting people with dementia and their carers in health and social care. NICE, England.

Ballard, C., Burns, A., Corbett, A., Livingston, G. and Rasmussen, J. (2013) Helping You to Assess Cognition: A Practical Toolkit for Clinicians. Alzheimer's Society.

○ Available at: www.alzheimers.org.uk/cognitiveassessment

Patients and carers' information and support:

Alzheimer's Society: www.alzheimers.org.uk

Dementia UK: www.dementiauk.org

Memory cafes directory: www.memorycafes.org.uk

Carers' Trust: www.carers.org

RCPsych patient information leaflet: www.rcpsych.ac.uk/healthadvice/problemsdisorders/dementiaandmemory problems.aspx

CHAPTER 31

Trauma and asylum

Laurine Hanna and Juliet Hurn

South London & Maudsley NHS Foundation Trust, London, England

RELATED CHAPTERS: anxiety (22), 'social' presentations (60)

Hakim Hussein, a 39-year old civil engineer, is seeking asylum. He fled Iran, after being tortured and witnessing his brother's execution. His GP refers him for nightmares and hearing his captors' voices, telling him he'll die. Hakim briefly tried an antidepressant, but declined psychology.

Assessing the impact of trauma – particularly in people from other cultures – needs patience and sensitivity. Spend time building Hakim's trust, and don't jump to diagnose Post Traumatic Stress Disorder (PTSD); normalise his responses to abnormal life events wherever possible.

TIP: Brilliant clinicians are usually unafraid of being kind.

Elizabeth Venables, Consultant psychiatrist

Preparation

1. Gather information – GP, old notes, collateral
- Need for interpreter – specific dialect?
- Past treatments
- PMHx, including traumatic injuries
- Progress of asylum claim
- Non-statutory organisation input.

2. Basic research on Hakim's home country/region
- Culture, including socio-cultural taboos which might affect disclosure
- Political situation/conflicts (Box 31.1).

3. Practicalities
- Arrange interpreter, checking Hakim's:
  - Preference on gender, dialect
  - Concerns, e.g. identification or repercussions, particularly in close-knit communities

Psychiatry: Breaking the ICE – Introductions, Common Tasks and Emergencies for Trainees, First Edition.
Edited by Sarah Stringer, Juliet Hurn and Anna M Burnside.
© 2016 John Wiley & Sons, Ltd. Published 2016 by John Wiley & Sons, Ltd.
Companion Website: www.psychiatryice.com

- Don't use family/friends as interpreters unless absolutely unavoidable
- Double assessment time (interpretation/sensitive issues) (Box 31.2).

Box 31.1 Asylum seekers and refugees: stressors (*Source*: Adapted from McColl et al. 2008.)

> *Pre-migration*
> - War, violence, genocide, imprisonment, torture
> - Losses: bereavement, home, social network, security, nutrition, healthcare.
> *Migration*
> - Arduous/dangerous journey to UK
> - People trafficking.
> *Post-migration*
> - Stigma, discrimination, ethnic minority status
> - Detention and dispersal process
> - Separation from family, children, social networks
> - Lack: social activities, money, accommodation, employment
> - Healthcare: more limited access; cross-cultural assessment/treatment barriers
> - Asylum decisions: stressful, often long delays.

Box 31.2 Working with interpreters

> *Speak to the interpreter beforehand:*
> - If they share Hakim's culture/religion, ask their advice about engagement
> - Have they worked in mental health before? Any worries?
> - They should:
>   - Translate exactly – no additions or omissions
>   - Interrupt you/Hakim if talking too much (interpret in "chunks", rather than lose detail)
>   - Clarify meaning if unsure
> - They shouldn't:
>   - *Edit* his replies – even if offensive or 'wrong' (e.g. delusions)
>   - Reduce long answers to a single word/sentence (but thorough summaries are helpful)
>   - Exclude you from conversations.
> *In the meeting:*
> - Sit so everyone can see each other (a triangle/semi-circle)
> - Speak *to* Hakim (not the interpreter)
> - Introduce everyone. Explain that confidentiality includes the interpreter
> - Speak clearly and slowly; pause between sentences to allow translation
> - No jargon.
> *Debrief afterwards:*
> - Was speech illogical, muddled, tangential or jumping between topics?
> - Cultural significance of anything you felt was unusual (could this be normal?)
> - Support them if upset about the content.

Assessment

> **PATIENT VIEW:**
> It was like a little voice inside me saying, "Please care" but because they're professionals, they can't show you that they care.
>
> **'Carlos'**

1. Approach

Trauma is hard to discuss – especially if Hakim has lost his confidence and ability to trust. Be sensitive and kind; assess over multiple meetings if needed.

- Explore 'safer' areas first: current situation and problems
- When you think he's ready, ask if he feels able to talk about what happened in Iran. Don't push him. He may only disclose parts of the story. Sexual assault is often disclosed late, or never.
- If he becomes highly distressed or lost in the trauma (e.g. dissociation, flashbacks), *ground* him: speak calmly and clearly, reminding him where he is, that he's safe. Ask him to focus on his surroundings, e.g. *Describe what you can see in this room/through that window* (encourage details) Couple this with relaxation strategies if required (p71).

Table 31.1 Stress-related disorders.

	Trigger	Timing	Symptoms
Acute stress reaction	Exceptionally stressful trauma (see below)	Immediately after trauma. Resolves within hours – days	Dazed, disoriented, unable to take in information Tearful, angry, anxious, despairing Overactive/withdrawn Dissociated
PTSD	*Exceptionally stressful* trauma • Experienced/witnessed • Perceived threat to life/physical integrity • E.g. serious physical/sexual assaults; childhood abuse; war, torture; accidents, disasters	Within 6 months, but can be delayed May become chronic	Avoidance of reminders Re-experiencing: • Flashbacks • Nightmares • Intrusive images/memories Hyperarousal: • Hypervigilance, exaggerated startle • Poor concentration, insomnia Emotional changes: • Numbness • Irritability/angry outbursts • Depression, anxiety, shame, guilt Other: • Pervasive feelings of threat/risk • Loss of self-confidence • Amnesia for parts of the event • Dissociation • Personality change (especially prolonged, repeated, or childhood trauma), e.g. mistrust, emptiness, withdrawal, disorganisation • NB: comorbid psychosis can be hard to distinguish from flashbacks and hypervigilance
Adjustment disorder	Less severe stressor, e.g. non-traumatic bereavement, migration, retirement	Usually within one month; resolves within six months	Varied, e.g. depression, anxiety, 'can't cope'. Symptoms don't meet thresholds for another disorder, e.g. too mild/brief for depression

TIP: I read somewhere: *never ask today what is better asked tomorrow* – it's served me well. The point being it's better to build rapport and relationship with someone *before* asking about child abuse or trauma.

Sarah Collins, Consultant Psychiatrist

TIP: *Debriefing* shortly after trauma (e.g. encouraging trauma 'processing') may worsen outcomes. PTSD symptoms in the first few months will often spontaneously improve. Practical support is most important.

2. Full history, remembering ...
- *Current social situation and difficulties*:
  - Housing; finances; social networks (mistrust, alienation, withdrawal?)
  - Immigration status: asylum claim, solicitor, appeals, litigation proceedings
  - Family: still in Iran? Contact/concerns?
  - Narrative of journey to UK
- *PTSD symptoms* (Table 31.1)
  - Trauma – if appropriate
  - Chronology – pre-/post-migration?
  - Effect on life
  - Past treatment – helpful? Contact with counselling or trauma services
- *Comorbidity*, e.g. anxiety disorders, depression, somatisation/chronic pain, psychosis, personality disorder
  - Relationship to PTSD, e.g. *Were you depressed before this happened?/ Would you be depressed if the flashbacks disappeared?*
- *PMHx*:
  - Trauma-related injuries, including brain damage $\pm$ STIs
  - Diseases prevalent in homeland, e.g. TB, HIV
  - Poverty-related issues, e.g. incomplete immunisation, malnutrition
- *Substance use:* common coping mechanism
  - Be aware of cultural preferences, e.g. khat (Somalia, Ethiopia, Yemen)
- *Personal history:* early/recurrent trauma increases vulnerability to PTSD
- *Pre-morbid personality*.

3. MSE, remembering ...
- Anxiety, dissociation, re-experiencing
- Affective or psychotic symptoms
- Cognitive deficits, e.g. from head injury
- Symptom interpretation.

4. Risk assessment, including
- Suicide/self harm
- Vulnerability to exploitation
- Risks if deported, e.g. further torture; suicide.

5. Physical assessment (you/GP)
- Full physical assessment/investigations
- $\pm$ GUM signposting.

TIP: Was Hakim happy with the interpreter? Share brilliant interpreters' contact details with your team.

Management

1. Deal with immediate risk
If Hakim needs admission (due to high risks), be sensitive: compulsory admission and treatment may remind of earlier trauma.

2. Psychoeducation
For some people, a PTSD diagnosis is a relief and explains their experiences; for others it makes no sense or feels stigmatising. Explain that certain symptoms can occur after trauma and ask whether he'd like you to describe them. Adapt your explanation to suit culture.
- *The brain's a bit like a filing cabinet. Most memories are processed and then filed away so you can open the 'drawer' and find them when needed, but shut the drawer and ignore them when irrelevant.*
  - *Extremely traumatic memories are so hard to process that you can't file them*
  - *Instead, they keep coming to mind as a recurring 'loop', and are triggered very easily, a bit like papers lying around in an office – it's hard to do anything without noticing or touching them.*
  - *This isn't a sign of 'madness', and avoidance isn't cowardly. Both are normal human response to extreme trauma*
  - *Some people need help to process and file away memories; they can then access them like any other memory*
- *People often lose confidence or feel they've become different, or separated, from other people*
- *Some coping strategies cause more problems, e.g. avoidance, withdrawal, ruminating, alcohol or drugs.*
Brief interventions can help, e.g. sleep hygiene (p72), relaxation (p71), exercise, routines.

3. Practical help (see resources on p202)
Prioritise this: if Hakim has some sense of stability/security he'll be better placed to undertake trauma-focused work. Signpost to sources of practical help and support, and consider whether an allocated CC might help link him in.
- Voluntary organisations:
  - Information about PTSD
  - Emotional support, supportive counselling
  - Advocacy
- Legal advice on finances, housing, and work:
  - The government provides asylum seekers with accommodation and a small, weekly cash payment ('subsistence') via the National Asylum Support Service (NASS)
  - *Failed* asylum seekers can access short-term housing and payment cards for food/toiletries
  - All children can access state education
  - Asylum seekers can apply for work if there's no asylum decision at 1 year
- Isolation:
  - Befriending service
  - Local refugee community groups (NB: Hakim may feel threatened or distressed by people from his homeland)
  - English classes
- Asylum process
  - Offer to liaise with his asylum case owner
  - Suggest he gives his solicitor your details if a medical report is needed.

4. Address co-morbidity

Depression, substance misuse (etc) may resolve with treatment of PTSD, but if severe, may need treating first.

5. Psychological treatment

Discuss with the team psychologist, including local provision of specialist services.
- Explore Hakim's reasons for declining psychology, e.g. anxiety; doesn't think talking can help; feels it's a sign of weakness.
- Acknowledge that facing the trauma in therapy feels frightening
- If he clearly doesn't want psychology now, focus on other areas of support
- Recognise cultural preferences for psychology styles e.g. if he doesn't want emotional work, he may prefer problem-solving or CBT
- Evidence-based trauma-focused treatments include:
  ○ CBT – includes anxiety management and *safe* re-exposure to traumatic memories and triggers, e.g. by recording a verbal narrative and listening to it
  ○ Eye Movement Desensitisation and Reprocessing (EMDR) – thought to encourage processing of traumatic memories through bilateral brain stimulation.

6. Medication

Recommended *after* psychology, but consider if:
- Hakim prefers medication
- Psychology doesn't resolve problems
- Co-morbid depression
- Severe PTSD symptoms (particularly hyperarousal/insomnia).

Find out why he didn't persevere with medication before, and offer information on antidepressants (p59–61).
- Start with an SSRI or (particularly if insomnia) mirtazapine
- Recommend continuing for at least a year.

If he doesn't improve, check adherence, discuss with your consultant, $\pm$ consider adding low dose olanzapine.

7. Also ...

- Discuss complex or atypical presentations with your team $\pm$ specialist services if available
- Check his GP is providing physical healthcare
  ○ Asylum seekers/refugees can access free healthcare
  ○ *Failed* asylum seekers can only access primary healthcare, except in immediately life-threatening conditions
- Recovery principles are helpful, especially for ongoing PTSD symptoms, e.g. helping Hakim focus on his goals; reminding him of his strengths/resilience.

PATIENT VIEW:

If doctors want to wake up a bit, it can make or break the team ... like head teachers in school. You're really powerful, full of potential. Psychiatry is fairly redundant – it's only a tiny bit of the jigsaw. But if you can get a clearer image of all the other pieces of the jigsaw and influence how everything's arranged ...

'Angela'

Take-home message

Spotting and treating PTSD is important, but remember that most people exposed to trauma don't go on to suffer mental illness. Social interventions may be more important than medication or psychology.

Reference

McColl, H., McKenzie, K. and Bhui, K. (2008) Mental health care of asylum seekers and refugees. *Advances in Psychiatric Treatment*, **14,** 452–459.

Further reading

NICE (2005) CG26: Post-traumatic stress disorder (PTSD): the management of PTSD in adults and children in primary and secondary care. NICE, England.

Farooq, S. and Fear, C. (2003) Working through interpreters. *Advances in Psychiatric Treatment*, **9**, 104–109.

Herbert, C. and Wetmore, A. (1999) *Overcoming Traumatic Stress: A Self-help Guide Using Cognitive Behavioural Techniques*, Robinson, London.

Summerfield, D. (2001) The invention of post-traumatic stress disorder and the social usefulness of a psychiatric category, British Medical Journal, **322** (7278), 95–98.

Royal College patient information leaflet: www.rcpsych.ac.uk/mentalhealthinfo/problems/ptsd/posttraumatic-stressdisorder.aspx

Charities/Third Sector

Refugee Council: help and support for asylum seekers and refugees
  ◦ www.refugeecouncil.org.uk
Asylum Aid – legal advice and representation
  ◦ www.asylumaid.org.uk
Medical Foundation for care of victims of torture – support and psychological services
  ◦ www.freedomfromtorture.org
Helen Bamber Foundation – network and resources if suffered human rights abuses
  ◦ www.helenbamber.org
Victim support
  ◦ www.victimsupport.org.uk

Government resources

Home Office website for asylum seekers: www.ukba.homeoffice.gov.uk/asylum
Asylum Advice UK: 0808 8000 630.

Military

SSAFA www.ssafa.org.uk (support for armed forces and families)
Combat stress. www.combatstress.org.uk

Mainly for professionals

UK Psychological Trauma Society: clinical network or UK Traumatic stress services
www.ukpts.co.uk

CHAPTER 32

Driving

Christina Barras

South West London & St George's Mental Health NHS Trust, London, England

RELATED CHAPTERS: outpatient clinics (18), bipolar affective disorder, BPAD (25)

Greg has BPAD, and is recovering from a manic episode. A colleague mentions that she regularly sees him riding his Harley-Davidson. He's booked into your clinic and you decide to raise the issue of driving.

Many people with mental health problems can safely drive, but some shouldn't, and it's often your (rather uncomfortable) responsibility to explain the relevant driving legislation. Driving may give Greg a sense of freedom, or enable him to work and connect with friends, so the possibility of losing his licence may be yet another devastating blow dealt by mental illness.

Box 32.1 Driver and Vehicle Licensing Agency (DVLA) regulations

The DVLA needs to know if a licence holder has a condition / is receiving treatment that may now, or in the future, affect their driving safety.
- Group 1: cars and motorcycles
- Group 2: large lorries and buses (similar standards usually apply to taxis). Standards are tougher than for Group 1, reflecting higher risks.

Notification is required if:
- Acute or chronic psychosis
- Hypomania/mania
- Severe anxiety or depression (with memory/concentration problems, agitation, behavioural disturbance, or suicidal thoughts)
- Alcohol or drug misuse/dependence (including prescribed e.g. benzodiazepines)
- Personality/behavioural disorders, if likely to be dangerous
- Dementia/organic brain syndrome
- Medication could affect driving.

Likely conditions needed to resume licensing (see DVLA guide for specifics):
- Period of wellness/stability of three to six months (up to three years for Group 2)
- Treatment adherence
- No medication side effects which could impair driving
- Good insight.

Psychiatry: Breaking the ICE – Introductions, Common Tasks and Emergencies for Trainees, First Edition.
Edited by Sarah Stringer, Juliet Hurn and Anna M Burnside.
© 2016 John Wiley & Sons, Ltd. Published 2016 by John Wiley & Sons, Ltd.
Companion Website: www.psychiatryice.com

Preparation

1. Gather information – notes
- Illness pattern and symptoms
- Historic driving offences/accidents
- Previous discussions about driving?
- Other risks, e.g. aggression, suicidality.

2. Gather
- Leaflet on mental illness and driving
- DVLA guidelines (Driver Vehicle Agency in Northern Ireland).

3. Discuss with:
- Consultant – any advice?
- CC – ask to attend, especially if Greg's likely to get angry.

Assessment

1. Approach
Start by checking how Greg is, and whether he has any issues to discuss. Then ask what he knows about driving regulations before bombarding him with information. This provides a starting point, both for content, and the emotional backdrop. You'll have a very different conversation if he's:
- Completely unaware
- Aware, but feeling worried or guilty that he's breaking the law
- Aware, but defiantly driving.

Hold the position that you *want* Greg to drive, *but* must follow the law:
- Emphasise working together towards the positive goal of being a safe driver – not a negative one of 'not crashing'
- This isn't personal. You're not against him/'on the DVLA's side'
- Rather than seeming powerful, *share* his sense of helplessness. Be clear that your hands are tied – it may help to show him the professional guidance
- Mention – but don't labour – that you want to keep him and others safe. If he doesn't believe he's risky, he may feel you're criticising his driving skills.
- Be hopeful: this is usually temporary.

The DVLA is more sympathetic to people self-disclosing, than those driving against medical advice – Greg can take control of this situation, if he wants to.

> **TIP:** The main thing I've learnt is that if you treat people with sincerity and respect, they will do the same. They may not agree with you, but will see that you're working with honour and integrity. In psychiatry, I think this is fundamental.
>
> **Ben Spencer, ST6**

2. Focused history, remembering ...
- *Recent psychiatric symptoms:* particularly relevant to driving (see MSE)
- *PMHx*: non-psychiatric conditions that may affect driving
  - E.g. epilepsy, TIAs, parkinsonism, diabetes, heart disease, visual impairment
- *Medication*: drowsiness and other side-effects

- *Substance misuse*: current use. Has he *ever* driven intoxicated?
- *Driving*
  - What does he drive? Make, model, colour, number plate ... ?
    - Valid tax, insurance and MOT (Ministry of Transport) test?
  - How often does he drive and why? E.g. commuting, leisure
    - Does he carry passengers?
  - Any worries about his driving? (Own/other people's comments)
    - Does he think his symptoms or medication affect him?
  - Can he remember anyone discussing driving before? (If so, what was said?)
  - Is he aware of DVLA rules (and that they apply to motorbikes)?
  - Driving convictions/cautions, speeding tickets
    - Accidents, near misses, road rage.

3. MSE, remembering ...

- Psychomotor agitation/retardation
- Tiredness, drowsiness, sedation
- Erratic behaviour, impulsivity
- Inappropriate behaviour, aggression
- Distractibility, including responding to hallucinations
- Elation, irritability, lability
- Delusions
- Thoughts of harm to self/others
- Hallucinations (including command)
- Poor concentration
- Poor problem solving
- Delayed responses
- Insight into illness, possible risks, next steps.

4. Risks

Would you be worried if he drove home *now?* Also check:
- Self-harm/suicide
- Recklessness/impulsive behaviour
- Aggression, including road rage.

Management

1. Deal with immediate risks

If Greg's driving is *immediately* risky (e.g. clearly unwell, intoxicated, or has 'parked' his motorbike in the wall of your building):
- Attempt discussion
- Advise him to stop driving for now
  - State safety concerns and legal position
  - Ask if he'd hand his keys to you/family
- If he won't listen, explain you must break confidentiality (unless this increases the risk, e.g. of violence)
- Discuss with your consultant and:
  - Inform the police, giving vehicle details if possible
  - Inform the DVLA (below)
  - Consider HTT/admission.

2. If not immediately risky

Explain Greg's legal duty to inform the DVLA he's driving, referring to DVLA guidelines (Box 32.1). Acknowledge he may not have known, and be prepared for him to be angry. Explain:
- If the DVLA withdraw his license, this is often temporary, especially if he continues with treatment
- Driving without informing the DVLA of medical conditions can result in …
  - A £1000 fine
  - Prosecution if involved in an accident
- His insurance probably won't cover him if there's an accident. He should inform his insurer of his illness and medications (premiums may increase).

If he agrees:
- Show him how to access the relevant DVLA form
  - Check if he'd like help completing it
  - Explain that you/a colleague may be asked for a medical report
- Use discretion to advise whether he's fit to keep driving whilst awaiting the DVLA decision. Discuss this with your consultant, but err on the side of caution.
- Offer written information and a further meeting to check progress.

If he disagrees (or lacks capacity, e.g. due to dementia):
- Try to persuade him to stop driving and contact the DVLA himself
- Ask permission to check whether carers are concerned
- If you think his driving poses significant risks, you must breach confidentiality and tell the DVLA
  - Explain your disclosure to Greg beforehand, if safe to do so
  - Discuss with your consultant ± Greg's GP
  - Complete the DVLA form or call their Medical Advisor to disclose concerns
- Offer to arrange a second opinion if he won't disclose because he disagrees with his diagnosis or its effect on his driving.

3. Documentation

Document your discussion, whatever the outcome.
- Update risk assessment
- Liaise with the GP, and write Greg a summary letter
- If you're asked to complete a medical report for the DVLA
  - Write honestly and straightforwardly
  - Offer to go over it with Greg before sending.

4. Ongoing care

After DVLA assessment
Greg may be allowed to keep his licence, possibly subject to regular reviews of medical fitness. If his licence is removed:
- Greg can appeal within 6 months
- He can request a second opinion if he disagrees with the medical report - discuss with your consultant
- Accepting treatment and getting/staying well increases the chance of him regaining his licence.

Problem-solve
If Greg can't drive, problem-solve:
- He may be eligible for a travel pass if he needs to travel for treatment – consult with his CC
- Consider vocational/occupational support.

What if … ?

… It's a grey area?

Sometimes, you'll be unclear about the level of risk or need to breach confidentiality (e.g. if Greg says he's stopped driving, but you suspect otherwise). Discuss with your consultant and Caldicott

Guardian (the Trust lead for confidentiality issues). You can also speak to the DVLA Medical Adviser without disclosing Greg's details initially.

Take-home message

Discuss driving clearly but sensitively. Recognise that losing a licence has major consequences, and the discussion may affect your therapeutic relationship.

References

DVLA information

Notification form for license holder: https://www.gov.uk/government/publications/m1-online-confidential-medical-information (car/motorcycle only: HGV/MPV licenses require a different form)
Guidance for professionals:
https://www.gov.uk/current-medical-guidelines-dvla-guidance-for-professionals
To speak to the DVLA medical adviser:
01792 782337 (professionals) / 0300 790 6806 (public).

DVA information (Northern Ireland)

http://www.nidirect.gov.uk/telling-dva-about-a-condition.

Further reading

GMC guidance

www.gmc-uk.org/Confidentiality_reporting_concerns_Revised_2013.pdf_52091821.pdf

Patient information

www.rethink.org/resources/d/driving-and-mental-illness-factsheet
www.mind.org.uk/information-support/legal-rights/fitness-to-drive/

CHAPTER 33

Discharge

Laurine Hanna

South London & Maudsley NHS Foundation Trust, London, England

> **RELATED CHAPTERS:** outpatient clinics (18), Care Programme Approach (19)

Rosie Poules, 53, has schizophrenia, and has been under your team for 15 years, but stable for 5 years. Your team manager wonders if she could be discharged, but Rosie's CC worries she'll react badly, and won't attend her GP for depot.

There's pressure with rising caseloads to discharge patients, and no magic formula to calculate how long someone should stay under secondary care. Discharge can be a welcome and positive step – *or* a source of arguments and anxiety. Where discharge is possible, make it safe and supportive: spot potential candidates, facilitate discussions, and plan for the practical and emotional challenges. Don't hang onto patients if they don't need you – this simply reinforces the idea that they are ill or dependent.

> **TIP:** *Manage expectations*: to help everyone focus on useful treatment and avoid fostering dependence, discuss treatment aims and likely time frames at early CPAs or clinic appointments. Regularly review whether the CMHT is the best or only way to meet someone's needs.

Preparation

1. Gather information – notes, CC, GP
- Progress during time in service
- Risks
- Rosie's view of discharge
- Does she meet local guidelines/criteria for discharge? E.g.
  ○ Specified period without relapse/admission
  ○ Medication optimised – GP could continue
  ○ Adequate psychosocial function; no longer needs MDT support.

> **TIP:** Teams don't always agree on the need for discharge, and the reasons can be complex, e.g. a CC may be very attached to a patient and find it hard to 'let go'. Discuss these issues in team meetings or targeted caseload reviews.

Psychiatry: Breaking the ICE – Introductions, Common Tasks and Emergencies for Trainees, First Edition.
Edited by Sarah Stringer, Juliet Hurn and Anna M Burnside.
© 2016 John Wiley & Sons, Ltd. Published 2016 by John Wiley & Sons, Ltd.
Companion Website: www.psychiatryice.com

Discharge *planning* meeting

For long-term patients, arrange this at least 3 months *before* discharge, inviting the GP and carers. It can help to structure the meeting as a formal CPA (Ch.19).

Emphasise the positives of discharge, which include:

* Getting on with life
* Independence
* A mark of success

Nonetheless, the losses and challenges of discharge can be anxiety-provoking. Explore and address these concerns *now* – otherwise, the coming months will be fraught with them, and *nobody* will feel confident or ready for discharge at the final meeting (Table 33.1).

Table 33.1 Common discharge concerns.

Concern from …	Concern	Options
Rosie	*Who will I talk to now?* (Loneliness/ emotional loss)	CC discussion with Rosie: explore and acknowledge meaning of their relationship
		Strengthen social network, e.g. proactively contact/enlist carers; build list of contacts
		Discuss/*try* possible activities e.g. evening classes, faith groups
		Signpost/refer, e.g. day centres, service user groups
	You think I'm well now – so I'll lose my benefits …	Explain: discharge *doesn't* mean she doesn't have mental health *needs*
		Discuss recovery: for some, voluntary/paid work is appropriate; for others, longer-term benefits are essential
		Signpost to benefits adviser/vocational worker
		Offer to write supporting letters, as needed
	What if I get unwell again?	Relapse prevention plan – CC will develop this with her
		• Identify early relapse signs
		• Clear plan, e.g. numbers to call, medication options
		• Re-referral is always available
	I don't know my GP/ they don't understand mental illness	Involve GP *before* fully discharged:
		• Contact GP to explain Rosie's care/concerns
		• Might hold discharge CPA *at* the GP surgery, with the GP $\pm$ practice nurse (especially if giving depot).
		• CC could accompany Rosie to the surgery to meet the GP, e.g. first appointment after discharge
		GP can always contact CMHT if stuck
Carers	*How will I cope if mum gets ill again?*	Adapt relapse prevention/crisis plan to carer
		Offer carer's assessment
		Signpost to carers' support organisations
	It takes ages to get a GP appointment – how will we get mum seen quickly?	Offer to contact the GP: can they add an alert to their system to respond promptly to worries?
		ED available if crisis
GP	*We don't look after serious mental illness/ very risky patients*	Check GP's concerns, e.g. risks you weren't aware of?
		Answer questions, discuss plans
		Offer advice:
		• Ongoing support, e.g. contact CMHT doctor/ED
		• When and how to re-refer
		• You or Rosie's CC could visit the surgery to discuss mental health/offer focused teaching
		Assure prompt team response to re-referral
	We don't prescribe depot/specialist medication	Education/advice, e.g. CPN could visit the practice nurse
		If you *can't* directly influence service arrangements, check options with team, e.g. depot or medication clinic?

The next months are key for:
- Consolidating her progress
- Relapse prevention and crisis planning
- Dealing with worries and problems
- Testing-out and building confidence in the discharge plan
- Ensuring a smooth handover to the GP, other agencies and social supports.

Plan the run-up to discharge, e.g.
- Gradually reduce frequency of CC contact
- Co-working period if transferring care to another agency
- Move prescribing to GP
- Address barriers to accessing GP care.

> **TIP:** Some people will *tell* you they don't want to be discharged ... Others show reluctance indirectly, e.g. by suffering crises when discharge is mentioned, or forgetting to collect medication from their GP. If so, reconsider worries and challenges: you've either missed something important, or underestimated their illness or the role your team plays for them.

Discharge CPA

1. Meeting
Invite everyone involved in Rosie's old and ongoing plan. See Chapter 19, and cover:
- *Current mental health* – plans to maintain health, manage ongoing symptoms
  - Negative symptoms may be missed after discharge unless highlighted now
- *Medications* – clarify practicalities, e.g. prescriptions, reviews, side effect management
  - Surgery confident and willing to administer depot?
- *Physical health*
  - Yearly health check (p50)
  - + Medication/SMI monitoring (Appendix A)
  - ± Rosie's specific needs
- *Psychosocial support*
  - Agencies *and* regular social contacts: contact details and roles
- *Risk*
  - Historic and current concerns
  - Risk management plan
- *Relapse planning*
  - Possible triggers
  - Relapse indicators
  - GP systems for spotting relapse, e.g.
    - Not collecting prescriptions
    - Not attending physical health check
  - Crisis plan (p315) in case of relapse
  - CMHT re-referral and routes back into care.

2. Documentation and handover
Document the discharge meeting, and ensure:
- Discharge letters: GP and Rosie (adapted from GP letter)
  - Include clear relapse prevention/crisis plans
- Relevant agencies informed of transfer of care, e.g. housing officer
- Other as required, e.g. risk assessment, diagnosis, HONOS (see Box 33.1 for older adults).

Box 33.1 Discharging older adults

> Be particularly alert to the following points with vulnerable, frail or ageing patients:
> - Comprehensive functional assessment (psychology/OT)
>   - Cognitive
>   - ADLs
> - Capacity: can they make informed decisions about care needs?
>   - Has anyone discussed end of life issues?
> - Adequate social support?
>   - Social services
>   - Non-statutory agencies, e.g. Alzheimer's Society
>   - Assistive technology needs, e.g. falls sensors, key-safe to ensure carer access
> - Carer stress and support, particularly older carers, e.g. spouse
> - Medical – highlight to GP:
>   - Physical comorbidities impact on mental health, and vice-versa
>   - Risks of polypharmacy, interactions, adverse reactions
> - Cognitive decline may affect prognosis of other illnesses (physical/mental)
> - Safeguarding issues – shared and addressed?

What if … ?

… One or more parties adamantly oppose discharge?

You might need to accept that ongoing care is more pragmatic than distress, disagreements and a near-certain re-referral in the near future. Possible compromises include:
- A 'trial' of discharge, to be reviewed after a certain period
- Less intensive input, e.g. infrequent clinic appointments.

… Rosie hasn't engaged with the team for a long time?

This is trickier. *For some patients, non-engagement is the main sign that they're very unwell, so should prompt assertive engagement ± MHA assessment, rather than discharge!* (See Ch.62) Approaches include:
- Gathering information, particularly risk and carer/GP concerns
- Proactive reviews, including announced or unannounced home visits
- Team discussions: discharge or continue trying to engage?
- Write to
  - Rosie: offer a 'final appointment'
  - Rosie + GP + involved agencies: explain reasons for discharge and discharge information, emphasising routes back into care and contingency plans.

Take-home message

Think about discharge early on. Plan, test and provide safety nets. Whether discharge is temporary or life-long, encourage people to try life *without* mental health services, whenever possible.

Further reading

Gask, L. and Croft, J. (2000) Methods of working with primary care. *Advances in Psychiatric Treatment*, **6**, 442–449.
Rethink offer training for GP surgeries to help improve care of patients with mental health needs:
www.ttcprimarycare.org.uk

CHAPTER 34

From admission to discharge

Katherine Beck and Abigail G Crutchlow

South London & Maudsley NHS Foundation Trust, London, England

---

RELATED CHAPTERS: Care Programme Approach (CPA, 19), ward rounds (35)

It's your first week on the ward. You have 18 patients, including two new admissions.

No matter how therapeutic, wards are artificial environments, separating people from the real world. The longer this continues, the more likely they'll see themselves as full-time 'patients', reliant on psychiatric services. By planning for discharge from the day of admission, you'll encourage independence, create safe and supportive discharge plans … and appease stressed-out bed managers.

PATIENT VIEW:

I was admitted … I actually have very fond memories of it [although] I was in a terrible space. There was a feeling of camaraderie within the staff team and they were nice to be with and that's what made the whole experience good.

'Angela'

Admission clerkings

Your clerkings reflect *you*, building your reputation as a thorough, compassionate and skilled clinician – or not. A decent clerking:
- Shows the person you care about them and their problems
- Helps the team understand their presentation
- Facilitates verbal presentations/discharge summaries.

PATIENT VIEW:

You're never going to get it right all the time, but just be aware that communicating well and kindly never stops being important. It never stops helping a person towards getting better.

'Patsy'

Psychiatry: Breaking the ICE – Introductions, Common Tasks and Emergencies for Trainees, First Edition.
Edited by Sarah Stringer, Juliet Hurn and Anna M Burnside.
© 2016 John Wiley & Sons, Ltd. Published 2016 by John Wiley & Sons, Ltd.
Companion Website: www.psychiatryice.com

Preparation

1. Gather information – notes, section papers, Care Coordinator (CC)
- Events before admission
  - Onset, triggers
  - Community plan/difficulties
  - MHA status
- PPHx: diagnoses, admissions, treatment
- Risks.

2. Ward staff
- How has this person presented since admission to the ward?
- Concerns, e.g. agitation, alcohol withdrawal.

Take someone with you if *any* concerns or *unknown* risks. If interviewing alone, ask a specific nurse to check on you frequently.

Assessment

> **PATIENT VIEW:**
>
> The assessment of illness needs to look at the deterioration in mental health compared to their normal functioning. Not who you become used to seeing in hospital.
>
> 'Ruquia'

Try to clerk new patients immediately, including overnight. This manages their needs and risks, while preventing a backlog of work for the doctor taking over.

1. Approach
Wards are stressful, disruptive places: there's limited freedom or privacy, and other patients may seem scary or unpredictable. People often feel frightened, angry or trapped – especially if detained or first-timers. So:
- Explain, reassure and be kind
- Encourage them to speak to their primary/named nurse if worried
- Address basic needs, e.g. hunger, desperate to call partner
- Don't lecture them if they want a cigarette. If this is their main stress-release, find out if they can smoke, and offer NRT if not.
- If they've just been fully clerked (e.g. in ED), check the information's correct and fill any gaps. *Don't* repeat the process – they'll think the previous doctor didn't listen, believe or document their story.
- Check what's been discussed already about leave. Some Trusts suggest informal patients voluntarily *stay* on the ward initially, e.g. 48–72 hours. This helps staff get to know them and manage risk.
  - Informal patients should *otherwise* expect to come and go freely
  - Detained patients - must wait for their consultant to grant leave
- If informal patients want to self-discharge, nurses will request a doctor's review first. If concerned, the doctor *may* briefly detain them, to enable a full assessment (Ch.38).

PATIENT VIEW:

I think the worst bit about being in hospital was when they shut that door behind me and I couldn't get out …. Seeing my dad look behind the door at me. And me screaming, trying to run to him. That was my first section.

'Patsy'

---

2. Clerking content (p32)

Complete your Trust's admission proforma, if available. Otherwise:
- Full history and MSE
- Physical assessment
- ± Collateral history: carers, CC, involved professionals, e.g. housing worker
  - General Practitioner (GP): clarify regular medication, PMHx, concerns
- Risk assessment
- Formulation/differential diagnoses
- HONOS (Health Of the Nation Outcome Scales; scores symptoms and disability)
- ± International Classification of Diseases (ICD) code.

3. Physical assessment (p37)

Complete an examination, baseline bloods, ECG, UDS and urine dip as soon as possible and within the first 24 hours. It's especially important where organic causes or physical comorbidity are more likely: older adults, people with a first episode psychosis, substance misuse or learning disability (LD).
- Always take a chaperone (regardless of gender)
- Allow more time for reassurance and explanation
- Break the assessment into chunks if they can't tolerate everything at once
- Needle-phobics: lay flat + local anaesthetic cream + friendly hand to hold.

If you *can't* complete the assessment immediately, see *What ifs … ?*

TIP: If you notice yourself moping after an assessment, pondering what a rubbish doctor you are and fumbling around for your contract to see how much notice you have to give, stop and ask yourself – is this always after the same patient? If yes, read up on countertransference.

Madeleine Kerr, Consultant

Admission plan

Address *immediate* care and risks, discussing your initial plan with the patient and nurses. Staff who already know the patient may predict how different ideas will pan out.
- **Admission status**: informal/detained
- **Leave**
  - Free to come and go? No leave?
  - Consider documenting: *If wishes to leave, contact doctor to assess under s5(2)*
- **Observation level ('obs')** – the degree of nursing checks (excluding physical obs). Follow local policy, using increased obs for increased risks, e.g. self-harm, aggression, absconding or chaotic behaviour. The nurses will guide you. Most people will be on general or intermittent obs:
  - *General* – minimum; hourly check
  - *Intermittent* – 4 irregularly-timed checks each hour (reduces behaviours like self-harm being scheduled between predictable reviews)

- ○ *1:1* – one colleague constantly with patient. Sometimes divided into *arm-length* or *within-eyesight* observations.
- ○ *2:1* – two staff constantly with the patient. Usual maximum, outside of PICU.
- **Physical health follow up**
  - ○ Physical observations if needed. Give precise instructions, including parameters to contact you (e.g. EWS score; specific BP reading, rather than "raised BP")
  - ○ Outstanding examination/investigations/results
- **Regular medication** – check with seniors/pharmacist, but as a *general* rule …
  - ○ Leave medication-free if:
    - New patient: the team can assess and choose medication *with* them
    - Non-adherent for a while (full review often needed)
  - ○ Restart meds if:
    - Well-known and concordant
    - *Recently* stopped medication which is known to work
    - NB: You'll sometimes restart a lower dose (e.g. clozapine, p241)
- **PRN medication (Appendix B.7):**
  - ○ Consider *this* person's likely needs over the next 24 hours
  - ○ Nurses know which medications are stocked ± what's helped previously
  - ○ Routinely prescribing rapid tranquilisation (RT) suggests you're on autopilot
- **Carers and contacts**:
  - ○ Highlight outstanding collateral histories and contact details (email/phone)
  - ○ ± Alert Community Mental Health Team (CMHT) and invite CC to ward rounds
- **Dependents**
  - ○ Children/elderly parents: contact social services urgently
  - ○ Pets: involve family/Royal Society for the Prevention of Cruelty to Animals (RSPCA)
- **Next review** – if needed before the next ward round, state who, when and why, e.g. *daily SHO review of suicidal ideation.*

With experience, you may suggest longer-term management.

PATIENT VIEW:

I remember being absolutely petrified when I first went in. In fact, the nurse who signed me in, I thought she was going to kill me … There was this process of three months on the ward … The first month where everyone's out to get you, to do you harm. The second month, it's like you're working it out. In the third month, you feel this resolution.

'Dominic'

Treatment phase

Whatever's happening with medication, there are things you should do for everyone.

PATIENT VIEW:

I just felt like I was in a holding pen and it was actually scary being around other ill people. It felt like the emotional and the human was neglected in face of the medical … So, the ward is a factory, designed to make sure you take medication, stay in the same place and don't harm yourself. You're infantilised because the staff turn in to almost police officers, or prison wardens … and it doesn't do them any good.

'Angela'

1. Approach

Good liaison with *everyone* throughout admission should prevent nasty surprises at the discharge meeting. It's easy to exclude patients from this – especially if they're withdrawn, psychotic or angry. This feels disempowering, and reinforces the message that they're in limbo, passively receiving 'care' whether wanted or not. The more involved they are in care planning, the more likely the admission will be useful to them. Get to know your patients and understand:

- Problems triggering admission
- Whether their current presentation suggests potential difficulties after discharge
- How they can help themselves
- How you can help
- How things are changing (document MSE weekly).

> **TIP:** Schedule in regular (if informal) sessions with patients, even on acute wards where you can easily just end up seeing them on a PRN basis. You can build valuable therapeutic relationships with most patients, in the worst of circumstances, and they will reward you.
>
> **Greg Shields, ST4**

2. SMART Goals (p72)

Goals provide focus and momentum, especially in long admissions. Set them in early meetings, ward rounds (Ch.35) or CPAs (Ch.19):

- Clinically, e.g. contain suicide risk; treat depression
- Personally, e.g. hopes for this admission and life more generally

    Wherever possible, support the patient to take the lead, rather than doing everything for them. If a key goal is symptom reduction, explain how you'll monitor this, e.g. self-report, MSE reviews, standardised tools.

3. Leave

The transition to discharge is ideally tested with increasing periods of leave, e.g. escorted, unescorted, overnight/extended leave. When asked to assess if an *informal* patient can take leave, check:

- *Notes and staff*
  - MHA status (if detained, is there s17 leave?)
  - Existing leave plans
  - Past episodes of leave
  - Risk history
  - Staff concerns, e.g. absconding, drug use, visiting an angry ex-partner
- *With the patient*
  - Their plans (duration, geography, purpose)? E.g. fetch clothes from home, attend college, visit the Queen …
  - Do they intend to return?
  - How will they handle problems, e.g. feeling paranoid, suicidal?
  - How can staff contact them? Do they carry a working mobile?
  - MSE: symptoms which could cause trouble by:
    - Drawing unwanted attention, e.g. sexual disinhibition
    - Making them approach or confront people
    - Placing them in danger, e.g. suicidal thoughts, impulsivity.

If you feel they *can* use leave, decide whether this should be unrestricted or initially tested out with some boundaries, e.g.

- Escorted (staff/relatives/friends)
- Specific duration (short periods are safer; longer periods build Trust)
- Certain places, e.g. hospital grounds, local shops, own home.

If you don't feel it's safe, explain why, and what needs to change, rather than just saying no. Should an informal patient still want to leave, assess under s5(2) (Ch.38).

Document clearly, and check progress with the patient, carers and staff, remembering that symptoms may resurface, off the ward.

4. Accommodation

Housing problems cause lengthy admissions, so establish any concerns with the patient, carers ± CC. You might suggest initial escorted home leave, allowing a colleague to help them check:

- Working keys
- Safe, secure, furnished and clean
- Gas, electricity, water
- Postal 'surprises', e.g. bills, rent arrears, eviction notices

Tackle problems early – it's frustrating to delay discharge because someone's home has become a crack den.

5. Test plans

Don't *assume* plans will work on discharge, especially if someone has problems with organisation, motivation or confidence. Test plans during admission, and deal with obstacles, e.g. attending a gym might uncover difficulties using buses, which can be overcome with initial staff support.

PATIENT VIEW:

When you discharge someone, have they got pathways? How do you connect them? What power do you have to help that person feel more able and more aware of what's out there?

'Amanda'

---

6. Pre-discharge

In the run-up to discharge, attention turns to:

- Stabilising medication
- Finalising accommodation plans
- Community risk management, e.g. self-harm, violence, vulnerability
- Relapse indicators and crisis plans
- Handover to GP/HTT/CMHT
- ± Need for Community Treatment Orders (CTOs; Table 15.1, p99).

Refer to the CMHT/HTT well *before* discharge, to let them discuss your referral or assess the patient on the ward.

Discharge

TIP: Discharge people when clinically ready, *not* because someone else needs their bed. Jumping to discharge patients in response to bed crises, teaches bed managers to pressurise *you* whenever beds are short. Politely outline your management plans, and refer them to your consultant if they're pushy.

1. Discharge meetings

Everyone should have a discharge meeting before going home. In brief admissions, this may be an informal discussion between the patient (± carer), a senior doctor and named nurse. Longer admissions require more formal meetings, often in ward rounds, and sometimes as discharge CPAs (Ch.19 or p224) – if so, invite people at least a week beforehand, e.g.

- Patient
- Carer(s)
- Key ward staff
- Community staff, e.g. CC, HTT representative, GP
- Relevant agencies, e.g. housing/probation/social worker.

If community staff can't attend, agree key issues with them *before* the meeting.

Bad meetings feel rushed and raise unexpected obstacles, which can't be resolved or which scupper discharge. Good discharge meetings are reassuring, reviewing progress and drawing together a clear plan in front of the patient and their team:

- Progress summary
- Ongoing concerns or symptoms - and plans to address them
- Current MSE
- Risks and management
- Social situation, e.g. housing, childcare, employment
- Medication
  - Duration
  - Effectiveness
  - Side effects
  - Ensure dosing's as simple as possible
  - PRN medications are generally stopped
- Community plan
  - Names and contact details of all involved
  - Responsibility for care, e.g. CMHT, GP
    - Seven-day follow up appointment
    - Prescribing and side effect monitoring
    - Bio-psycho-social interventions
  - How family/carers can link in and provide support
  - Crisis plan
- Questions and concerns.

PATIENT VIEW:

I came out of hospital and I saw it on the care plan! I had *psychotic reactive something*. I've no memory of them saying to me, "You've got this condition." Nobody else is gonna tell me. None of my friends told me. Not my parents ... 'Cos they're definitely too frightened to tell you.

'Isaac'

---

2. Discharge paperwork

Immediate tasks

Consider writing the patient a bullet-point list of the key discharge / crisis plan (p315) points. This may help them remember appointments and essential messages while awaiting their copy of the discharge summary. They may also need:

- Med 3 certificate - a "fit note" if they need further time off work (p87)
- *TTO/A (To Take Out/Away) Medication*: complete and send the TTO form to pharmacy as soon as possible, so there isn't a lengthy wait for medication.
  - Some forms summarise the admission, diagnosis and discharge plan
  - Maximum medication supply is usually 7–14 days

- ◦ If overdose is a risk, consider a shorter script *or* hand medication to carers/HTT
- ◦ Ensure the GP ± CMHT receive a copy and know who will continue prescriptions

If you organise these tasks during / immediately after their discharge meeting, they won't have to hang around waiting. It's a small thing, but it makes a big difference to people.

Discharge summary

Complete this promptly to keep everyone in the loop and stop your paperwork piling up. Increasingly, you're expected to send/email/fax this to the GP within a day/week. Some Trusts split it into:

- Part 1: admission clerking and plan (sent promptly after admission)
- Part 2: progress on ward and discharge plan (sent promptly after discharge).

Summaries need only take 30 minutes at discharge if you write up admission clerkings as early as possible, and summarise lengthy admissions every week or month. Some wards only write short summaries of the key details: this can be useful with well-known patients, but risks losing important information.

TIPS:

- Read colleagues' summaries and discuss different formats with your consultant in supervision. Establish the 'best' format *before* you start writing/dictating
- Draw a discharge summary template and complete it during admission clerkings to avoid missing anything important
- Don't write '*see previous discharge summary*' when you should write information: it's extremely frustrating for future readers, especially if they can't *access* previous summaries.

Other

Ask the ward clerk about other administrative discharge tasks, e.g.

- HONOS
- ICD code.

3. Say goodbye

It's odd not to say goodbye, especially after long admissions. Always take time to wish people well.

TIP: Start thinking about the ethics of psychiatric practice, and don't be afraid to point out when something doesn't accord with them. We get too used to working in some dreadful environments, and seeing awful things happen to patients.

Greg Shields, ST4

What if ... ?

... The person's being *readmitted*?

When readmitting someone who's absconded or experienced problems on extended leave, *focus* your assessment:

- Summarise background information
- Recent events and reason for readmission
- MSE
- Risk assessment
- Physical health examination (±UDS).

The plan is as for any newly admitted patient, though leave is usually suspended until further review.

... You *can't* complete the admission clerking?

You may need to postpone your assessment if the patient:

- Adamantly refuses
- Is highly agitated
- Is asleep.

Check the admission observations and staff impressions of physical and mental state – then weigh your clinical concerns against the patient's wish to be left alone or sleep. If no immediate concerns, you may be able to postpone the clerking, summarising their notes, completing an MSE from a distance, and highlighting items in your plan. If on-call, ask the nurses to contact you when the patient's awake or more amenable. If concerned, you may need to wake them, or insist on a brief assessment.

... Physical assessment is urgently needed but refused?

You may be deeply worried about someone's physical state, e.g. suspected delirium, NMS, overdose. Clearly explain the problem, and consider offering oral sedation to facilitate the assessment if they're frightened or aroused (obviously, not if GCS is already lowered!).

Assess capacity (p102). If they lack capacity, you can investigate and treat in their best interests under the MCA. As a *last resort*, you can ask nurses to restrain someone while you take bloods. If so:

- You *cannot* imagine how frightening this is for patients
- It's risky for patients and staff
- Explain your rationale to the team
- Prepare all equipment and ensure everyone knows their role beforehand
- Someone must reassure the patient and explain what's happening throughout
- Ask another doctor or experienced nurse to assist you
- Prioritise the most essential bloods, in case movement dislodges the needle.

Remember that restraint may affect blood results, e.g. raised CK.

... The patient is suddenly discharged?

Some patients self-discharge (Ch.38) or are discharged by Tribunals (Ch.49). There's rarely time to hold a discharge meeting, but you should provide TTOs and contact the CMHT/GP to arrange a seven-day follow-up. The paperwork is the same.

... The patient doesn't want to be discharged?

Meet with the patient and a senior nurse, dropping the idea that you need to discharge them. Explore their concerns about going home, e.g.

- Overlooked/undisclosed problems
- Misunderstanding about the plan.

Explanation and reassurance often suffice, but you may need to discuss delaying discharge or changing the plan with your consultant. People with personality disorders, may have particular problems around discharge (p286).

Take-home message

Plan for discharge early, and keep everyone involved to make it as smooth as possible.

Further reading

Patient information on what to expect throughout an admission, provided by King's Health Partners in association with Rethink: http://www.mentalhealthcare.org.uk/psychiatric_wards.

CHAPTER 35

Ward rounds

Katherine Beck

South London & Maudsley NHS Foundation Trust, London, England

---

RELATED CHAPTERS: admission to discharge (34), CPAs (19)

Your first ward round is this afternoon. The ward manager gives you a list of patients for review.

Ward rounds are usually once or twice a week, and take a few hours. They're the place where team decisions are made, thus a good place to learn about management (Box 35.1). Rather than being visited at their bedside, patients usually attend a conference room, and can feel understandably overwhelmed by the crowd of MDT representatives. Some consultants use ward rounds to gain updates, before reviewing patients in a more relaxed manner, one-to-one.

Box 35.1 Ward round aims

- Presentation of new admissions
- Patients/carers give their views and ask questions
- Staff feedback on progress
- Formal consultant and MDT review
- Review and update of plans, e.g.
  - Medication changes, side effect management
  - Review results and consider need for further tests
  - Offer psychological input, social support, occupational health activities
  - Review leave and MHA status
- CPAs
- Discharge planning

PATIENT VIEW:

The other thing I find totally bizarre is the ward round. There are, what: fifteen professionals? Thirteen you'll never see again and have no interest in your case. You're usually jammed into a room which is too small and hot. The psychiatrist speaks to you from on high and can say whatever they like to you, and no one will challenge what they say. I've had terrible things said to me. It's totally inappropriate and totally oblivious to the vulnerability of the person. It's worse than a job interview.

'Krish'

Psychiatry: Breaking the ICE – Introductions, Common Tasks and Emergencies for Trainees, First Edition.
Edited by Sarah Stringer, Juliet Hurn and Anna M Burnside.
© 2016 John Wiley & Sons, Ltd. Published 2016 by John Wiley & Sons, Ltd.
Companion Website: www.psychiatryice.com

Preparation

1. Check your team's expectations
There are different approaches to ward rounds, so ask your ward manager or consultant beforehand:
• Who organises it, e.g. nurse, ward clerk, you?
• How should you present new patients? (Duration, level of formality)
• Are specific appointment timings allocated? If so, how are these decided?
• Which patients are reviewed? How is this decided?

> **TIP:** Tell your consultant you'd like to complete a Workplace Based Assessment on alternate ward rounds.

2. Plan the ward round (if it's *your* job)
• List patients needing review ± allocate time slots
• Plan CPAs or large meetings near the start, as fewer people will be kept waiting should everything run late
• Ask patients who they'd like to attend. Inform them and carers of timings.
• Consider inviting the CC/CMHT representative, or (if discharging) the HTT.

3. Read the notes
• Ensure all jobs from the last ward round have been completed
• Be prepared to present each patient. You'll need:
  ◦ Admission circumstances, key background history
  ◦ Progress since last ward round
  ◦ Investigation results/physical examination findings
  ◦ Current MSE
  ◦ Current medications.

4. Other
• Bring
  ◦ Current drug and physical obs charts, s17 leave forms
  ◦ New admission clerkings
  ◦ Blank drug charts and s17 forms
• For brownie points, prepare tea, coffee and biscuits.

During ward round

> **TIP:** Always remember what's happening *outside* the ward round: "When's the doctor going to see me ... ?"
>
> Piers Newman, RMN

1. Approach
Try to make the process easier for patients and carers. Your consultant should lead, but consider how you can help, e.g.
• Ask unnecessary staff to step out (just have a 'core team' present)

- Invite carers or advocates to sit beside the patient
- Introduce everyone
- Give the patient time to talk at the start – and respond to comments – rather than silently listening while everyone talks about them.

PATIENT VIEW:

I was in a ward round and listening to these observations of the nurses and they were saying, "She's really quiet, we have to go and get her out of her room." And I was like, *I'm here!* I was literally thinking I was being really good and not making any problems by staying in my room. It was very strange being talked about as if you weren't there.

'Kim'

---

2. Documentation
You'll usually need to:
- Document the ward round
- Make a list of your jobs as you go.

If typing notes on a computer, *expect the system to crash.* Try saving all entries as a single word-processing document, then cutting and pasting entries into the notes afterwards. This also makes it easier to keep track of your jobs. Consultants have their own preferences for the structure of reviews, but the following may help:
- *Title:* ward round – date and time
- *Attendees:* name and roles, including patient and carers
- *Patient's name*
- *Admission date*
- *MHA status:* informal/section X
- *Progress/feedback:*
  ◦ Patient
  ◦ Family
  ◦ Nursing
  ◦ Other
- *Ward round discussion,* e.g. medication review, goals
- *MSE*
- *Capacity to consent to treatment* (yes/no + why)
- *Risks*
- *Impression* diagnosis $\pm$ progress (e.g. improving/deteriorating)
- *Plan* (including)
  ◦ Current medication (including PRN)
  ◦ Obs level (p214–215)
  ◦ Leave allowance and conditions
  ◦ Further investigations/jobs
  ◦ Next review date.

3. Talking
Be prepared to give your opinion, but be wary of jumping in at every opportunity: show-offs are annoying. Ward rounds are a chance to build skills and knowledge, as well as gaining on-the-job teaching. Ask questions of the MDT, not just your consultant.

After

Update all patient records and complete your jobs list. Gently prompt your consultant to complete s17 leave forms, if not done during the round.

What if ... ?

... It's a CPA?

The care of patients with complex needs should be coordinated under the CPA (Ch.19). CPA meetings should be held for inpatients:

• Whenever their care plan or circumstances significantly change, e.g. admission, discharge, transfer between wards
• Every 6–12 months in long admissions.

To maximise attendance, invitations should be sent one to two weeks in advance.

> **TIP:** Watch Video 6 on this book's companion website to see a discharge CPA in action

Take-home message

Planning is everything. That, and biscuits.

CHAPTER 36

Common side effect management

Katherine Beck[1], Noreen Jakeman[2], and Sarah Stringer[3]

[1] South London & Maudsley NHS Foundation Trust, London, England
[2] Lewisham & Greenwich NHS Trust, London, England
[3] King's College London, London, England

RELATED CHAPTERS: clozapine (37), opiate overdose (66), stiff, feverish patients (67), lithium toxicity (69)

Tom, 40, has schizoaffective disorder. You restarted his regular medications on admission, 3 weeks ago: an antipsychotic, mood stabiliser and antidepressant. He's asked to see you about side effects.

Medication side effects ruin people's lives – and any hope of adherence. As a rule of thumb, the more drugs on the chart, the higher the side effect load – particularly at higher doses. You'll commonly see:
• Extrapyramidal side effects (EPSE) (Table 36.1)
• Sedation
• Weight gain
• Sexual side effects.

PATIENT VIEW:

I've had no end of problems with my medication. I've been violently sick. I've collapsed at home ... I've fainted ... it's just a nightmare. I'm not happy. I can't function. They keep giving me medication that makes me feel sick. A glass of fruit juice might be better than what I'm being put through.

'Dee'

EPSE are most common with first generation antipsychotics (FGAs) but also occur with second generation antipsychotics (SGAs). Movement disorders can also be caused or exacerbated by other drugs, including lithium, valproate, antidepressants, promethazine and metoclopramide.

PATIENT VIEW:

I said, "Look, I can't bear these side effects!" And they said, "Well, that's because you're not taking it properly." That's all they said to me.

'Imran'

Psychiatry: Breaking the ICE – Introductions, Common Tasks and Emergencies for Trainees, First Edition.
Edited by Sarah Stringer, Juliet Hurn and Anna M Burnside.
© 2016 John Wiley & Sons, Ltd. Published 2016 by John Wiley & Sons, Ltd.
Companion Website: www.psychiatryice.com

Table 36.1 EPSE key information.

EPSE	Onset after start/increase antipsychotic	Presentation
Acute dystonia	<1 week (PO) Minutes–hours (IM/IV) *Or on reducing anticholinergic*	Sustained, painful muscle spasm: • Torticollis • Trismus • Blepharospasm • Oculogyric crisis (eyes roll up) • Opisthotonous (arched neck and back) • Jaw dislocation • Laryngospasm Frightening and dangerous – go straight to management (Table 36.6, p232) N.B. *Tardive dystonias* are delayed-onset spasms (months–years)
Akathisia	Hours–weeks	Unpleasant, inner feeling of restlessness/compulsion to move • May increase risk of suicide/aggression
Parkinsonism	Days–weeks	Pill-rolling tremor Rigidity Bradykinesia
Tardive dyskinesia (TD)	Months–years	Involuntary, choreoathetoid movements: face, lips, tongue, trunk and extremities • 50% are irreversible • Worst at rest • May disappear with voluntary movement or distraction

Preparation

If Tom has acute dystonia, go straight to management (Table 36.6).

1. Gather information – nurses, notes, drug chart
• Which side effects have staff noticed?
• Current medications: start dates; recent changes/omissions
• DHx: previous side effects, reasons for changing
• Substance misuse history ± recent UDS
• Observe Tom discreetly, e.g. walking down the ward. Movement disorders are easier to spot while someone's not concentrating on their movement.

2. If you suspect EPSE, fetch a firm, armless chair for the examination

Assessment

1. Approach
Think broadly: where there's one side effect, there may be more.
• Tom might not disclose embarrassing problems unless asked directly, e.g. erectile dysfunction, gynaecomastia, galactorrhoea; urinary incontinence with antipsychotics

- He may not *notice* TD unless others have commented on it, or may hide it by chewing gum or talking behind his hand.

Stigma is important – side effects can mark people out as 'patients', however well controlled their illness.

TIP: If unsure whether a complaint could be a side effect, look it up.

---

2. Focused history, remembering ...

- *HPC:* see Table 36.2
- *PMHx and systems review, especially*
  - Cardiovascular risk factors
  - Diabetes
  - Neurological problems
- *Substance misuse*: alcohol, drugs, smoking, caffeine
- *Over the counter (OTC) medication*
- *Has medication helped at all?* (current MSE?).

PATIENT VIEW:

I could hardly walk ... Oh, I forgot all about how horrible! People must have thought I was drunk. I fell asleep and I was travelling all night. I could have been raped. Maybe I was! Because I was in this deep sleep that anyone could do anything to me. I think [risperidone] is killing me and it's making me very day-dreamy. I leave saucepans on all night, I wake up at 3am thinking, *sniff sniff*. Oh my God, my vegetable soup's been on all night, my lovely vegetables that I peeled so carefully!

'Sarah'

---

3. Physical examination

Complete a relevant physical examination, including physical obs, Body Mass Index (BMI) and waist circumference. Genital examination is generally unhelpful in sexual dysfunction. Check for nipple discharge on clothing in galactorrhoea (± ask patient to privately 'milk' their breast tissue).

Complete a full neurological exam if you suspect EPSE, following Table 36.3. Ask Tom to:
- Remove shoes and socks (so you can see his toes)
- Spit out any gum
- Tell you if he has tooth/denture discomfort (resembles/exacerbates TD).

It's sometimes hard to distinguish parkinsonism from idiopathic Parkinson's Disease (PD). Look for clues (Table 36.4), but if unsure, refer to neurology for single photon emission computed tomography (SPECT) imaging. If Tom has PD *and* EPSE, he'll need joint management with neurology.

PATIENT VIEW:

It can be exceptionally annoying to want to read the newspaper or play Scrabble and not be able to because either my legs don't want to sit still or there is what feels like thick fog or cotton wool in my head [...] When I was on the depot kind of haloperidol I found that if I was walking around I would want to lie down and if I was lying down my legs would want to walk around. I could never get my body comfortable and I was intensively aware of it all the time.

Janey Antoniou

Experiences of Mental Health In-Patient Care, p35

Table 36.2 Common side effects – history.

Complaint	Check …

All side effects	• Effect on:
	  ◦ Life/function
	  ◦ Mood, confidence or self-esteem
	• Relationship to:
	  ◦ Medication(s)
	  ◦ Underlying illness, e.g. apathy, low mood

EPSE	• *Any* unusual movements
	• Stiffness, shakiness, restlessness
	• Mental/physical slowing
	• Sleep
	  ◦ Akathisia disrupts
	  ◦ Parkinsonism causes problems turning
	  ◦ TD disappears during sleep

Sedation	• Check against medication timings:
	  ◦ Most drowsy?
	  ◦ Most alert?
	• Sleep pattern (insomnia often key)
	• How much of his day is spent asleep/drowsy?

Weight gain	• ↑ Appetite • Current diet • ↓ Exercise, e.g. due to sedation, stiffness • Clothing – tighter, looser? Different belt notch?

Sexual	• Any sexual problems *before* medication?
	• ↓ Libido
	• Loss of orgasm
	• Problems present when masturbating?
	• Breast growth/'leaking'
	• Effect on sexual relationships
	• *Men:*
	  ◦ Erection problems: getting or maintaining (Box 36.1)
	  ◦ Presence of morning erections
	  ◦ Ejaculation problems: premature, delayed, absent
	• *Women:* are periods regular? Exclude pregnancy.
	• Evidence of breast cancer/osteoporosis (chronic hyperprolactinaemia)

Box 36.1 Erectile dysfunction: organic, psychological or mixed aetiology?

Organic
• Older
• Gradual onset
• No erections in the morning or when masturbating alone
• Cardiovascular risk factors
Psychological
• Younger
• Sudden onset
• Associated with depression/anxiety
Alcohol use exacerbates both types ('brewer's droop').

Table 36.3 EPSE examination.

Position + test	Area ± instructions	Signs	A	P	TD
Inspection	*Sitting as still as possible: feet flat on floor, legs slightly apart. Hands on knees (1 minute), then hung unsupported down the sides of the chair (1 minute).*				
	Forehead and eyes	Fixed expression ("mask-like facies")		✓	✓
		↓blink rate		✓	✓
	Mouth	Brow wrinkling, ↑blinking			✓
		Puckering, lip-smacking, pouting			✓
		Grimacing, smiling			✓
		Opening and shutting			✓
		Tongue darting in and out			✓
		Jaws: clenching, chewing, nibbling, lateral movement			✓
	Arms and hands	Tremor: regular, repetitive, rhythmic		✓	✓
		Choreoathetoid movements, including wrist and finger flexion and extension ("guitar"/"piano-playing" movements)			✓
	Legs and feet	Leg swinging; crossing and uncrossing		✓	✓
		Foot stamping; jiggling		✓	✓
		Choreoathetoid movements, e.g. ankle and toe flexion/extension, toe wiggling			✓
		Foot tapping/squirming			✓
		Heel dropping			✓
		Lateral knee movements			✓
	Neck, shoulders, hips	Twisting, rocking, squirming, pelvic thrusts			✓
Questions	After 1 minute: *Do you feel restless or fidgety? Do you feel the urge to move or walk about?*	"Yes" to either question	✓		
Tongue	*Open your mouth and let your tongue lie still*	Restless tongue			✓
	Stick out your tongue	Can't hold tongue protruded (± writhing)			✓
	Raise your tongue	Drooling		✓	
Tone	Test limbs	Stiffness, resistance		✓	
	Head: gently hold his head between your hands, fingers on the back of his neck; rotate x3	Stiffness, resistance		✓	

(continued overleaf)

Table 36.3 (*continued*)

Position + test	Area ± instructions	Signs	A	P	TD
Finger movements	*Tap your thumb with each finger as fast as possible … Now the other hand.*	Finger bradykinesia		✓	
		Worsening facial movements			✓
Glabellar tap	*Please don't blink.* Stand behind him so he can't see your finger. Steadily and quickly tap between his eyebrows until blinking stops.	>5 blinks/infraorbital muscle twitches		✓	
Stand still for >1 minute					
Inspection	Legs and feet	Shuffling/tramping movements	✓		
		Rocking from foot to foot	✓		
		Walking on the spot/pacing	✓		
Questions	*After 1 minute:* *Do you feel restless or fidgety?* *Do you feel the urge to move or walk about?*	"Yes" to either question	✓		
Tremor	*Hold your arms out in front, palms down*	Tremor hands ± rest of body		✓	
Arm drop	*Please copy me.* Hold arms out at shoulder height, then let them drop to your sides	Slowed fall		✓	
		Quiet slap of arms on sides			
		No rebound bounce			
Gait	*Walk to the end of the room and back*	↓Arm swing		✓	
		Stiff, stooped or shuffling gait		✓	
		Propulsion and retropulsion		✓	
		Turning difficult (*en bloc* turning)		✓	
		Worsening finger/facial dyskinesias			✓
		Walking subjectively lessens distress	✓		

Table 36.4 Clues to help distinguish PD from EPSE.

	EPSE	PD
Age	<60	>60
Resting tremor	Symmetrical	Asymmetrical
Family history PD	X	✓ (especially <40y)
Symptoms appear after …	Started or ↑ antipsychotic	Years of unchanged antipsychotic
SPECT imaging	Normal	Abnormal

4. Investigations

Ensure all routine investigations are up to date (Appendix A) and see Table 36.5.

PATIENT VIEW:

The doctors told him when he takes the medication, he's going to get diabetes. Yeah, before they gave him the medication they told him that diabetes is around the corner. And when he took it, he got diabetes and then, the company that gave him that psychiatric medication was the same company that made the medication for his diabetes.

'Derek'

Table 36.5 Common side effects – investigations.

Complaint	Check …

All side effects	• Drug chart:
	   ° Can doses be lowered?
	   ° Could timing change to improve side effects?

EPSE	• UDS • TFTs – if restless + possible hyperthyroidism • Serum caeruloplasmin – if suspect Wilson's disease, e.g. choreiform movements, cognitive impairment, jaundice, liver signs, Kayser-Fleischer rings • FHx – Huntington's disease (choreiform – discuss with neurology) • SPECT – possible PD
Sedation	• Sleep diary
Weight gain	Always consider the risk of more general *metabolic syndrome* (↑ weight, BP, raised lipids, glucose) and cardiovascular risk. • BMI + waist circumference • BP • Fasting glucose, lipids • ECG
Sexual	• BP • ECG • Prolactin levels (≥1h after sleeping/eating) • Fasting glucose, lipids • TFTs – hypothyroidism can lower libido • LFTs, U & Es – liver/kidney failure can cause sexual dysfunction • Pregnancy test: in amenorrhoeic women • DEXA scan if chronic hyperprolactinaemia/amenorrhoea

Table 36.6 Common side effects – initial management options.

Problem	Common culprits	Management options
Acute dystonia	FGAs	Act quickly: painful, frightening ± dangerous, e.g. jaw dislocation, breathing problems: • Procyclidine 5–10 mg 　○ Emergency: IM (onset within 5–10 minutes) 　○ Less severe: PO • Continue procyclidine PO (e.g. 5 mg bd/tds) for a week, gradually reducing over two to three weeks (longer if depot) • Consider stop/↓ antipsychotic; change to SGA • Check for hypocalcaemia if ongoing problems
Akathisia	FGAs Aripiprazole	• ↓ Antipsychotic or change to SGA (best = clozapine > quetiapine > olanzapine > risperidone; aripiprazole worst) • Try propranolol 30–80 mg
Parkinsonism	FGAs (NB: valproate/lithium commonly cause tremor)	• Exclude Parkinson's disease (PD) – Table 36.4 • ↓ Dose • Change FGA to SGA • Try anticholinergic, e.g. procyclidine 5 mg – review within 3 months • Propranolol for lithium/valproate tremor
Tardive dyskinesia	FGAs	• The longer this continues, the more likely it'll be irreversible • *Stop* anticholinergics, e.g. procyclidine • ↓ Antipsychotic or change to SGA (quetiapine or clozapine best). • *Don't* ↑ antipsychotic dose (only temporarily decreases TD) • Try tetrabenazine if these fail
Sedation	SGAs (clozapine >olanzapine >risperidone >quetiapine) Mirtazapine, TCAs Benzodiazepines Promethazine Lithium Valproate	• If recently started medication, reassure that it may wear off • Sleep hygiene (p72) and regular exercise • Consider ↓ responsible medication or ↑ *more slowly* • Change timings, e.g. 　○ Change mane to nocte dosing 　○ If 'morning hangovers' take medication earlier in the evening (e.g. 8pm, not 10pm)

Weight gain

SGAs
(clozapine > olanzapine > risperidone)
Mirtazapine
Lithium
Valproate
Promethazine

- Splitting doses can help
- Switch to less sedative medications e.g. aripiprazole, amisulpride, sulpiride; SSRIs
- Avoid combining sedative medications

- Monitor BMI, waist circumference, BP, lipids, glucose
- Psychoeducation: diet and exercise
- Involve dietician early
- Set weight targets
- Involve CC, e.g. meeting while walking; organise gym membership
- Consider ↓ dose or switching to a more weight-neutral medication, e.g. aripiprazole, lurasidone amisulpride, sulpiride; SSRIs
- Consider *adding* aripiprazole

Sexual dysfunction

FGAs
Amisulpride, risperidone
Most antidepressants; all SSRIs
(especially paroxetine)

- Exclude/treat organic causes, e.g. hypertension, diabetes, obesity, excess alcohol
- If prolactin >2500ml/L, check visual fields and refer to endocrinology (?prolactinoma)
- Reassure and monitor *if* likely to improve:
  - Early in treatment
  - Once underlying illness resolves, e.g. depression, psychosis
- If no better, decrease doses or switch to less problematic medications, e.g.
  - Aripiprazole, clozapine, quetiapine, olanzapine, lurasidone
  - Mirtazapine, agomelatine
  - Venlafaxine causes less erectile dysfunction
- Aripiprazole can be added to other antipsychotics to decrease prolactin (~5 mg mane)
- Consider
  - Relationship counselling/sensate focus therapy
  - Psychosexual clinic referral
  - Sildenafil – though currently restricted NHS usage

Management

1. Explain
Whatever the problem, explain how problems relate to medication. Actively involve Tom in management planning, including deciding which side effects he'd rather cope with, if some are unavoidable, e.g. weight gain versus EPSE. If problems don't resolve with the steps below, seek expert advice, e.g. pharmacy, neurology, endocrinology, dietician.

2. Management
See Table 36.6 and Appendix B1 for relative side effect profiles. See Ch.37 for clozapine-specific side effects.

3. Follow-up
Add an alert to the drug chart and notes. Ensure Tom's doctors review problems, if out-of-hours.

> **TIP:** *'Beginner's mind'* can provide a valuable source of valid questions before the cynicism of experience sets in. What seems unorthodox today is tomorrow's innovation and today's enthusiasms can (often) turn out to be fads.
>
> John Joyce, Consultant

Take-home message

Side effects are common, disabling and often treatable. See them as an early warning system for future problems – not least, non-adherence.

References

EPSE rating scales:
Abnormal Involuntary Movement Scale (AIMS) – assesses for TD
Guy W. (1976) *ECDEU Assessment Manual for Psychopharmacology*, revised edn, Washington, DC, US Department of Health, Education, and Welfare.
Barnes Akathisia Scale (BARS) – assesses for akathisia
Barnes,T. R. E. (1989) A rating scale for drug-induced akathisia.*British Journal of Psychiatry*, **154**, 672–676.
Modified Simpson-Angus Scale (MSAS) – assesses for parkinsonism and akathisia
Simpson GM, Angus JWC. (1970) A rating scale for extra pyramidal side effects. *Acta Psychiatrica Scandinavica* **212** (supplement): 11–19.

Further reading

Hardcastle, M., Kennard, D., Grandison, S. and Fagin, L. (2007) Experiences of Mental Health In-Patient Care. Narratives From Service Users, Carers and Professionals. Routledge, Oxford.
Taylor, D., Paton, C. & Kapur, S. (2015) *The Maudsley Prescribing Guidelines in Psychiatry*, 12th edn, Wiley-Blackwell, Chichester.

CHAPTER 37

Clozapine

Stephanie Young[1] and Noreen Jakeman[2]

[1] South London & Maudsley NHS Foundation Trust, London, England
[2] Lewisham & Greenwich NHS Trust, London, England

> **RELATED CHAPTERS:** psychosis (23, 24), common side effect management (36)

Peter Ryan is 27, and was admitted to hospital informally to start clozapine. He's tried several oral antipsychotics, but remains distressed by the demons who chant at him.

Clozapine can transform people's lives, both by treating intractable psychosis *and* inflicting unpleasant and dangerous side effects. It's primarily used for Treatment Resistant Schizophrenia (TRS), which affects around 20% of people with psychosis. TRS is defined as:
- An inadequate response to two full trials of antipsychotics
  - At recommended doses for at least 6–8 weeks each
  - Including at least one second generation antipsychotic (SGA).

Clozapine can help with tardive dyskinesia, negative symptoms or if other antipsychotics aren't tolerated. It also decreases suicide rates and patients on average live longer than those given other antipsychotics. Nonetheless, well-meaning clinicians often avoid discussing clozapine, forgetting the *patient* should weigh side effects and blood tests against their ongoing symptoms. Offer eligible people an early trial, whilst accepting it can be a tough drug to take.

PATIENT VIEW:

After a while I said, "OK – clozapine." So they put it up to *four hundred* – and you know I'm already having trouble with *three*. That was very depressing because I want a life and I want my brain to think … We were on that ward together and we were both put on clozapine, but she's gotten on with it better than I have. She wasn't on as much as me, which I think probably does make a difference.

'Sarah'

Preparation

1. Call
- Pharmacist – guidance through local procedure
  - Which clozapine monitoring service is used?
- CMHT – have they started the registration process?

Psychiatry: Breaking the ICE – Introductions, Common Tasks and Emergencies for Trainees, First Edition.
Edited by Sarah Stringer, Juliet Hurn and Anna M Burnside.
© 2016 John Wiley & Sons, Ltd. Published 2016 by John Wiley & Sons, Ltd.
Companion Website: www.psychiatryice.com

2. Notes
- Confirm TRS diagnosis
- Previous antipsychotics: doses, duration, adherence, efficacy, side effects
- Previous clozapine: side effects, residual symptoms, reasons for stopping
  - Draw a timeline, correlating doses $\pm$ plasma clozapine measurements ('clozapine levels') with side effects and efficacy
- Physical co-morbidity, recent investigations.

Assessment

Clerk Peter as usual.

1. Psychiatric History, remembering…
- *HPC:* current problem/symptom list
- *PMHx:* cardiovascular, diabetes, seizures, blood/bone marrow disorders, constipation/bowel obstruction
- *DHx:* other medications
  - Few *serious* interactions, but discuss with pharmacy if SSRIs, carbamazepine, phenytoin, ciprofloxacin, erythromycin, chemotherapy or depot antipsychotics
- *Smoking status:* Box 37.1.

2. MSE, remembering…
- Baseline positive and negative symptoms
- Insight, including views on clozapine:
  - Dislikes medication/thinks it unnecessary
  - Side effect worries
  - Difficulties with regular tablets/blood tests.

3. Risk Assessment, including…
- Suicide
- Violence
- Clozapine side effects (see Table 37.1).

4. Baseline physical
- *Full examination, especially:*
  - BP, HR, temperature
  - BMI, waist circumference
  - Cardiovascular examination
- *Investigations (check clozapine monitoring service requirements):*
  - FBC – essential
  - $\pm$ U&E, LFTs, fasting glucose and lipids, troponin, CK, CRP
  - ECG, including QTc (< 440 ms in men; < 470 ms in women). Clozapine doesn't greatly $\uparrow$ QTc, but risks increase when combined with other antipsychotics, e.g. if cross-tapering.

Box 37.1 Clozapine and smoking

Cigarette and cannabis smoking rapidly (two to three days) induce the clozapine-metabolising cytochrome P450 enzyme system:
- ↓Smoking = ↑plasma clozapine = at constant dose ... side effects ± toxicity
- ↑Smoking = ↓plasma clozapine = at constant dose ... relapse?

With patients:
- Explain smoking effect (NRT *doesn't* affect clozapine dose requirements)
- Record and check smoking status regularly
- *Ask them to tell you/CC if changing smoking habit.*

Staff providing smoking cessation advice *must* understand the implications for clozapine dosage.

Management

1. Discussion

Meet with Peter ± carers. Ask the ward pharmacist to attend – they can answer tricky questions and may have patient information leaflets or DVDs. Cover:
- Why clozapine is being considered
- Potential benefits (relate to Peter's troublesome symptoms)
- Common and serious side effects (Table 37.1)
- Mandatory blood tests
  - Weekly for 18 weeks
  - Then fortnightly until the end of the first year
  - Then monthly (if WCC stable)

Table 37.1 Clozapine side effects.

Common	Severe but rare
Sedation	Risk of a 'weakened immune system'
Weight gain	• Neutropenia:
↑Glucose and lipids; ↑risk of diabetes	○ 2–3 people in 100 (2.7%)
Tachycardia	○ Half occur within the first 18 weeks
Hypotension (advise to stand up	○ Risk isn't dose-related
slowly, especially initially)	• Agranulocytosis:
Hypertension	○ <1 in 100 people (0.8%)
Hypersalivation	○ Usually within the first 18 weeks
Constipation	○ Death is rare, thanks to monitoring
Fever	(<1 in 10,000)
Nausea	Pneumonia (associated with reflux/saliva
Gastro-oesophageal reflux	aspiration)
Bed-wetting	Thromboembolism (kills 1 in 4500 patients)
Fits (usually at high doses)	Cardiomyopathy
	Myocarditis
	Bowel obstruction (constipation can kill)

- Peter's questions and concerns
- Whether he's happy to start clozapine, or needs more time/information.

Clozapine can be given against his will, under the MHA, but the need for blood tests may begin a long-term battle. Wherever possible, consent is the best way forward.

> **TIP:** Treat infections or constipation aggressively – they're *never* minor problems in clozapine patients. Signs of infection may also be confused with developing myocarditis/cardiomyopathy.

2. Registration

The pharmacist will guide you through the practicalities of registering Peter. The monitoring service checks the initial FBC and national database for any history of neutropenia on clozapine. If these are OK, they'll give permission to prescribe. Pharmacy can only dispense clozapine once the monitoring service has received a normal FBC each week, and given a 'green' result.

3. Prescribe and monitor

Find your Trust's clozapine titration protocol
- Reduce or stop existing antipsychotics first
- Prescribe clozapine as per the titration chart (bd dosing after Day 1)
  - Even tiny doses can be fatal in clozapine-naïve patients – hence cautious titration
  - If he misses a dose during titration, check with pharmacy and write a new chart:
    - <48h – can usually continue titration from the last dose he *received*
    - >48h – re-titrate from the beginning
- He needs a weekly FBC – essential to handover to covering doctor if you're off work
  - Other tests: check clozapine monitoring service's advice (and Appendix A.5)
- Follow protocols for checking physical obs while titrating
  - Once the dose is stable, check obs at least weekly on the ward (e.g. with FBC)
- It may take a few weeks to reach the 'right' dose, based on efficacy, side effects and plasma clozapine measurements (Box 37.2)
  - Usual dose 200–450 mg/day
  - Maximum 900 mg/day
- *After titration, if Peter misses a dose ...*
  - <48 hours – continue the prescribed dose
  - >48 hours – re-titrate from the start (though pharmacy may advise a *faster* titration). Check that his last blood test is still valid before prescribing.

Box 37.2 Clozapine plasma measurements

- It's hard to prescribe safely without clozapine plasma measurements
- Steady state takes up to seven days of stable dosing
- Take trough sample for plasma clozapine measurement, 10–12 hours post-dose
- *Remind staff and patient to postpone morning dose until morning blood test is taken*
- Plasma clozapine is related to dose, but is higher in non-smokers and women
- Official therapeutic range 0.35–0.50 mg/L
  - If someone responds satisfactorily at a lower plasma clozapine, be glad and *don't increase the dose!*
  - Higher plasma clozapine concentrations *may* be appropriate, but ...
    - May worsen MSE
    - Increase the seizure risk (consider prophylactic valproate, lamotrigine or gabapentin)

- If you get a high plasma clozapine level (>1.0mg/L), repeat the blood test. If confirmed, consider cautious dose reductions, e.g. 25mg/day steps.
- Norclozapine is the principal plasma metabolite of clozapine. Its half-life is longer than clozapine's, so measurement is useful for assessing adherence.
  - The average plasma clozapine:norclozapine ratio across the dose range is 1.3
  - A ratio <0.5 suggests recent poor adherence in the last few days …
  - … *Or* that the patient metabolises clozapine particularly quickly, e.g. some young male smokers

TIP: It can be difficult to dispute 'clozapine toxicity' as the cause of death at an inquest, with the associated implication that clozapine dosage was inappropriate. This is because blood clozapine and norclozapine often rise after death, e.g. clozapine x5; norclozapine x4. If you have regularly (e.g. yearly in apparently successful therapy) measured plasma clozapine in life, this places you in a much stronger position to answer questions about the possible role of clozapine in a death.

Robert Flanagan, Consultant Clinical/forensic Toxicologist

4. Monitoring

Clozapine may have reduced Peter's symptoms and improved his insight – but it's important to recheck his understanding, questions and worries; this may help with longer-term adherence.

Monitor closely for side effects (Ch.36), and ensure someone takes responsibility for ongoing physical health monitoring (Table 37.1). Address problems, e.g.

- *Hypersalivation* – try hyoscine 300mcg, sucked and swallowed nocte
  - Hyoscine patches may help
  - NB ↑risk constipation
- *Constipation* – high fibre diet ± regular laxatives
- *Nausea* – anti-emetic (not metoclopramide/prochlorperazine – due to risk of EPSE)
- *Nocturnal enuresis* – no fluids at bedtime
  - Manipulate dosing schedule
  - Desmopressin may help if severe, but monitor for hyponatraemia
- *Fever* – antipyretic and check FBC
  - If persists >38.5°C, stop clozapine and contact monitoring service.

5. Follow-up

Many Trusts run nurse-led clozapine clinics, which oversee monitoring and liaise between the clozapine monitoring service and hospital pharmacy. They may provide linked services, e.g. psychoeducation and monitoring of physical health, MSE and side effects. Contact the clinic and introduce Peter to the staff *before* discharge, to smooth the transition. He'll still need CMHT follow-up and a CC. Advise Peter to seek help for *any* signs of constipation or infection (especially chest infection).

TIP: Visit your local clozapine clinic. Understanding the practicalities of how it works makes your job easier.

What if … ?

… His white cells drop?

You'll receive an *amber* result from the clozapine monitoring service. Although you can continue to prescribe clozapine, they'll advise extra blood tests, and close monitoring for fever, sore throat, mouth ulcers or 'flu-like symptoms. *If you get a red result, stop clozapine immediately, look for signs of infection and transfer to ED if unwell.* Follow your clozapine monitoring service's guidance. Two consecutive red results prevent re-challenge with clozapine. Discuss alternatives with pharmacy, remembering that other antipsychotics (e.g. olanzapine) may lower white cells.

... Peter has benign ethnic neutropenia (BEN)?

If he's of African or Caribbean origin, Peter may have a higher proportion of *marginated* neutrophils – these sit next to vessel walls, rather than circulating freely, but still function normally in fighting infection. This means his neutrophils and white cell counts may *appear lower* than average, even before starting medication. It doesn't preclude a trial of clozapine, but a small (and harmless) drop in his neutrophils may be hard to distinguish from true clozapine-induced neutropenia. Discuss with haematology, pharmacy and the clozapine monitoring service – they may adjust the ranges for red/amber/green.

... He becomes tachycardic?

Tachycardia is common and usually benign, but may indicate:
• Myocarditis/cardiomyopathy – both occur most commonly during titration
• Pulmonary embolism
• Infection.
On the telephone:
• Ask if Peter looks/feels unwell – attend urgently, if so
• Request repeated obs, including a *manual* pulse and BP, and total EWS.
On the ward:
• Review clozapine titration and obs charts
  ◦ HR: steadily risen since clozapine was started = worrying
  ◦ HR: increased, but normalised after each increased dose = reassuring
• History and examination for PE, infection, cardiac cause
  ◦ Myocarditis: palpitations, chest pain, hypotension, shortness of breath, fever, extreme fatigue, 'flu-like symptoms
  ◦ Cardiomyopathy: cardiac failure, sweating, palpitations, breathing problems
• ECG – compare with baseline
• ±Screening bloods, e.g. FBC, U&E, CRP, troponin, D-dimer
• If no worrying features, consider other causes of tachycardia, e.g.
  ◦ Stress/agitation
  ◦ Substance misuse, caffeine, nicotine
  ◦ Other medications, e.g. salbutamol
  ◦ Omitted medications, e.g. beta-blockers.
Action:
• Discuss all concerns with the medical registrar or cardiologist
• *Resting tachycardia with chest pain/heart failure = stop clozapine, transfer to ED*
• Significant/persistent ↑HR
  ◦ Omit clozapine
  ◦ Meanwhile, consider need for alternative medication, e.g. benzodiazepines
  ◦ Notify Peter's team to urgently review and investigate
• Mild ↑HR but otherwise normal
  ◦ Give the last dose of clozapine that *didn't* raise HR (but rewrite the whole chart)
• Asymptomatic and obs normalised: give due dose of clozapine
• NB: Ask cardiology about adding a beta-blocker if Peter has ongoing, symptomatic but benign sinus tachycardia.

... Peter stops clozapine once discharged?

This is a common scenario for CMHT trainees. Using a motivational interviewing approach (p74), explore Peter's reasons, e.g. side effects, blood tests. Check if *any* benefits, e.g. quality of life, fewer demons' voices. Check for relapse indicators and discuss options with your consultant:

- Continue clozapine in *some* way, e.g.
  - Easier blood tests, e.g. local anaesthetic cream
  - Treat side effects (Ch.16 general; p239 clozapine-specific)
  - Reduce clozapine, e.g. in 25–50 mg steps
- *Re-titrate if >48 hours without clozapine*
  - Liaise with pharmacy and the clozapine monitoring service regarding retitration and ongoing monitoring (may now need weekly FBCs, even if he'd reached monthly testing)
  - Decide how best to dispense and organise physical obs. He may need admission if the CMHT/HTT can't offer daily BD monitoring for the next 2 weeks
- If relapsing/increasing risks:
  - Clozapine can help – discuss rapid re-titration with pharmacy
  - *Have a low threshold for HTT support or admission*
  - You may need to supplement clozapine with another antipsychotic whilst titrating: seek senior and pharmacy advice
- If Peter refuses clozapine or is too chaotic to restart:
  - Consider alternatives. Which antipsychotic helped *most* before clozapine? Could this offer some stability, while addressing his concerns about clozapine?
  - Admission may be needed ± clozapine restarted under the MHA.

Always think: *what's happened to the unused tablets?* Retrieve them, as they pose a high risk of fatal poisoning to Peter or any contacts who might 'borrow' them.

PATIENT VIEW:

Apparently, if you omitted to take [clozapine] two days straight you'd be sent back in... I was always so scared they'd take me in, I never told them. I remember taking it because they were giving me the blood test the next day, so I took it... and I collapsed.

'Sarah'

... He has residual symptoms?

If you've reached the maximum tolerated dose, discuss options with Peter and the team:

- Clozapine augmentation, e.g. add amisulpride, risperidone
- Accept a degree of treatment resistance, using whichever antipsychotic helped the most
- Strengthen psycho-social treatments.

Take-home message

Clozapine is the most effective antipsychotic, and first choice in TRS. For some, it's the route to recovery. For others, it's no better than anything else. But unless they've tried it, they'll never know.

Further reading

Flanagan, R.J., Spencer, E.P., Morgan, P.E., Barnes, T.R.E. and Dunk, L. (2005) Suspected clozapine poisoning in the UK/Eire, 1992–2003. *Forensic Science International*, **155**, 91–99.

Mortimer, A.M. (2011) Using clozapine in clinical practice. *Advances in Psychiatric Treatment*, **17**, 256–265.

Taylor, D., Paton, C. & Kapur, S. (2015) *The Maudsley Prescribing Guidelines in Psychiatry*, 12th edn, Wiley-Blackwell, Chichester.

CHAPTER 38

Self-discharge and section 5(2)

Abigail G Crutchlow

South London & Maudsley NHS Foundation Trust, London, England

---

RELATED CHAPTERS: admission to discharge (34)

Sally was admitted informally to Triage. She's now packed her bags and wants to leave.

People often change their minds about admission, not least because wards can be frightening or disturbing, especially for first-timers. You must assess:
- **The risks if Sally leaves**
- **Whether to detain her under the MHA.**

Preparation

1. On the telephone
- If you'll be delayed or Sally's actively trying to leave, ask the RMNs to consider holding her under s5(4) – this lasts 6 hours.

2. On the ward
- *Briefly greet Sally on arrival*
  - Introduce yourself, apologise for any delay, and acknowledge her frustration
  - Explain that you must read her notes – estimate how long this'll take
- *Staff and notes* – admission clerking, past week's events, last ward round, risk assessment
  - Working diagnosis/current symptoms
  - Does she have leave? Is she using it? Any problems?
  - Risks if discharged
  - Current plans for discharge/self-discharge.

Assessment

1. Approach
Don't start trying to persuade Sally to stay – you'll end up in conflict. Instead, assume she has good reasons to leave – you want to understand them, and ensure she's safe and supported.

2. Focused history, remembering ...
- *HPC:* Why she wants to go home, e.g.
  - Feeling unsafe/unsettled
  - Missing family, friends, children
  - Worried about people, home, belongings, pets
  - Dissatisfied with treatment

Psychiatry: Breaking the ICE – Introductions, Common Tasks and Emergencies for Trainees, First Edition.
Edited by Sarah Stringer, Juliet Hurn and Anna M Burnside.
© 2016 John Wiley & Sons, Ltd. Published 2016 by John Wiley & Sons, Ltd.
Companion Website: www.psychiatryice.com

- ○ Conflict – staff, patients
- ○ Cravings, e.g. cigarettes, alcohol, drugs, food
- ○ Worsening psychosis
- ○ To harm herself/confront someone
- *If she leaves …*
  - ○ Would she return?
  - ○ Where will she go? What will she do?
  - ○ Who's at home?
  - ○ Can she imagine any problems? How would she handle these?

3. MSE, remembering …

- Intoxication/withdrawal
- Active symptoms, e.g. psychosis, depression
- Thoughts of harm to self/others
- Insight:
  - ○ Why was she was admitted? Have these problems resolved?
  - ○ What help does she want?
  - ○ Would she *seek/accept* help if needed? Explore …

> **TIP:** The MCA is irrelevant, as Sally *wants* to leave. DoLS (p103) is occasionally appropriate if someone *complies* with admission, but *lacks capacity* to agree to it.

4. Risk assessment

What are the risks if discharged?
- Self-harm
- Violence
- Harm from others, self-neglect, accident
- Disengagement/non-adherence.

5. Collateral

If Sally plans to stay with someone, ask to speak to them, e.g. family/hostel staff. If she refuses, you can still listen to their concerns without sharing her information. Feeling you should breach confidentiality due to high risks suggests you should consider using s5(2).

Management

1. Problem solve

Whether Sally can leave or not, try to address her problems, e.g. facilitate family contact, or a smoking break; mediate between her and other patients, organise an alcohol detox (p254–256). She may now be happy to stay, or await assessment by her consultant/HTT.

2. Decision-making

If Sally *still* wants to leave, decide whether she should:
- Self-discharge
- Go on leave
- Be detained on s5(2)

Discuss your plan with the nurses *before* finalising it with Sally. If they disagree or you're uncertain, contact your senior. In office hours, contact Sally's registrar/consultant – they'll be annoyed if you discharge her without discussion.

> **PATIENT VIEW:**
>
> It's the collaboration – I have to take responsibility for a degree of wellness, I have to take the steps that will enable me to maintain a degree of stability.
>
> **'Imelda'**

3. Discharge

If it's safe for Sally to go home, she can self-discharge. Beforehand, check:
- Ward consultant/on-call senior agreement
- She's going somewhere safe, and can get in (if not, could she stay with a friend?)
- Carers agree.

Depending on your concerns, organise follow-up within the next 7 days (GP/CMHT/HTT). Plan any medication management, e.g. give TTOs to Sally/HTT; HTT to prescribe. Write a crisis plan (p315) with Sally and share this with carers. Document your plan and risk assessment.

> **TIP:** If there's a risk of overdose, limit TTOs and double-check: *should* you be discharging her?

4. Leave

If Sally's low risk and happy to return, a period of leave may help. Be guided by the nurses, who might suggest initial escorted leave. Meanwhile, contact Sally's consultant for early review.

Consider offering *day patient status*, i.e. sleeping at home but spending daytime on the ward. If so:
- Check local protocols, otherwise Sally may lose her bed and be unable to return!
- Agree whether she'll attend the ward for specific times (e.g. 9am–5pm), or specific reasons (e.g. medication, ward rounds, meals, activities).
- Ensure staff can contact her
- Review medication timings so she can receive them *on* the ward.
- *Consider* giving a limited medication supply to take at home, e.g. she won't want to take sedatives at 5pm. Ask pharmacy if unsure.
- Sally should return to the ward or contact staff if problems
- Document the plan and risks.

5. Section 5(2)

You can detain Sally under s5(2) – a doctor's holding order – *if* she:
- Won't stay informally
- Appears to suffer from a mental disorder
- Poses risks to self/others should she leave hospital.

Discuss with seniors if unsure.

S5(2) lasts up to 72 hours, to enable a full MHA assessment *as soon as possible*. It:
- Only applies to inpatients (not ED – see Table 50.2, p312)
- Isn't renewable (i.e. it's bad practice to use two s5(2)s "back-to-back")
- Doesn't allow treatment. If Sally needs medication for agitation:
  ○ Try to use PO with her consent
  ○ Restraint and IM are given under the MCA or common law (Table 74.1, p443), but an urgent MHA assessment is needed.

Complete s5(2) paperwork (you are the 'nominated deputy' – on the form). Take a nurse with you to explain your decision; consider a larger team if Sally's likely to react aggressively.

Document your plan. If on-call in the early evening/weekend, ask your registrar to assess as soon as possible. At night, you can usually handover to the team in the morning, unless the MHA assessment is urgent.

TIP: Don't over-sedate! Seniors may race in to assess Sally and find her fast asleep.

TIP: Young people and borderline patients are often emotionally dysregulated and struggle to self-soothe because they were never enabled to do it in early life. They may want control to be taken away so they feel safe, e.g. by acting in a way which makes sectioning them seem the right thing to do. If they're treated in a very restrictive way whenever they're distressed, it reinforces the idea that they can't control their own emotions, making it harder to learn self-soothing. In this way, placing them on a 5(2) can be very detrimental to their already fragile sense of self. Often speaking with them, hearing their narrative and validating their distress can diffuse the situation.

Stephen Kaar, ST4

What if ... ?

... She's detained but wants to leave?
She can't, unless her consultant has granted s17 leave. Contact them to ensure they're aware of her needs and suggest Sally appeals her section if appropriate (p303).
... She absconds ('goes AWOL')?
Follow Trust policy. The nurses usually handle this, but may request your help with the italicised points:
- Gather information – presentation and risks
- Try to contact her – find out where she is and ask her to return
- *Contact carers* – if she's consented to information sharing or the risks warrant it
  ○ They may know where she is and convince her to return
- *If a specific person is at risk of harm, ask her consultant whether to breach confidentiality, and if so, who should make the call*
- *If she's on a forensic section (s35, 36, 37, 47 or 48) contact the MHA office/a forensic psychiatrist for advice*
- Contact the police, summarising her case, physical description, and anywhere she's likely to go. They can:
  ○ Conduct a 'welfare check' (if informal) – visit her address to check she's OK. *Clarify the level of risk, and what to do if she doesn't answer,* otherwise they may break her door down.
  ○ Return her to hospital (if detained)
- Complete an incident form, update the risk assessment
- Check in with the police every shift.
On Sally's return, you should:
- Explain concerns
- Explore reasons for absconding
- Problem-solve
- Assess MSE, risks, physical health (self-harm, UDS, breathalyser)
- Consider the need for s5(2) if informal
- Suspend leave and consider ↑obs if detained, e.g. 1:1, 2:1

Take-home message

Your job isn't to convince everyone to stay. Address concerns, make a safe plan, negotiate where possible, and use s5(2) when you've no other choice.

Further reading

Department of Health (2015) Mental Health Act 1983: Code of Practice. The Stationary Office, Norwich.

CHAPTER 39

Seclusion reviews

Katherine Beck

South London & Maudsley NHS Foundation Trust, London, England

RELATED CHAPTERS: aggression (74), Video 5 (see companion website)

You've been called to PICU to review Alex Walker. He's 20 and in 'seclusion' after assaulting another patient.

Seclusion (supervised confinement) means isolating a severely disturbed patient in a designated room, to *prevent harm to others*. It mustn't be used:
- **If other interventions might work**
- **For longer than needed**
- **Because you lack staff**
- **As a 'treatment', punishment or threat**
- **To manage self-harm/suicide risk.**

Seclusion can feel distressing, undignified and punitive – both for the secluded patient, and other patients on the ward. Read your Trust's seclusion policy.

Box 39.1 Seclusion

- One patient, in a lockable room.
- Continuous observation from outside, ideally by a nurse of the same gender
- Low stimulus environment
- No moveable furniture/'weapons'/ligature points
- En suite bathroom facilities
- Easy communication with staff, e.g. buzzer/intercom
- MDT review of need to continue seclusion – facilitated by the Emergency Response Team (ERT):
  - Doctor attends within first 30 minutes
  - Reviews are then two-hourly (nursing) and four-hourly (medical)
  - Registrar/consultant reviews if longer seclusion, e.g. >8 hours continuous, or >12 hours over two days

PATIENT VIEW:

One time I was in this seclusion room going a bit out of my mind, but this nurse really got through to me. She spoke loudly, clearly and slowly to me, she explained exactly what she was doing and why she was doing it before she did it.

'Thomas'

Psychiatry: Breaking the ICE – Introductions, Common Tasks and Emergencies for Trainees, First Edition.
Edited by Sarah Stringer, Juliet Hurn and Anna M Burnside.
© 2016 John Wiley & Sons, Ltd. Published 2016 by John Wiley & Sons, Ltd.
Companion Website: www.psychiatryice.com

Preparation

1. On the telephone
- When's the medical review due?
- Agree to attend 15 minutes before the ERT arrive to read the notes.

2. On the ward
- *Background history, especially*
  - MHA status (if informal, organise urgent MHA assessment)
  - Reasons for seclusion; risk history
  - Doctor's view at last review
  - PMHx/substance misuse
  - DHx: neuroleptic naïve/response to previous medications
  - Advanced statement of Alex's preferences for management if aggressive?
- *Drug chart*
  - *All* medication over the past 24–48h (within British National Formulary maximum doses?)
  - Any medications refused, omitted, spat out?
  - Medication due in this review? If so, what? (PRN/regular)
  - If there's a T2 or T3 form (p101–102) but the necessary medication isn't listed, discuss emergency treatment with a senior (under s62).

3. Listen to the ERT handover and establish ...
- Progress since seclusion began and last review
- Staff views on ending/continuing seclusion
- If unsafe to enter, how you'll speak to Alex, e.g. intercom
- Whether physical obs ± medication should be offered *before* you talk to Alex. Combining them with the interview is quicker, but may irritate or confuse him.
- Topics which upset Alex – avoid these initially
- How the decision will be made to continue or end seclusion, e.g.
  - You and the lead nurse step out to discuss *or*
  - The whole team exits, closes the door, then decides

> **TIP:** You're *always* last in – and first out of – the seclusion room. This stops you obstructing the ERT, or being accidentally 'secluded' ...

Assessment

You need to decide whether Alex is:
- Medically fit
- Ready to leave seclusion.

1. Observe Alex before entering
- Alert and able to follow instructions?
- Intoxication/withdrawal
- Injuries, physical illness, breathing problems/respiratory rate (RR)
- Defecation/urination in the room (confusion, hostility, disinhibition, fits?)
  - If urinating in a bottle, ask someone to save this (UDS ± dip).

2. Approach
- Maintain your safety (p19); stand back if any history of spitting
- Even if you've met Alex, don't assume he recognises you. Introduce yourself and explain that you'll ask a few questions ± examine him.
- Start by checking for worries or questions.

3. Physical review, remembering ...
- Physical obs (nurses)
- Pain, physical problems; injuries, e.g. from restraint or self-harm
- Eating/drinking (if not, why not?)
- Screen:
  - Over-sedation, confusion/delirium
  - NMS
  - Acute dystonia
  - Intoxication/withdrawal syndromes
- Physical examination as appropriate (minimum = check pulse for arrhythmia).

4. MSE, remembering ...
- Cooperative *or* hostile/aggressive/sexually disinhibited
- Able to hold a conversation *or* shouting, swearing/mute
- Irritable/scared/labile
- Delusions, especially related to aggression, e.g. persecution by staff/patients
- Thoughts of harm to self/others. Does he 'need' to protect himself?
- Hallucinations (especially commands)/frightening experiences
- Cognition: grossly oriented?
  - Concentration?
  - Able to follow instructions?
  - Can he remember your name and job?
- Why does he think he's in seclusion?
  - Views of triggering incident
  - Remorse/intent to repeat?
  - How would he handle similar situations?
  - Can he imagine any problems if he left seclusion?
  - Willing to take medication? (Gain consent if possible.)
  - Does he understand the behaviour needed to end seclusion?

TIP: Leave discussions about the reasons for seclusion until last – it's *most* likely to cause agitation.

5. Plan next steps
- Check for questions/concerns
- Explain that you'll discuss the plan with the nurse in charge.

Management

1. Immediate decisions
Terminate seclusion
End seclusion if Alex no longer presents an immediate risk to others, e.g. calm, cooperative and (ideally) regrets violence. You must also end seclusion if he needs transfer to ED. Consider:
- Risks – to particular patients, staff
- Risks – to Alex, e.g. retribution from other patients

- Initial nursing plan, e.g. 2:1, move to 'extra care' area, main PICU
- Changes to drug chart (regular or PRN).

You should also terminate seclusion if Alex needs urgent medical care – plan transfer carefully with the nurses, as he may pose risks to medical patients and staff.

Continue seclusion

If Alex remains aggressive *or* highly unpredictable (e.g. calm one moment but aroused the next), you'll need to continue seclusion. Decide:

- Behaviour required to end seclusion
- Any medication changes (PRN/regular)
  - When to administer the next dose (now/next review)
  - Omit/decrease medication if over-sedated.

If you disagree with the nurses, explore their concerns: they have to cope with Alex's behaviour once you've gone. If you can't agree, discuss with seniors.

2. Feedback to Alex

Explain the plan to Alex, particularly the reasons for continuing or ending seclusion.

- Praise and encourage calm or cooperative behaviour
- If seclusion must continue, give specific examples of behaviour which:
  - Prompted this decision
  - Will end seclusion.

3. Debrief

Attend the staff debrief.

- Ask whether the nurses would have liked you to do anything differently
- Check timing of next medical review + whether SHO, registrar or consultant.

4. Documentation and handover

Document:

- Reasons for continuing/ending seclusion
- Physical status and MSE
- Any medication given
- Complete the medical section of the seclusion notes.

If on-call, tell seniors when their reviews are due, unless this 'heads-up' will wake them. Try to observe a couple of senior reviews.

What if ... ?

... You're asked to decide if seclusion should be *started*?

Senior nurses usually make this decision, but may involve you if you're present during an aggressive outburst. Consider the risks, based on Alex's current behaviour and past history when similarly aroused. Review recent events and interventions, and consider alternatives to seclusion:

- Verbal de-escalation
- 'Time out' (e.g. 15 minutes to calm down in his room)
- Physical separation from particular patients
- 1:1/2:1 obs
- Oral PRN
- Rapid tranquilisation (p442–444)
- PICU.

If there are no sensible alternatives, seclusion is necessary.

PATIENT VIEW:

If you can show you care, you'll get that back from someone. People with mental health problems are very clued in. They know when you're feeling miserable. You come along with your bad day and they come and upset you more and you react … and the next thing they know, they're being put in the seclusion room.

'Shola'

… He's asleep?

Sleep is therapeutic – it might not help to wake Alex every few hours. Check for physical health concerns, e.g. head-banging, head trauma. Observe him through the door including RR. You may need to wake him if:

- He slept through the previous review
- Your local seclusion policy *insists* patients are woken each review
- Observation alone can't assure you he's OK.

Take-home message

Check local policy and work closely with nursing staff to ensure seclusion is used appropriately.

Further reading

Department of Health (2015) The Mental Health Act 1983: Code of Practice. The Stationery Office, Norwich, Chapter **26**, pp300–308.

CHAPTER 40

Alcohol misuse

Lisa Conlan, Isabel McMullen, and Cheryl Kipping
South London & Maudsley NHS Foundation Trust, London, England

RELATED CHAPTERS: illicit drugs (41), drug-seeking (58), delirium tremens (77)

Karim Patel, 54, was admitted overnight via ED, following an overdose. He vaguely reported 'social drinking' every evening. This morning, you've been called to review his increasing agitation.

Consider alcohol use in *all* newly admitted patients, even if they deny drinking alcohol. Don't assume:
- Abstinence due to age, ethnicity or religion
- *'Social Drinking'* is low-risk drinking.

Admissions are opportunities to offer advice about alcohol and prevent alcohol-related complications, e.g. fits, delirium tremens (DTs), Wernicke's encephalopathy (WE). Attend as soon as possible – Karim is distressed and may be withdrawing; staff are worried and need support.

Preparation

1. Notes
- Informal/detained
- Past and present substance misuse
- Substance misuse team involvement
- If Karim denies drinking, do clues suggest otherwise? E.g.
  - ↑ MCV, LFTs/GGT
  - PMHx/physical signs associated with alcohol use
- Other diagnoses, e.g. psychosis, depression
- Risks.

2. Nurses
- Describe Karim's presentation and *changes* since admission
- Obs – ask staff to repeat
- UDS
- Breathalyser (if available): are levels high, falling or absent?
- Scores on alcohol assessment tools, e.g.
  - AUDIT: Alcohol Use Disorders Identification Test (Appendix C2)
  - SADQ: Severity of Alcohol Dependence Questionnaire (Appendix C3)
  - CIWA-Ar: Clinical Institute Withdrawal Assessment of Alcohol Scale, Revised (Appendix C4)
- Immediate risks, e.g. absconding, physically unwell, aggression.

Psychiatry: Breaking the ICE – Introductions, Common Tasks and Emergencies for Trainees, First Edition.
Edited by Sarah Stringer, Juliet Hurn and Anna M Burnside.
© 2016 John Wiley & Sons, Ltd. Published 2016 by John Wiley & Sons, Ltd.
Companion Website: www.psychiatryice.com

Assessment

1. Approach
To get accurate answers, ask about alcohol pragmatically, explaining how you'll use information, e.g. addressing discomfort, physical health or medication choice.
- Be non-judgmental: drinking isn't evidence of weakness or immorality
- Respect Karim's choice to continue, reduce *or* stop drinking
- Avoid lectures and scare-stories
- Asking about a 'typical day' gathers information efficiently, e.g. morning drinking (withdrawal), total units, social isolation.
- Always go through the last 5 days (whether typical or not) to understand *recent* consumption
- Ask what Karim *likes* about alcohol *before* exploring problems or negatives
- If his history's vague, think *confusion*, rather than *difficult* or *drunk*
  - If not confused, he may be evasive because of your manner or past negative experiences with professionals.

TIP: The 'gold-standard' alcohol-screening tool is the AUDIT. Check every patient's score (range 0–40):
- >8 suggests increasing risk (hazardous) drinking
- >20 suggests dependence

2. Focused history, remembering ...
- *All current substance misuse: T(R)APPED* (p34–35)
  - Calculate daily and weekly alcohol units (Box 40.1)
  - NB: benzodiazepines, GBL/GHB (p464) are cross-tolerant with alcohol
  - When was his last drink?
  - Is he drunk, OK or withdrawing?
  - Addictions team input? Keyworker details and current plan.
- *PPHx:* especially relationship to alcohol
  - E.g. depression, self-harm, anxiety, alcoholic hallucinosis, memory problems
- *PMHx:* especially alcohol-related problems
  - E.g. fits, DTs, peptic ulcers, pancreatitis, cirrhosis
- *Forensic history*, e.g. fighting, drink-driving.

Box 40.1 Alcohol units

- Volume in litres x % Alcohol By Volume (ABV) = units
  - E.g. 1 pint (568ml) of 5% lager = 0.568 x 5 = 2.84 units
- 'Home measures' vary hugely. Check bottle size and how long one lasts/how many Karim buys each week
- Recommended limits (with two drink-free days/week):
  - Women 2–3u/day (binge ≥6u single session)
  - Men: 3–4u/day (binge ≥8u single session)
- Quick reference guide – Appendix C1

3. MSE, remembering ...
- Intoxication/withdrawal symptoms
- Slurred/muddled speech
- Psychosis
  - Delirium/DTs (especially visual hallucinations)
  - Alcoholic hallucinosis (auditory hallucinations when sober and alert)

- Confusion/cognitive impairment
  ○ DTs, WE, hepatic encephalopathy, infection
  ○ Head injury (falls/fights)
  ○ Alcohol-related cognitive impairment
- Current motivation to change.

4. Physical assessment, remembering...

- *Examination*
  ○ Physical sequelae of alcohol use
  ○ Alcohol withdrawal/WE (Table 40.1)

Table 40.1 Alcohol–related presentations.

Problem	Timing	Signs and symptoms
Wernicke's encephalopathy (WE)	*Anytime* Risk factors include: • Withdrawal • Glucose administration • Malnutrition/low BMI • Poor diet, skipping meals • Decompensated liver disease/ comorbid acute illness • Vomiting • Memory loss/ blackouts • >6u/day • Comorbid drug use • Homelessness	Only 20% of cases show the *classic triad*, so assume WE if any of: • *Confusion* • *Ataxia* • *Ophthalmoplegia* (usually lateral gaze paralysis, i.e. VI palsy) • Nystagmus • Hypothermia + hypotension • Memory disturbance • Unconsciousness **Medical emergency: transfer to ED!** If untreated, may die or develop Korsakoff's dementia (permanently unable to lay down new memories)
Uncomplicated withdrawal syndrome	*After last drink:* Onset 4–12h Peak 24–48h Ends by day five to seven	• Tremor • Sweating • Nausea / retching / vomiting • Headache • ↑ HR (> 90bpm) • ↑ BP (> 90mmHg diastolic) • Restlessness, agitation, anxiety, mood changes • Insomnia • Craving • Mild pyrexia
Fits	*After last drink:* 6–48h	Generalised tonic-clonic
Delirium tremens (DTs) (Ch.77)	*After last drink:* Onset 1–5 days Peak 2–4 days Ends by day 7–10	• *Prodrome: restlessness, fear, insomnia* • Withdrawal symptoms + ○ Fluctuating confusion ○ Hallucinations (visual, auditory, tactile) ○ Delusions ○ Affective changes, e.g. lability, terror, anger ○ Gross tremor ○ Dilated pupils ○ Early: ↑HR, BP, RR, temperature ○ Later: cardiovascular collapse **Medical emergency: transfer to ED!**

- *Investigations*
  - FBC, U&E, LFTs, glucose, GGT, INR, prothrombin time
  - In severe/complicated dependence: ↓Hb, platelets, WCC, Na$^+$, K$^+$, Mg^{2+}; ↑MCV; ↓/↑glucose
- UDS
- ECG.

5. Risk, especially:
- Self-harm/suicide
- Violence, absconding
- Physical health risks / WE / DTs
- Safeguarding (children / vulnerable adults).

Management

1. At admission
Deal with medical emergencies (Ch.65)
DTs (Ch.77) or WE need urgent transfer to ED. While awaiting transfer, give:
- Reassurance
- Oral fluids (advise ED *no* IV fluids containing glucose before thiamine)
- Pabrinex 1 pair of ampoules IM stat (give 2 pairs if suspected WE)
- ± Chlordiazepoxide e.g. 50 mg stat if withdrawing.

Monitor and treat withdrawal
If alcohol-dependent, consider the need for detoxification (detox). If still drunk, ask staff to start qds physical obs, and watch for withdrawal. Follow your Trust's protocol if available, otherwise, the guidance below may help.

If staff <u>aren't</u> trained to use CIWA-Ar: use a fixed dose regimen
The admission SADQ score can guide a fixed dosed regime of chlordiazepoxide (Table 40.2). Ensure a medical review within the next 12–24 hours, and at least qds physical obs. Don't be afraid to change the dose if over-sedated/under-treated. Mild dependence rarely needs chlordiazepoxide.

If staff <u>are</u> trained in CIWA-Ar: initial symptom-triggered, then fixed dose regimen (better control):
- *Day 1:* monitor CIWA-Ar and physical obs 1–2 hourly for the first 24 hours
  - Chlordiazepoxide 25–50 mg prn, every 1–2 hours (max 250 mg/24h), depending on CIWA-Ar score, e.g.
    - Mild (score 0–9)/asleep = 0 mg
    - Moderate (score 10-14) = 25 mg
    - Severe (score 15+) = 50 mg
    - NB: Give first dose *now* if withdrawing
- *Day 2–5:* at 24 hours, calculate the total chlordiazepoxide given (*baseline dose*).
  - Seek specialist advice if >250 mg
  - Reduce by roughly 20% of the *baseline* each day, until day five (e.g. Table 40.3)
    - Divide into 4 doses, with greater weight on evening and night doses
  - Stop prn chlordiazepoxide.
Don't be afraid to continue symptom-triggered dosing over day two if poorly controlled on day one, physically ill, or he's already received lots of PRN by your review on day two. Contact a senior or the Addictions team if unsure about the dosing – it can be quite confusing at first, especially if you're familiar with different protocols.

Table 40.2 Example fixed dose alcohol detox regimens (using chlordiazepoxide).

Daily alcohol consumption	15–25 units		30–49 units		50–60 units
SADQ score	Moderate: 15–25		Severe: 30–40		Very severe: 40–60
Day 1	15 mg qds	25 mg qds	30 mg qds	40 mg qds*	50 mg qds**
Day 2	10 mg qds	20 mg qds	25 mg qds	35 mg qds*	45 mg qds**
Day 3	10 mg tds	15 mg qds	20 mg qds	30 mg qds	40 mg qds*
Day 4	5 mg tds	10 mg qds	15 mg qds	25 mg qds	35 mg qds*
Day 5	5 mg bd	10 mg tds	10 mg qds	20 mg qds	30 mg qds
Day 6	5 mg nocte	5 mg tds	10 mg tds	15 mg qds	25 mg qds
Day 7	*Stop all benzos*	5 mg bd	5 mg tds	10 mg qds	20 mg qds
Day 8		5 mg nocte	5 mg bd	10 mg tds	15 mg qds
Day 9		*Stop all benzos*	5 mg nocte	5 mg tds	10 mg qds
Day 10			*Stop all benzos*	5 mg bd	10 mg tds
Day 11				5 mg nocte	5 mg tds
Day 12				*Stop all benzos*	5 mg bd
Day 13					5 mg nocte
Day 14					*Stop all benzos*

*Needs close monitoring
**Needs close monitoring + specialist advice
Source: NICE 2010. Reproduced with permission of NICE

Table 40.3 Example chlordiazepoxide symptom-triggered.

Day	Total (mg)	9am	12pm	5pm	10pm
1	200	= *Total of PRN doses every 1–2 hours*			
2	160	40	30	40	50
3	120	30	20	30	40
4	80	20	15	20	25
5	40	10	5	10	15

Notes:
- Slow the reduction if withdrawal reappears
- Detoxes may need extending beyond day five if severe dependence or comorbid benzodiazepine/GBL/GHB misuse (seek specialist advice)
- If elderly/liver disease, consider using shorter-acting benzodiazepines (e.g. oxazepam), to prevent accumulation and respiratory depression
  - Chlordiazepoxide 15 mg = oxazepam 15 mg = diazepam 5 mg
- Encourage oral fluids – dehydration predisposes to arrhythmias
- Metoclopramide for nausea; paracetamol for pain; antihistamine for itch
- No unescorted leave/baths during the detox assessment phase (seizure risk).

Thiamine

WE is caused by acute thiamine (Vitamin B_1) deficiency – explain the risks and prescribe high potency B vitamins (Table 40.4). Pabrinex triggers anaphylaxis *extremely* rarely, but ensure adrenaline 0.5 mg IM is prescribed and available.

Table 40.4 Thiamine indications.

Detox needed	Any signs of WE	Pabrinex	Vitamin B Compound strong 1 tablet PO tds + Thiamine 100 mg PO tds
No	No	–	✓
Yes	No	IM 1 pair od 5 days (Give IV if in general hospital)	✓ After Pabrinex course
Yes	Yes	Transfer to ED ≥2 pair IV tds 3–5 days Then 1 pair od 3–5 days (or until no further improvement)	✓ After Pabrinex course

Other

- Prescribe diazepam 10 mg PR PRN for withdrawal seizures
- If agitation continues, reassess and consider other causes, e.g. head injury, WE.
- Monitor for ↓RR if combining a detox with PRN medications for agitation.
- If also receiving opiate substitute prescribing, seek specialist advice.

2. During admission

Medications

- Ensure prn benzodiazepines are struck-off once stabilised on regular chlordiazepoxide
- Be alert to drug-seeking behaviour; avoid using benzodiazepines for agitation
- Continue vitamin B for at least 2 weeks; longer if malnourished or ongoing drinking.

Address drinking

Use an MI approach (p74). If you have a substance misuse in-reach nurse, they can engage with Karim during his admission. If he's keen to stay abstinent, discuss options with addictions, e.g. acamprosate or naltrexone (reduce cravings); disulfiram (causes unpleasant reaction if he drinks alcohol).

Discuss and address his reasons for drinking, e.g.

- Insomnia: sleep hygiene (p72)
- Anxiety: relaxation exercises (p72)/Cognitive Behaviour Therapy (CBT) (p68)
- Unresolved bereavements/childhood abuse: consider psychotherapy
- Social issues, e.g. unemployment, loneliness, boredom.

He may be interested in accessing help from local addictions services and/or self-help or mutual aid groups, e.g.

- Alcoholics Anonymous (AA)
  - www.alcoholics-anonymous.org.uk
- SMART Recovery
  - www.smartrecovery.org.uk

PATIENT VIEW:

I've found AA very helpful. Whilst I can see that it's not for everyone, and not the only path, it's surely worth a mention. Provide people with the information to make an informed decision. It's free, it helps people.

'Ricky'

Address comorbidity

Monitor mood and suicidality. Alcohol's depressant effects take a while to lift (NICE suggests waiting 3–4 weeks before considering an antidepressant). Abstinence is the most powerful antidepressant, but consider medication or psychological therapy, where appropriate.

Formally assess cognition. Cognitive impairment may need a neuropsychiatric referral, package of care or specialist placement, e.g. if Korsakoff's syndrome (Table 40.1).

Optimise physical health, referring to specialists as appropriate.

PATIENT VIEW:

The difficulty is being told, "We can't treat you unless you've had your alcohol treated." As if the two are utterly separate issues, without there being a sense of one impacting upon the other. There was no cohesive provision of a service that recognises I'm drinking because my mental health is so excruciatingly painful.

'Sheila'

Leave

Before Karim has unaccompanied leave, discuss whether he plans to remain abstinent or continue drinking. Abstinence is ideal, but realism is needed. Discuss with him:
- Triggers for drinking, and how he'll manage these, e.g.
  ○ How he'll spend his time – can he keep busy and avoid pubs/off licences?
  ○ Who he'll see – can/should he avoid certain peers?
- ± Ways to limit drinking, *if* he intends to drink
  ○ Try to negotiate limits, and discuss strategies, e.g. alternating between alcoholic and soft drinks.
You should also explain what he should expect when he returns, particularly if intoxicated, e.g.
- Medical review, increased observations, omitting medication
- Reasons for this, i.e. keeping him safe (not punishing him!)
Unplanned discharge in response to drinking isn't appropriate. If your team plans to discharge Karim if he drinks, this should be negotiated with him, and his risks fully explored. Only carry through such a plan if *safe*, and after discussion with carers, the ward ± community team.

TIP: Should someone return from leave clearly drunk, don't *enforce* a breathalyser. It's likely to inflame the situation, and doesn't add much. Close monitoring and clinical review are essential.

Cheryl Kipping, Dual Diagnosis Specialist Nurse

Carers

Emphasise that Karim is ultimately responsible for his drinking, though carers may provide support *or* need support themselves. Al-Anon is an organisation providing support to family and friends of people suffering with alcohol dependency:
- www.al-anonuk.org.uk
- 020 7403 0888
If Karim's visitors bring alcohol onto the ward, discuss this with them and Karim. Set boundaries and consider searching their bags before visits. Clarify that they won't be allowed onto the ward (or will be asked to leave) if staff think they're intoxicated or bringing alcohol with them.

3. At discharge
- Don't give benzodiazepines or night sedation as TTOs
- Repeat advice on lower risk drinking

- Prescribe ongoing B vitamins if he's malnourished or will keep drinking heavily
- Recognise the risks associated with relapse, e.g. suicide, self-harm, violence.
  - You can't keep Karim in hospital indefinitely to manage risk
  - Everyone involved should understand that drinking raises his risks
  - Police should be called if violent when drunk
  - Discuss DVLA guidelines (Ch.32)
- Don't *automatically* refer Karim to the substance misuse team: if he's not ready, he won't go.

Take-home message

Alcohol withdrawal is treatable and often avoidable: have a low threshold for monitoring, offering detoxification and thiamine.

Reference

NICE (2010) Alcohol use disorders: sample chlordiazepoxide dosing regimens for use in managing alcohol withdrawal. NICE, England.

Further reading

NICE (2011) CG 115 Alcohol-use disorders: diagnosis, assessment and management of harmful drinking and alcohol dependence. NICE, England.

Lingford-Hughes, A.R., Welch, S., Peters, L. and Nutt, D.J. (2012) British Association for Psychopharmacology updated guidelines: evidence-based guidelines for the pharmacological management of substance abuse, harmful use, addiction and comorbidity: recommendations from BAP. *Journal of Psychopharmacology*, **26** (7), 899–952.

Taylor, D., Paton, C. & Kapur, S. (2015) *The Maudsley Prescribing Guidelines in Psychiatry*, 12th edn, Wiley-Blackwell, Chichester.

Keyes, M. (2012) Under the Duvet. Penguin, London.

Galloway, J. (1991) The Trick is to Keep Breathing. Vintage, London.

E-learning course on screening and brief advice www.alcohollearningcentre.org.uk/eLearning/IBA/

CHAPTER 41

Illicit drugs

Isabel McMullen, Lisa Conlan, and Cheryl Kipping

South London & Maudsley NHS Foundation Trust, London, England

RELATED CHAPTERS: alcohol misuse (40), drug-seeking (58), opiate overdose (66), delirium tremens (77)

Chrissie, 35, was clerked by the duty doctor while you were in teaching. She's become increasingly upset, telling the nurses she's hearing voices and has missed her usual morning dose of methadone 60 mg. They found some cannabis on her at admission. You've been called to review.

Don't keep Chrissie waiting – if withdrawing, she'll become increasingly uncomfortable and frustrated. Attend swiftly if you suspect alcohol or GBL withdrawal, as these can be fatal. Only prescribe opiate substitutes if clear evidence of dependence: opiate withdrawal is unpleasant, but opiate *overdose* kills. Polysubstance misuse is very common: don't hesitate to seek specialist advice, especially when multiple drugs are involved.

Preparation

1. Notes
- Informal/detained
- Past and present substance use
- Currently under substance misuse services?
- Other diagnoses, e.g. psychosis, depression, personality disorder
- Risks.

2. Nurses
- Describe Chrissie's presentation and *changes* since admission
- Obs + UDS (Box 41.1)
- Immediate risks, e.g. absconding, physically unwell.

3. Substance misuse team
Addictions services usually work office hours. If nearing 5pm, get their details from Chrissie and call them *before* interviewing her – a delay may leave her withdrawing overnight. Her dispensing pharmacist can provide information on evenings and weekends. Gain *written* confirmation of:
- Current methadone/buprenorphine prescription
- Formulation, dose, frequency of administration

Psychiatry: Breaking the ICE – Introductions, Common Tasks and Emergencies for Trainees, First Edition.
Edited by Sarah Stringer, Juliet Hurn and Anna M Burnside.
© 2016 John Wiley & Sons, Ltd. Published 2016 by John Wiley & Sons, Ltd.
Companion Website: www.psychiatryice.com

- Date and time of last script ± supervised consumption
- *Clarify whether she took each of the last three days' doses – tolerance is lost quickly!*
- Stop community prescription until further notice.

Don't take this information from the GP unless *they* are the prescriber.

Assessment

1. Approach

In addition to the points covered in Ch.40 (alcohol):

- Chrissie may *over*estimate her use to encourage substitute prescribing
- All withdrawal states are horrible and require compassion
- Clarify slang and unfamiliar drugs, especially 'legal highs' (drugs not yet classified under the Misuse of Drugs Act):
  - www.DrugScience.org.uk / www.TalkToFrank.com
  - www.neptune-clinical-guidance.co.uk

PATIENT VIEW:

Sometimes you wish you had a broken leg and crutches, and that people would know that you're ill as well.

'Vicky'

---

2. Focused history, remembering...

- *ALL current substance misuse: 5 day history; TRAPPED* (p34–35)
  - *Street* (illicit) methadone (using 'on top' of methadone script?). Note that this may be watered down, so 'doses' may not be accurate.
  - Intravenous drug use (IVDU)
    - ± Sharing injecting equipment, e.g. needles, spoons, filters
  - Time and amount of last use
  - Is she high, OK or withdrawing?
- *Substance misuse plan:*
  - Team, keyworker
  - Methadone/buprenorphine script: dose, prescriber, dispensing pharmacy, supervised consumption; weaning off or continuing long-term?
  - Other management, e.g. psychology, housing
- *PPHx* and links with substance misuse, e.g. psychosis and cannabis
- *PMHx*, e.g. complications of injecting/smoking
- *Forensic history*, e.g. offending while intoxicated/to fund her habit.

TIP: Although there's no safe methadone equivalent for heroin (you must prescribe based on objective withdrawal signs), it's still useful to know how much heroin Chrissie's using. If she doesn't know heroin weights, ask how many *bags* she uses, how many *fixes* (doses) each bag provides, and the daily cost. Prices and purity vary, but at the time of writing, London £10 = 1 bag of heroin = 0.1–0.3 g. Dependent use is commonly 0.25–2.0 g/day

---

3. MSE, remembering...

- Intoxication/withdrawal
- Suicidal thoughts/plans

- Psychotic symptoms *aren't* opiate-related, so consider …
  - Other drugs
  - Functional psychosis (some evidence opiates can mask psychosis)
  - Pseudohallucinations
- Motivation to change.

4. Physical assessment
- *Examination:* complete a full physical – drug users often have poor physical health.
  - Opiate intoxication: drowsy, ptosis, small/pinpoint pupils, ↓RR
  - Opiate withdrawal:
    - Restlessness, shivering, piloerection, aching bones/muscles
    - Lacrimation, rhinorrhoea, sweating, diarrhoea, vomiting
    - Dilated pupils (>4 mm)
    - Tachycardia, yawning, sneezing
- Evidence of other drug intoxication/withdrawal (Appendix C6)
- Recent drug use, e.g. track marks
- IVDU complications:
  - Check sites (including groins) – cellulitis/abscess
  - Septicaemia/osteomyelitis /infective endocarditis
  - DVT/PE
  - Ulcers, necrosis, gangrene
- *Investigations:*
  - UDS (Box 41.1) ± breathalyzer
  - Routine bloods, gamma-GT
  - ± Hepatitis, HIV, TB testing
  - ECG – many drugs cause arrhythmias; methadone can ↑QTc.

Box 41.1 UDS detection times

> Time and extent of last use affect detection. Tests aren't 100% sensitive, won't pick up 'legal highs', and can be cheated, e.g. with polydipsia.
> - Heroin ~1–2 days
> - Amphetamine ~2 days
> - Cocaine ~2–3 days
> - Methadone ~7–9 days (may be prescribed *or* illicit)
> - Buprenorphine ~8 days
> - Cannabis ~1 week (light use); up to 45 days (heavy daily use/high body fat)
>   - Once positive, you can't monitor recent cannabis use until the UDS is negative again

5. Risks, remembering …
- Physical/psychiatric complications of drug use
- Self-harm, suicide, violence
- Safeguarding (children / vulnerable adults)

Management

1. At admission

Prescribing
Methadone is a synthetic, long-acting opiate, prescribed as a heroin substitute in dependency. Its effects resemble heroin's but lack the same "high". Methadone can decrease risks and offer stability as part of a careful treatment programme, but the key message is *methadone kills; withdrawal doesn't.*

Always follow Trust guidelines, and seek specialist substance misuse advice when unsure, the patient's pregnant, or also using alcohol, benzodiazepines or GBL/GHB.
• Prescribe naloxone in case of overdose, 0.4 – 2 mg IM/IV prn for *all* opiate users (Ch.66).
If *not* prescribing methadone, explain your reasons to Chrissie clearly.
While any evidence of opiate intoxication
• Don't prescribe *any* opiates/benzodiazepines
• Nurse 1:1 with 30 minute physical obs + GCS
• Give naloxone if RR <8 (p406)
• As intoxication wears off, monitor for withdrawal.
If she's not intoxicated with anything and you've written confirmation that she's been supervised taking her prescribed methadone dose daily for the last three days:
• You can prescribe her usual community dose
• If there's any uncertainty, be cautious, e.g. if she's missed one to two days, start at a lower dose and titrate up
• If she's missed ≥3 days' doses, titrate as below (tolerance drops quickly).
If evidence of recent opiate use (e.g. UDS) and objectively withdrawing
• Follow Trust protocols. If these are unavailable …
• Monitor with an objective scale, e.g. COWS (Appendix C5)
• Give low dose methadone *liquid* (never tablets), e.g. 5–10 mg of 1 mg/1ml solution
   ○ Onset is within 30 minutes; peaks at 2–4h. Can accumulate as long half-life.
   ○ Monitor response 4-hourly
   ○ Give further doses *only* if objective withdrawal, e.g. COWS score >20
   ○ Omit if drowsy or intoxicated
   ○ Don't exceed 30 mg/24 h without specialist advice
• Change to regular methadone (bd) and *stop* prn as soon as possible
• Check ECG (methadone can prolong QTc, especially with other psychotropics).

General measures
Beyond opiates, alcohol, GBL and benzodiazepines, there aren't any evidence-based treatments for withdrawal. It may help Chrissie to know what to expect, e.g.
• *Heroin:* withdrawal peaks 32–72 h after last use; mostly subsides by day five
• *Methadone:* withdrawal peaks four to six days after last dose; lasts 10–12 days
• *Cannabis:* withdrawal peaks on day two to three and generally subsides by day seven. Unsettled sleep and vivid dreams may continue for two to three weeks.
• For other drugs, see Appendix C6.
To minimise distress, treat withdrawal from *any* substance symptomatically (Table 41.1).

2. During admission

Address substance misuse
If Chrissie is already receiving methadone from the team, invite her keyworker/doctor to ward rounds and jointly develop care plans. If she *isn't* under the addictions team, explain that

Table 41.1 Withdrawal – symptomatic management.

Problem	Associated drug	Options
Insomnia	Many, e.g. cannabis, methadone	Sleep hygiene; nocte sedative* e.g. zopiclone 7.5 mg
Agitation	Many, e.g. crack, cannabis	Relaxation exercises; low dose benzodiazepine*
Diarrhoea	Opiates, alcohol	Loperamide
Nausea/ vomiting	Opiates, alcohol	Metoclopramide
Pain ± fever	Opiates, cannabis, alcohol	Paracetamol/ibuprofen
Stomach cramps	Opiates	Mebeverine or metoclopramide
Muscle cramps	Opiates	Topical rubefacients
Nicotine withdrawal	Tobacco	NRT

*Avoid with methadone/buprenorphine. Agree short, fixed usage (e.g. 3 days) to prevent abuse

methadone/buprenorphine prescribing can only continue post-discharge by referring to them (*not* her GP). Liaise early with addictions to guide prescribing and create a joint plan.
* Use an MI approach (p74)
* Psychoeducate
* Input by inreach worker from addictions team/ward staff with specialist training
* Self-help/mutual aid groups, e.g.
    ○ Narcotics anonymous: www.ukna.org / Cocaine Anonymous: www.cauk.org.uk
    ○ SMART Recovery: www.smartrecovery.org.uk

Consider drug use potential while on leave
Make a pragmatic MDT plan, involving Chrissie and recognising *her* issues, e.g. whether her drug use:
* Affects any underlying mental illness
* Places her or others at risk
* Will continue after discharge.
Before leave, explain to Chrissie that her tolerance may have dropped, so using opiates on leave could kill, especially if combined with (prescribed) methadone, alcohol, benzodiazepines, or other 'downers' (CNS depressants).
    UDS testing can be useful on return from leave, but should be negotiated beforehand as part of her care plan, so it's not a surprise.
* Affirm negative tests (positively reinforce her abstinence)
* Positive tests should have clear consequences, e.g. trigger a care plan
* Support staff if she returns intoxicated. Consider risks, and review plans with her when sober.
If Chrissie brings drugs onto the ward, other patients may be at risk. Support nurses to address this, e.g. searches after leave; supervised visits/excluding certain visitors; involve police ± drug dogs.

Medications
Don't refuse analgesia simply because Chrissie misuses opiates. For severe pain, monitor objectively and discuss with the addictions service or local pain team.
Drug interactions:
* Methadone prolongs the QTc, so avoid other QTc prolonging drugs, e.g. citalopram
* Methadone levels are altered by drugs which inhibit or induce CYP3A4 (causing increased sedation or withdrawal, respectively). These include some SSRIs – so check before prescribing, and explain the need for consistent use.
* The Maudsley Prescribing Guidelines details prescribed and illicit drug interactions.

Address comorbidity
* Assess ± treat mental illness, e.g. depression, anxiety disorder, psychosis
* Optimise physical health, including STI testing
* Address social problems, especially where they trigger drug use/mental illness
* Offer carers support and information, e.g.
    ○ Families Anonymous: www.famanon.org.uk
    ○ Adfam: www.adfam.org.uk
    ○ Some substance misuse services also run family/carer groups.

3. At discharge

Addictions team appointment
* Arrange an Addictions team appointment for the afternoon of discharge/ next morning
* Give Chrissie her last morning dose on the day of discharge and fax confirmation of this (time, date, dose) to the substance misuse team. She should usually attend the team immediately.

- *NEVER give methadone or buprenorphine as TTOs.*
Reinforce harm minimization messages at the discharge CPA
- Opiates
  - ○ Methadone must be stored securely and out of reach of children
  - ○ Tolerance will be decreased – overdose from street opiates is more likely
  - ○ If she *does* use heroin, smoking is safer than injecting
- IV drug use
  - ○ Give details of local needle exchanges
  - ○ Advise on safer injecting, e.g. www.nta.nhs.uk/uploads/hrdvd5.pdf
- Cannabis/amphetamines/cocaine
  - ○ Highlight the link between these and psychosis
- Ensure carers know how to handle overdose, e.g. call 999, place in recovery position/start BLS. (Some addictions services provide naloxone and teach carers how to use it, in case of OD).

Take-home message

Always confirm the methadone prescription before prescribing. If in doubt, start low, go slow.

What if … ?

… She wants to leave?
Assess as you would anyone asking to self-discharge (Ch.38). Don't let drug use distract you from other concerns, e.g. suicidal thoughts. If her wish to leave is prompted by withdrawal, symptomatic treatment may change her mind.

… She's on buprenorphine?
This is a partial agonist, but there's a risk of precipitated withdrawal. Seek specialist advice.

… She's on an injectable methadone/heroin prescription?
Consult specialists!

Further reading

Winstock, A.R., Ford, C. and Witton, J. (2010) Assessment and management of cannabis use disorders in primary care. *British Medical Journal*, **340**, c1571.

Budney, A.J., Hughes, J.R., Moore, B.A. and Vandrey, R. (2004) Review of the validity and significance of cannabis withdrawal syndrome. *American Journal of Psychiatry*, **161**, 1967–1977.

Department of Health England and the devolved Administrations (2007) Misuse and Dependence: UK Guidelines on Clinical Management. London: Department of Health (England), the Scottish Government, Welsh Assembly Government and Northern Ireland Executive www.nta.nhs.uk/uploads/clinical_guidelines_2007.pdf.

National Institute for Health and Clinical Excellence (NICE) guidelines:
  - ○ CG120 Psychosis with Coexisting Substance Misuse (2011)
  - ○ CG51 Drug Misuse: psychosocial interventions (2007)
  - ○ CG52 Drug Misuse: opiate detoxification (2007)
  - ○ Methadone and Buprenorphine for the Management of Opioid Dependence (2007) Technology Appraisal 114.

National Institute for Drug Abuse. US website with useful research and detailed explanations around drugs of abuse. http://www.drugabuse.gov.

CHAPTER 42

Pregnant patients

Anna M Burnside

East London NHS Foundation Trust, London, England

> **RELATED CHAPTERS:** Bipolar affective disorder (BPAD) (25), pregnancy (29), puerperal psychosis (78)

Your colleague admitted Josie Soler, 25, to your ward overnight. She's currently manic, but 24 weeks pregnant, so he left her medication-free.

Pregnant patients cause anxiety, as staff see them infrequently and may worry they'll inadvertently harm the baby. Worries aside, this is an important window for psychiatric and antenatal care, which can improve Josie's postnatal outcomes. Work closely with her obstetric team and your nearest perinatal psychiatric service, especially around prescribing and the need for Mother and Baby Unit (MBU) placement.

Preparation

1. Notes ± CC
- Is the CMHT aware that Josie's pregnant?
  - Does her Care Plan address her wishes during pregnancy?
  - Has she been referred to perinatal psychiatry?
- PMHx: problems affecting pregnancy or drug choice
- DHx:
  - Current medications
  - Medication exposure since conception
- Risk events when unwell; pre-existing child protection concerns.

2. Staff
- Behaviour, particularly attempts to leave or abnormal thoughts about the pregnancy
- Evidence of substance misuse/withdrawal.

Assessment

1. Approach
Listen carefully, identify her worries and reassure where possible. Common concerns are:
- Harm to the baby while in hospital
  - Harm from violent patients or staff use of restraint
  - Medications
  - No antenatal care
- Social services removing the baby.

Psychiatry: Breaking the ICE – Introductions, Common Tasks and Emergencies for Trainees, First Edition.
Edited by Sarah Stringer, Juliet Hurn and Anna M Burnside.
Companion Website: www.psychiatryice.com

Reassure her that staff will keep her safe on the ward. Explain you're medically trained, and will work closely with specialists to organise safe treatment and antenatal care; you'll always seek expert advice when out of your depth. Social services *will* be involved, but always aim to keep families together.

Josie may feel judged as a 'bad mother', especially when asked about substance misuse, thoughts of harm or delusional beliefs about the baby. Explain that you ask all pregnant women about these things, as they're actually very common, and you can help when you know about them.

PATIENT VIEW:

Don't just put everything down to a person's being crazy and they don't know what they're talking about because there's sense in amongst that so-called crazy way of talking.

'Viv'

---

2. Focused history, remembering ...
- Pregnancy: wanted/unwanted/accidental?
  - Antenatal care so far
- *PMHx:* including obstetric history
- *PPHx*: post-partum problems; psychotropics previously used in pregnancy
- *Substance misuse*: drugs, alcohol, smoking
- *SHx*: partner, family. Are other children safe? Is there a history of domestic violence?

3. MSE, remembering ...
- Mood
- Thoughts of harm to self/foetus
- Psychotic symptoms (especially focused on the foetus)
- Insight, especially medication preferences/refusal.

4. Physical assessment, remembering ...
- Full examination, including BMI and BP
  - Don't examine her pregnant uterus if unconfident
- Blood tests (guided by obstetrics)
- Urine dipstick (infection/diabetes; protein may suggest pre-eclampsia)
- UDS
- ECG.

5. Risk assessment, remembering ...
- Self: self-harm, suicide, neglect, dehydration, harm from other patients
- Foetus: exposure to teratogens; harm from Josie's behaviour
- Neonate: neglect, infanticide.

Management

1. Immediate management
Manage as usual, with special attention to antenatal care and medication.

Liaison with Antenatal and Social Services
Mania makes Josie's pregnancy high risk. Liaise closely with antenatal services, using her existing team if available.
- Discuss how to share information and care plans, e.g. e-mail, fax
- Midwife: involve local midwifery leads for mental health and safeguarding

- ◦ Antenatal checks/scans – due/outstanding?
- ◦ Can they attend the ward if needed?
- ◦ Contact details for advice (the nurses will appreciate this)
- Obstetrician: advice on physical health care plan
  - ◦ Outstanding tests (avoid repetition between services)
  - ◦ Frequency of physical monitoring/blood tests
  - ◦ Parameters to trigger concern
  - ◦ Contact details if concerns (including out-of-hours).

Involve Children and Families Social Services early, highlighting safeguarding issues, support needs, and worries about any other children.

Perinatal Psychiatry
Discuss Josie's case with the perinatal service: they assess and manage women with mental health problems during pregnancy and in the year post-partum. They may offer in-reach, telephone advice, or assessment for a Mother and Baby Unit (MBU).

Medication
Even if you've done a literature review, don't make medication decisions alone – ask your consultant, pharmacist and perinatal psychiatrist. Unless impossible, discuss choices *with* Josie ± her partner ± pharmacist.
- Medication risks are usually outweighed by the risk of mania to Josie ±baby
- An antipsychotic is probably safest in acute mania (Table 29.1, p186).

Agitation
Plan ahead in case of agitation or aggression.
- Avoid restraint or medication (high risk)
- Emphasise verbal de-escalation ± physical isolation
- When restraint is unavoidable
  - ◦ Use the least restrictive option for the shortest time
  - ◦ Restrain Josie on a large beanbag or cushions, lying her on her left side (not flat) to avoid inferior vena caval compression
- When medication is unavoidable use low dose oral medication
  - ◦ If IM required: low-dose lorazepam/promethazine are probably safest, unless about to deliver. Some Trusts use antipsychotics – discuss with perinatal, obstetrics and pharmacy *first*.

Other issues
- Facilitate contact with her children if safe and they won't be unduly distressed
  - ◦ Lack of contact often makes mums refuse voluntary admission
- Encourage smoking cessation ± NRT
- Dietary advice: avoid soft cheese, pâté, liver, vitamin tablets containing vitamin A
- Discuss drug/alcohol problems with the addictions team and pharmacy.

2. Issues during admission
- Involve Josie's family
- Psychological input (e.g. CBT, sleep hygiene) may minimise medication use
- Drug levels change as pregnancy progresses: levels can guide dose adjustment
- Facilitate antenatal care
- Transfer to an MBU, if possible.

3. At discharge
There are three possible outcomes, depending on the risks, local provision, MSE and timing of labour:
- Discharge home, e.g. with HTT ± perinatal/CMHT input
- Transfer to delivery suite

- Transfer to MBU, either for final weeks of pregnancy or post-delivery.

Whichever happens, arrange a meeting with all involved to plan delivery and discharge. Include the midwife, pharmacist, perinatal psychiatry representative, Children and Families social worker ± Child Safeguarding Lead. Address:

- Contact details of all involved professionals:
  - ◦ CMHT (including consultant and CC)
  - ◦ GP
  - ◦ Midwife ± safeguarding midwife
  - ◦ Consultant obstetrician
  - ◦ Health visitor
  - ◦ ± Translator
- Identified problems/needs, including whether Josie's likely to deteriorate during or after the birth
- Medication
  - ◦ Before/during delivery
  - ◦ Post-partum (breast-feeding?) – see http://toxnet.nlm.nih.gov/newtoxnet/lactmed.htm
- Labour plan
  - ◦ Josie might visit the labour ward beforehand if helpful
  - ◦ Bag and TTOs packed, ready to go to the delivery suite
  - ◦ If labour starts while on leave, to call 999 and your ward
- Post-delivery
  - ◦ Psychiatric review (liaison/perinatal psychiatry)
  - ◦ Whether Josie will return to your ward/MBU
  - ◦ Psychiatric team to liaise with labour ward staff regarding her ability to care for the baby
  - ◦ Contraception discussion
- Contingency planning: who would Josie like to look after the baby, if she can't, for any reason?

What if … ?

… She refuses antenatal care?

If she lacks capacity and antenatal care can be justified for her own health and welfare, it can be given in her best interests, under the MCA. If the care can only be argued for the sake of the foetus (or she has capacity but refuses input), discuss with Trust lawyers, the Child Safeguarding lead *and* Children's Social Services. A case conference may be needed. Keep assessing her wishes, since these may change as mania resolves.

Take-home message

Pregnant women present complex problems and need specialist input and advice. Relapse in the post-partum period is common and women can become extremely ill with alarming speed, placing them and their child at high risk of harm.

Further reading

NICE (2014) Antenatal and postnatal mental health: clinical management and service guidance.

Taylor, D., Paton, C. & Kapur, S. (2015) *The Maudsley Prescribing Guidelines in Psychiatry*, 12th edn, Wiley-Blackwell, Chichester.

Viguera, A.C. and Cohen, L.S. (1998) The course and management of bipolar disorder during pregnancy. *Psychopharmacology Bulletin*, **34** (3), 339–346.

CHAPTER 43

Inpatients with forensic histories

Penelope Brown

South London & Maudsley NHS Foundation Trust, London, England

RELATED CHAPTERS: forensic (28), aggression (74), violent threats (80)

Mike's 66, and has a history of schizophrenia and alcohol misuse. He was last in hospital 12 years ago, after release from prison for murder, and remains on life licence. He's been admitted with a psychotic relapse.

Although past behaviour predicts future behaviour, don't let a forensic history *define* your patients. That doesn't mean you should be complacent or minimise Mike's risk – even if he's elderly, frail or the offence was many years ago. Instead, try to see him as a whole person, including the offence *and* his life since. Management is essentially as usual, but with specific attention to risk, liaison and legalities.

PATIENT VIEW:

When people look at your file, all they see is your past, and they judge you. They rejected me based on what I did in the past. They didn't give me a chance.

'Edmund'

Preparation

1. Notes and CC
- Reasons for relapse and admission; CMHT's concerns
- Transferred from community, another hospital, police station, court, prison?
- Legal status:
  - Informal/detained. Is his section civil (Table 15.1, p98–99) or 'forensic' (Appendix E3)?
  - Community restrictions, e.g. CTO, restriction order (s41), probation?
  - *Life licence* means he received a life sentence but was released early and is liable for recall if he breaches the conditions of his licence. He'll have a parole officer who can clarify the conditions.
- Risk:
  - Risk history, current risk assessment, forensic reports, HCR-20
  - Symptoms linked to offending
  - Index offence
    - Context: MSE at time, triggers, premeditated/impulsive
    - Victim characteristics

Psychiatry: Breaking the ICE – Introductions, Common Tasks and Emergencies for Trainees, First Edition.
Edited by Sarah Stringer, Juliet Hurn and Anna M Burnside.
© 2016 John Wiley & Sons, Ltd. Published 2016 by John Wiley & Sons, Ltd.
Companion Website: www.psychiatryice.com

○ Details of offending since index offence
○ Inpatient risks, e.g. assaults, previous PICU admissions.

2. Nurses

Explore staff concerns, which may be absolutely appropriate, or a reaction to the index offence. Taking time to understand their concerns can contain anxiety and ensure appropriate – not heavy-handed – management.

Assessment

1. Approach

Before seeing Mike with a trusted nurse, review the safety tips (Ch.6).

Whilst it's not uncommon for psychiatric patients to come into contact with the law, very few have committed serious offences. Although you may feel angry, scared, or even disgusted by serious offending, don't act on these emotions, e.g. by avoiding Mike or behaving punitively. Notice your feelings, and use them to understand how people react to him in everyday life.

Listen to your gut feeling. If something feels 'wrong', take a break and work out what's going on.

TIP: I can't emphasise this enough: communication styles affect risk. If certain words, gestures or mannerisms set off individual patients, recognise and avoid these. Many 'incidents' are essentially because patients feel chronically let down or disrespected – or staff appear disinterested. Be respectful, interested and honest, and never promise anything you or your team can't deliver.

Cameron Russell, Forensic CMHT AMHP

PATIENT VIEW:

All their life, especially black people's lives, they've been oppressed ... and it's regurgitated on the ward. They're talking to you like a dog and you've got no control over your own life ... and when you try and express yourself, they're always looking at you from this psychiatric point of view and like you don't know what you're talking about. You're not feeling well anyway, but people are treating you like that and it's only a matter of time for some people to kick off. And as a result the control and restraint comes in and that's just a horrendous experience for those people who've suffered it.

'Herman'

2. Full history, remembering ...

• *HPC:* problems/story of relapse
  ○ Triggers, e.g. stress, non-adherence, substance misuse
  ○ Coping (especially with feelings of threat), e.g. withdrawal, carrying weapons, confronting people
• *Substance misuse*: increases risky behaviour
• *Premorbid personality*: especially antisocial/impulsive traits
• *Forensic history:*
  ○ Index offence: what happened and why? Remorse? Consequences?
  ○ Charges or convictions since
  ○ Current charges/police contact/need to attend police station or court?

3. MSE, remembering ...
- Agitation, aggression; intoxication/withdrawal
- Irritability, suspiciousness, fear
- Persecutory delusions, passivity
- Feeling threatened or disrespected
- Thoughts of violence ± sexual fantasies
- Thoughts of self-harm
- Hallucinations (especially commands)
- Insight into his CMHT's concerns. Views on illness, admission, treatment.

4. Physical examination, remembering ...
- Signs of substance misuse/withdrawal
- UDS

5. Risk assessment
If current circumstances (e.g. MSE, drinking, behaviours associated with violence) resemble those during past assaults, he may be at high immediate risk of violence. Consider:
- Vulnerability of particular patients/staff
  - E.g. gender, ethnicity, historic problems with Mike
- Known triggers and warning signs of aggression
- Can he access/fashion 'weapons' (i.e. from his own possessions, objects on the ward)?
- Special skills, e.g. martial arts training
- Risk of *retributive* violence from others, especially if confrontational/provocative

Management

All the usual principles apply.

1. Immediate management
Initial safety
- Observation level: intermittent/1:1/2:1. Contact PICU early if transfer's likely.
- Protect vulnerable patients, e.g. close observation, separating them and Mike
  - You *can't* tell them Mike's history
- Remove potential weapons, e.g. pool cues or balls
- No leave before consultant review
- Update the risk assessment, highlighting any knowledge gaps.

PATIENT VIEW:

Being on two-to-one, it's terrible. They watch you do everything. You can't go to the toilet without being watched.

'Craig'

Liaison
Your team may need to contact:
- Probation officer ± Victim Liaison Officer (VLO)
- Police – if Mike's due to be interviewed, under investigation, or on bail

- Court – if facing charges/ongoing court case
- MAPPA (Box 8.1, p42)

VLOs are assigned by probation to victims of the most serious crimes. They update victims on patient progress and leave conditions, and can represent victims' views at Tribunals.

Legalities

Forensic sections (s35, 36, 37, 38, 45, 47, 48) are equivalent to civil sections, but used when people have been charged or convicted of an offence (Appendix E3). *Restriction orders* (s41 or 49) are *added* when someone poses grave risks to the public. From your point of view:

- Contact your MHA Office for detailed advice
- If Mike's been *recalled* under a restriction order, explain the reasons to him
- Only the Secretary of State (via the Ministry of Justice) can grant leave or discharge for restricted patients. This can prolong admission, causing frustration – part of your role is recognising and managing this frustration.
- Your seniors may need to write legal reports, and will appreciate your *thorough* admission clerking/part 1 discharge summary.

2. Issues during admission

- Ensure his CC is contacted early to plan longer-term management, e.g. need for supported or 'forensic' accommodation
- Address substance misuse issues, as these increase his risks
- If Mike must attend court, ensure dates and details are in the ward diary. Ask staff to help him contact his solicitor, if needed.
- As noted, leave and discharge may need to be agreed by the MoJ. Tribunals rarely grant discharge without successful trials of leave.
- Update risk assessment and management plans. You can help update an HCR-20 if supervised by someone trained in using this tool.
- Consider contacting the forensic team for
  - Advice on:
    - Legal terms, processes or protocols
    - Writing legal reports
    - Risk management
    - Accessing specialist services, e.g. psychological treatments for personality disorders
  - Specialist assessment, e.g. of psychopathy, dangerousness
  - Specialist management, e.g. transfer to medium secure unit/forensic team caseload

3. Discharge issues

The team/CC should alert MAPPA to Mike's imminent discharge. As a rule of thumb, the CC, registrar or consultant should refer anyone with a history of serious sexual or violent offences – or at least discuss this with the local MAPPA coordinator.

Work closely with the receiving CMHT, to make Mike's discharge as smooth as possible. Ensure he has TTOs, a 7-day follow-up with a specific person, and a written crisis plan. The CC should update the VLO, if involved.

TIP: Some 'forensic patients' spend long periods in prison or hospital, becoming institutionalised. This can make discharge particularly difficult for them, as they're used to the structure and routine of hospital. Discuss anxieties about leaving hospital with them before discharge, checking they feel adequately supported in case of future problems.

Penelope Henderson, Forensic Consultant

What if ... ?

... Mike's been recently arrested for assault?
Your team should liaise with the police and court:
* Tell police where he is, both for interview, and to explain that he can't attend the police station
* If the police ask if he's fit for interview (Box 70.2, p424), defer to your consultant
* Facilitate court attendance
* Confirm any bail restrictions.

Your seniors need to know any legal restrictions, especially if he's ready for leave or discharge before any court hearing, e.g. bail restrictions preventing him going home.

... Mike's restricted (s41 or s49) and needs emergency transfer to a general hospital?
Discuss first with ED, in case he *can* be managed on site. If he needs emergency transfer, organise this as quickly as possible (Ch.65). There's likely to be a local policy, and you should inform the RC/on-call consultant and follow any existing plans concerning the need for escorts. Document your assessment clearly, including reasons why the emergency can't be managed on the psychiatric unit. Your cover letter to ED must explain his MHA status and clearly highlight any risks. For further guidance:
* www.justice.gov.uk/downloads/offenders/mentally-disordered-offenders/mhcs-guidance-s17-leave.pdf

Take-home message

Risk assessment and information sharing with other agencies is key in managing forensic patients, but don't forget the basics.

CHAPTER 44

People with learning disabilities (LD)

Rory Sheehan

North London Training Scheme for Psychiatry of Intellectual Disability, London, England

RELATED CHAPTERS: LD and behavioural change (59), adult safeguarding (63)

Oliver is 28 and has obsessive-compulsive disorder (OCD), autistic spectrum disorder (ASD) and a mild LD, with a full-scale IQ of 56. He was admitted over the weekend with severe self-neglect, secondary to excessive checking rituals. He's refused all physical interventions and withdrawn to his room, seeming frightened and tearful in communal areas.

Adjustments should be made – where possible – to help people with LD access mainstream care, rather than expecting them to attend 'special' services. Unfortunately, general adult wards can be frightening and overwhelming places, magnifying communication or functional difficulties, and making people seem less capable than usual. Problems include:

- Loss of familiar faces, environment, routines
- Noise and constantly changing staff and patients
- Other patients – unpredictable, scary or bullying
- Limited staff LD experience.

Oliver's mild LD is easier to overlook than more severe forms: he's likely to be mobile, have no obvious chromosomal/genetic syndromes, and may appear to understand, when he's actually struggling. His ASD may disable him more than you'd expect from his IQ score alone (Table 44.1).

TIP: When presenting to colleagues, describe Oliver as having (not being) a learning disability (i.e. "He's LD" is offensive).

Preparation

1. Notes
- Admission clerking and physical assessment
- Usual community care package/home environment
- Current medications.

2. Nurses:
- Ask them to describe his behaviour (rather than interpret it, at this stage)
- Functional level
- Concerns and problems.

Psychiatry: Breaking the ICE – Introductions, Common Tasks and Emergencies for Trainees, First Edition.
Edited by Sarah Stringer, Juliet Hurn and Anna M Burnside.
© 2016 John Wiley & Sons, Ltd. Published 2016 by John Wiley & Sons, Ltd.
Companion Website: www.psychiatryice.com

Table 44.1 Degrees of LD.

LD	IQ range	Communication level	Approximate level of function
Mild	50–69	Conversational language, though development may be delayed	• Struggle academically, but can usually read, write, count • Self-caring • Usually live and work independently ($\pm$ support) • Not always diagnosed (especially older adults, who won't have been formally assessed at school)
Moderate	35–49	Varies from simple to no speech; may learn basic sign language, e.g. Makaton	• Limited academic progress, but some people read, write, count • Likely to need support with Activities of Daily Living (ADLs) • Can often do simple practical work with supervision • Usually fully mobile • May need supported accommodation / to stay with family
Severe	20–34	Simple or no speech. Might learn *objects of reference* to communicate, e.g. picking up a cup when thirsty	• Can do simple tasks with assistance • Reduced/absent self-care and mobility • Likely to live in the family home or 24-hour-supported placement
Profound	<20	Very limited verbal communication	• Can't self-care: require full-time support • High rates of medical problems, e.g. epilepsy, immobility, visual/hearing impairment, incontinence • Identifiable cause more likely

3. Carer $\pm$ CC

• Oliver's baseline, compared with current presentation
• How much does Oliver understand?
• Communication tips
• Any idiosyncracies, e.g. sensory preoccupations, specific interests.

Ask Oliver whether he'd like to see you alone or with a carer; document consent to have someone stay with him.

Find a quiet room with few distractions to help him focus on the interview. Set aside at least double the time you'd usually allocate and ask staff to only interrupt you with emergencies.

Assessment

1. Approach

Speak *to* Oliver – even if his carer's present. If the carer takes over, ask them to let Oliver speak, or politely request some time alone with Oliver. If you don't understand Oliver, ask him to repeat himself, then ask permission to clarify things with his carer.

- Ask Oliver to say if he doesn't understand
- Use ordinary, simple words
- Short sentences. One idea per sentence. Pause between sentences.
- Be alert to signs you're patronising him
- Try to gauge his understanding throughout the interview
- Stay concrete, avoiding metaphors, euphemisms or abstract language, e.g.
  - *Do you want to die?* (not *Do you feel you don't want to be here anymore?*)
  - *Does your leg hurt?* (not *How does your leg feel?*)
  - *Do you ever wet yourself?* (not *Do you have accidents?*)
- Enhance communication with objects, drawings $\pm$ facial expressions and gestures (but recognise that his ASD may make him struggle to interpret body language)
- Oliver may agree with everything, either because he wants to please you, or is embarrassed to say he doesn't understand. Avoid leading questions (e.g. *You're not suicidal, are you?*), and double-check answers by asking the opposite question, e.g.
  - *Are you happy?* (A: *Yes*)
  - *Are you sad?* (A: *Yes*)
- Check understanding, e.g. *Can you tell me what we've been talking about?*
- *Repetition* doesn't prove understanding.

ASD-specific:
- Direct eye contact, physical contact or close proximity may be distressing
- Sit slightly to one side of Oliver, giving him plenty of personal space
- Limit/avoid direct eye contact
- If he has a favourite object, make sure he has this and look *at* it or just past him.

2. Focused history, remembering...

Oliver's already been clerked, so don't drag him through a detailed history. Be prepared to fill any gaps through collateral histories and old notes, especially if he's stressed when unsure.
- *Start with his experiences on the ward* (the change of environment may be difficult)
  - How's he getting on with other patients?
  - Can you change anything to make him happier here?
- *Clarify problem list/psychopathology and effect on life*
  - OCD points (Ch.56)
  - ASD points (Table 44.2)
  - LD: ADLs, activities, hobbies, work; things he enjoys/needs help with
- *Screen:* comorbid depression/other anxiety symptoms
- *DHx:*
  - Does Oliver take medicine every day? Any problems with taking it?
  - Side effects (give common examples)
  - Does it help?

3. MSE, remembering...

- Non-verbal communication
- Restricted/repetitive behaviours
- Overt compulsions
- Obsessions/covert compulsions. These are distressing and driven by anxiety, but can be hard to distinguish from ASD-related restricted preoccupations/need for order.
- Reciprocal conversation (to-and-fro conversation, or just monologues/answers?)
- Mutism
- Unusual syntax, neologisms, loss of prosody
- Responding to abnormal experiences?
  - If he's interested in sensory phenomena (e.g. lights, particular textures, smells) and internal experience (thoughts or feelings) he may *look* like he's responding to hallucinations.

Table 44.2 Autistic Spectrum Disorders.

Diagnosis: problems present before age 3, in at least 2 domains

Reciprocal social interaction	Language and communication	Repetitive and restricted behaviours
• Difficulty interpreting other people's feelings • Poor eye contact • Unusual postures/ body language • Failure to develop peer relationships • Prefers solitary play • Lack of imaginative world • May not seek comfort	• Speech delayed $\pm$ limited/ absent • Repetitive language and idiosyncrasies, e.g. pronoun reversal, echolalia • Tendency not to use non-verbal gestures e.g. pointing • Can take meanings literally and not recognise jokes or sarcasm	• Strong adherence to routine • Dislike of change • Intense and narrow interests • Focus on small parts of an object • Compulsive behaviour, e.g. ordering objects • Stereotyped and repetitive motor mannerisms • Self-injury, e.g. head-banging, skin-picking

4. Physical health assessment

Offer a full health check. You may need to do this in chunks, or wait until he trusts you, or carers can help. Unlike people with moderate-profound LD, there are no specific guidelines for people with mild LD, so health needs may be more easily missed.

- Systems review
- Pain can cause markedly disturbed behaviour, e.g. dental abscesses, ear infection, tummy ache, constipation (Table 59.1, p366)
- Investigate for physical problems early, as these commonly present late
- Consider screening tests to identify acute infection, e.g. CRP
- Demonstrate examination/investigation techniques on carers first
- Mild sedation for blood tests if very anxious.

5. Risk assessment, remembering ...

- Risk from others: especially bullying, exploitation
- Self-harm: stereotyped behaviour/if distressed
- OCD-related, e.g. self-neglect, poor oral intake
- Safeguarding? (Ch.63) If in residential care, how did he become so neglected? Were all steps taken to prevent this?

6. Capacity

Assess capacity for treatment decisions (p102–103). Oliver's LD/ASD *don't* mean he automatically lacks capacity, though he may need simplified information and more time to make decisions. If lacking capacity, the MHA/MCA may be needed (for use of DoLS on the ward, see p291).

Management

Offering extra care and attention to patients with disabilities isn't only kind, but a legal obligation under the Equality Act 2010. All the usual NICE guidelines apply to treatment.

1. At admission

Practical

- Offer the quietest bedroom on the ward (move other patients if needed)
- *Show* Oliver around the ward – he may struggle with verbal directions

- Reverse changes/losses if possible, e.g. carer contact, fetch favourite sensory object
- Facilitate contact with friends, as Oliver may find it hard, outside his usual environment
- Give Oliver choices whenever possible, then extra time to make decisions.

Medical
- Don't assume his presentation is due to his LD – you'll overlook treatable mental or physical health problems (this error is called 'diagnostic overshadowing')
- Treat OCD as for someone without LD, e.g. SSRIs +/or CBT
- Medications: start low, go slow (as you would for older adults). Oliver may be sensitive to side effects, *and* struggle to describe them (both due to his LD *and* ASD).

Liaison/MDT
- Request the Health Action Plan/Hospital Passport within 24 hours (if available)
  - Contains health care needs information, including communication needs
  - Available from GP, social worker or carer
- LD social worker (if allocated): current care package, care or housing issues. Plan discharge from the point of admission to avoid lengthy stays.
- Community support packages (e.g. keyworker) remain unchanged during short admissions – include them in ward management. Even if unable to attend usual activities (e.g. college), Oliver will appreciate familiar faces.
- LD community team
  - If under their care: they'll provide useful information and send a representative or CC to ward rounds
  - If not under their care, discuss whether he's appropriate for their team.

Admin
- Complete HONOS-*LD* – an adapted version of HONOS (p115)
- The more severe the LD, the harder it is to diagnose problems, as people struggle to describe experiences. Discuss using adapted screening questionnaires with the LD service, e.g. Glasgow Depression Scale.

2. During admission
As you get to know Oliver, optimise his care and help him get involved in ward life.

Practical
- Implement routine (ASD) $\pm$ pictures (LD) to help this ('visual timetable')
- Don't do everything *for* Oliver. Assess what he can do himself and when he needs help. This may change as he settles in, so stay flexible, and praise his achievements, e.g. joining patient meetings.
- Monitor for teasing, bullying, or exploitation by other patients, e.g. persuading Oliver to 'lend' (give away) money. Encourage him to report problems.
- Involve IMCA/IMHA/ward advocate
- Use accessible leaflets to help explain things (see Resources, p280)
- Carers' needs – address stress and support needs, e.g. local carers' groups.

MDT
- Best interests meeting if capacity issues
- OT: address functional problems on the ward or at home. Some community LD teams provide in-reach OT
- Social worker: ongoing liaison about Oliver's care package, accommodation, benefits
- Psychotherapy may need modifying, but don't assume it's *too hard* for Oliver. Most psychologists have some LD experience, but speak to the LD team's psychologist if needed.

Medical
Address non-acute health needs and link Oliver in with services as needed, e.g.
- Optician, dentist, hearing tests, chiropodist, neurology review of epilepsy … ?
- Talk about relationships (don't assume he isn't sexually active). He may need sex education, contraceptive advice or GUM testing.
- Check GP guidelines on physical healthcare (see resources). An annual health check is required if moderate-profound LD, and particular syndromes need specific tests (e.g. yearly thyroid testing in Down syndrome)
- Teach self-examination (testicular; breast for women)
- Women: cervical/mammogram screening

Inpatient Referral
There are relatively few specialist units serving people with moderate-severe LD and complex comorbidity or challenging behaviour. If Oliver's needs really *are* too complex for a general adult ward, discuss referral with the tertiary service.

3. At discharge
In addition to the usual advice …
- Medication: simple prescribing (e.g. once-daily), dossette boxes, carer dispensing and simple written/photo instructions. Trial the system on the ward before discharge
- Written/pictorial advice on seeking help
- Follow-up via generic/LD CMHT
- 117 aftercare (same as for patients without LD, p99)
- Add alerts to the notes, e.g. around communication difficulties and solutions
- Assign someone to complete a 72-hour telephone follow-up
- HONOS *LD*.

What if … ?

… You suspect ASD, but it hasn't been diagnosed?
The local community LD team is best-placed to diagnose, with:
- A thorough developmental history
- Standardised psychometric tools
  - Autism Diagnostic Interview-Revised (ADI-R)
  - Autism Diagnostic Observation Schedule (ADOS).

There's no cure for ASD, but management involves a multi-disciplinary team approach with psychiatrists, SALT, OTs, and psychologists. Co-morbid psychiatric illness is common and treatable, e.g. ADHD, anxiety and depressive disorders.

… He has a severe LD?
See Ch.59. Discuss with the community team and carers: if your ward can't meet Oliver's needs, it may be better for him to receive extra community support in his usual environment, or transfer to a specialist ward.

Take-home message
Communication is *key* for people with LD.

Further reading

Hoghton, M. and the RCGP Learning Disabilities Group (2010) A Step by Step Guide for GP Practices: Annual Health Checks for People with a Learning Disability. RCGP, London.
www.rcgp.org.uk/bookshop/eresources/free-eresources/a-step-by-step-guide-for-gp-practices-annual-health-checks-for-people-with-a-learning-disability.aspx

Accessible (easy-read) materials

www.Booksbeyondwords.co.uk
www.easyhealth.org.uk

Charities

www.mencap.org.uk – Mencap
www.learningdisabilities.org.uk – Foundation for people with learning disabilities
www.autism.org.uk – National Autistic Society
www.downs-syndrome.org.uk – Down's syndrome association
www.fragilex.org.uk – Fragile X society.

CHAPTER 45

Emotionally unstable personality disorder (EUPD)

Jane Bunclark and Juliet Hurn

South London & Maudsley NHS Foundation Trust, London, England

RELATED CHAPTERS: Community EUPD (26) self-harm (51), self-harm on ward (71)

Karen has EUPD – borderline type – and was admitted informally yesterday after an overdose. Despite laughing and joking with peers, she insists she's suicidal and has threatened to leave because 'nobody cares'. Her named nurse suggests you discharge Karen, as she's 'time-wasting'.

The conflicts of EUPD can intensify during admissions, and the potential for staff splitting increases. Notice your own reactions, communicate clearly and *plan* the admission; avoid knee-jerk reactions and open-ended or unstructured inpatient stays.

TIP: Spending long shifts with demanding patients can cause strong, unconscious dynamics to build within staff and patients. This is never more important than with patients with borderline personality. Think: *why is this member of staff asking me to treat this patient this way? What's the relationship between the patient and the staff? What's the emotion the patient is projecting and why?*

Stephen Kaar, ST4

Preparation

1. Gather information – notes, CC/CMHT, ward staff
- Admission circumstances and CMHT views
- Presentation on ward, interaction with staff and patients
- Community plan, including inpatient plans/contracts
- Previous admissions – reasons, duration, helpfulness
- Risks
- Staff views; knowledge from past admissions.

2. Remind yourself of psychological mechanisms in EUPD
(Ch.26, Table 26.1)
- Notice staff counter-transference (p78–79) including *splitting*.

Psychiatry: Breaking the ICE – Introductions, Common Tasks and Emergencies for Trainees, First Edition.
Edited by Sarah Stringer, Juliet Hurn and Anna M Burnside.
© 2016 John Wiley & Sons, Ltd. Published 2016 by John Wiley & Sons, Ltd.
Companion Website: www.psychiatryice.com

3. See Karen with an experienced nurse

Assessment

1. Approach
Remember that Karen may be very sensitive to shame/rejection.
- Allow plenty of time, but say how long you have; rushing will feel dismissive
- Set the tone for treatment throughout this admission: compassionate but boundaried
- Monitor your reactions and avoid showing irritation/disapproval.
- *Consider* gently explaining how her problems/reactions might relate to EUPD (p170).

> **TIP:** Be mindful of the transference. Instead of then feeling bogged down by hostility, despair, or impotence, use it to inform your understanding of how it feels to live in their skin. When all else fails, stay completely calm when with them, and then let off a little steam with your colleagues. None of us are saints, and there's always a limit to how much you can patiently absorb. This doesn't make you a bad person. Be understanding to yourself as well as your patients.
>
> Lizzie Hunt, ST4

2. Focused history, remembering...
- *HPC:* overdose circumstances, triggers and function
  - Karen's understanding of the admission, e.g. *"I wasn't safe on my own"*
  - Her experience on the ward so far, e.g. environment, relationships, treatment
  - Her expectations of the admission, staff, you ... ?
  - What does she want to happen now?
- *Comorbidity*, e.g. depression, PTSD
- *Substance misuse*
- *SHx*: support network; helpful *or* strained relationships
- *DHx*: medications and how she thinks they help.

3. MSE, remembering...
- Rapport, transference/psychological mechanisms
- Depressed, cheerful, irritable; labile
- Suicidal/self-harm thoughts
- Pseudohallucinations/hallucinations
- View of admission and treatment plans.

4. Risk assessment, remembering...
- *Self-harm/suicide* (see Ch.51)
  - Usual pattern
  - Current episode – different/more serious?
- *Other risks to self:* vulnerability, e.g. sexual exploitation
  - Abuse/domestic violence
- *Risks to others*: children, e.g. neglect, abuse.

5. Physical health, including
- Self-harm-related, e.g. scars, cigarette burns
  - Overlooked overdose?
- Sexual health (contraception/GUM).

Management

1. At admission

Long admissions are usually unhelpful, or even damaging, e.g. preventing Karen from relying on her existing coping strategies/supports; problems with escalating self-harm and staff splitting. If a 'crisis' admission *is* needed, aim to keep it short. The key issue is encouraging Karen and staff to consider the *purpose* of admission, e.g.
- Support during a chaotic time
- Re-establishing some stability, e.g. through a consistent ward environment
- Helping Karen reflect, remember her resources and re-establish self-responsibility.

> **TIP:** Some patients only want to talk about suicide/harming themselves. Change the game by saying, "I understand you feel like hurting yourself at the moment, but I'm here to see how we can help you with your problems. So let's leave aside your thoughts of suicide for a moment and talk about the problems in your life ... "
>
> **Daniel Harwood, Old Age Consultant**

Planning the admission

Don't make unrealistic promises, e.g. about curing problems or staying 'until better'. Always check your consultant's and CMHT's views, especially regarding timescales. Involve a few key staff (e.g. CC, ward manager), and reinforce the community plan wherever possible:
- Encourage Karen to suggest 1–2 admission goals, e.g.
  - *Have a safe place while I'm feeling terrible*
  - *Learn better ways to cope with suicidal thoughts*
  - *Start to tackle alcohol problems*
- Discuss how to achieve them (use SMART goals, p72) e.g.
  - Daily sessions with named nurse
  - Attend daily ward groups
  - Gather information on debt management/alcohol services
  - Discuss medication
- Include a reasonable timescale, e.g. two to ten days
  - Consider explaining that long admissions can worsen problems, by preventing her from problem solving, relying on her family/friends/CMHT ± making her feel trapped.
- Discuss discharge planning – how will Karen know she's ready?
- Explain boundaries to increase safety and stability – *not* to punish her, e.g.
  - Frequency of doctor meetings/1:1 time with nurses
  - Ward rules, e.g. no alcohol
  - Consequences, e.g. aggression will require police involvement, consideration of discharge
- Crisis/contingency planning, including staff responses, e.g.
  - *If I want to cut myself, I will ...*
    - *Ask to speak to my named nurse (who can help me use other coping strategies)*
    - *Listen to my music*
  - *If I want to leave hospital, I will ...*
    - *Re-read my treatment goals*
    - *Ask for some escorted leave to give me 'time out'*
- Type the plan and give Karen and staff a copy, but remember this *isn't* a legal contract! Uphold it where possible, but stay flexible and be prepared to rethink/renegotiate issues.

Medication
- Confirm current medications with prescriber(s)
- Don't alter medications (even if you disapprove of them) without discussing with the CMHT and Karen
- Think carefully before starting new medication. Avoid sedatives/benzodiazepines.
- Remind Karen that medication isn't a cure for EUPD, but may help modestly
- Review medication safety, given the overdose.

You and the team
Discuss Karen's presentation with the team (± ward psychologist), e.g. in ward rounds or staff support group. Recognising transference/counter-transference will help you understand Karen's behaviour, and stop you exacerbating it.
- Remember:
  - The core features of EUPD (e.g. her inconsistent behaviour) are *part and parcel* of the disorder (p166–167: Table 26.1 & Box 26.1)
  - Karen's admission serves a *purpose* – it's not an imposition or annoyance
  - Psychodynamically speaking, the ward may temporarily offer a soothing containment that she didn't experience with parents
- Suggest regular staff support sessions and treatment plan reviews
- Involve your consultant if things become fraught.

2. During admission

> **TIP:** *Any* interaction is about trying to be therapeutic, whether a brief pass in the corridor or a full interview. The aim with personality disordered patients is to bring them back to a relationship of mutual respect and the idea we can cooperate to find a solution.
>
> **Duncan McLean, Consultant Psychiatrist and Psychotherapist**

Don't be over-ambitious: you can't 'cure' EUPD during an admission. Focus on containment, Karen's goals and practical help.
- Be consistent without being rigid (a difficult balance):
  - Keep referring to the admission plan
  - Review discharge plans
  - Advocate against changing named nurses/wards
  - Try to uphold your own agreement around frequency of reviews.

Psychological work
A crisis admission won't allow in-depth work, but you might arrange/encourage:
- Psychoeducation about EUPD, coping strategies, problem-solving
- Motivational work, e.g. alcohol use
- Ward groups, e.g. art therapy, discussion groups
- Recovery work: reviewing strengths, goals, support networks
  - Remind Karen that EUPD symptoms usually improve over time
- Links with the ward psychologist ± planning community therapy.

Ongoing communication
- Explain to Karen that requests made in anger/frustration/distress will usually be 'parked' and reviewed as soon as she's calmer.
- Encourage reflection, e.g.

○ *What triggered that?*
○ *What might the consequences be if you do that?*
- Avoid making major decisions or transitions (e.g. discharge) when she's highly distressed – this is often counter-productive (e.g. immediate re-admission after walking in traffic).

Leave
- Encourage Karen to take responsibility for leave
- Avoid making leave a reward or punishment for certain behaviours (e.g. self-harm) – this removes her sense of self-responsibility
- Escorted leave may be offered if risks increase
- Offer a 'check in' meeting after leave to see how it went
- Involve carers as needed, especially when moving to overnight leave. This can help shift Karen's attachment away from the ward.

Other
- Don't let the EUPD label blind you to new pathology, e.g. depression, hypomania
- Maintain links with the CMHT/CC. Invite them to ward rounds; involve them in care planning.
- Document clearly.

3. At discharge
Plan the discharge date and try to stick to this; avoid discharging just before a weekend, as Karen may feel abandoned/unsupported.

Discharge CPA
- Review the original plan and the extent to which goals have been met
- Praise and encourage Karen for the work she's done
- Clarify community follow-up, including
  ○ *Continuing* work towards unmet goals
  ○ Community review *earlier* than seven days may offer Karen containment
- Reinforce crisis plans.

Medication
- Provide short TTOs (four to seven days) to minimise overdose risks
  ○ Stop PRN medications. If unavoidable, agree a clear CMHT review date.
- Ensure clear plans for repeat prescriptions.

PATIENT VIEW:

I felt very vulnerable and one psychiatrist asked, "Do you always feel like this at discharge?" Quite rightly so, I did. When I got out, everything just felt loud. I felt like someone had a megaphone next to my ear. And it was hard. So then I'd self-harm or take a major overdose to get back into hospital cause that's where I felt safe.

'Denise'

What if ... ?

... Karen threatens to harm herself on the ward?
Remain kind, calm and matter-of-fact. Offer 1:1 time (with yourself/named nurse) to talk things over.
- Remind her of the crisis plan/alternatives to self-harm

- Review safety, e.g. access to sharps
- If she chooses to self-harm, staff will try to help her regain control/minimise damage
- Discuss with seniors, but try to avoid:
  - Increased observations and restraint, except when significant risk
  - Restricting leave – this *can* be experienced as punitive or withdrawing Karen's responsibility.

... Karen self-harms on the ward?

See Ch.71.

... Karen wants to self-discharge?

See Ch.38, remembering:
- If Karen's combative/highly distressed, suggest talking once calmer
- Rather than making assumptions (e.g. that she wants a reaction from you), explore her motivation
- If reasons are interpersonal/emotional, let her air these, e.g. *The nurses don't care about me, so I might as well go*
- Explore risk rationally, rather than responding to your own anxiety
- Review the treatment plan and discuss whether she thinks her goals have been met
- Discuss alternatives, e.g. escorted/unescorted leave
- If she's fairly safe to leave, liaise with her CMHT and reiterate the crisis plan
- If concerned about her safety:
  - Discuss with seniors
  - Remember that detaining people with EUPD is often unhelpful, but if needed, use s5(2) whilst seeking advice.

... Karen won't leave the ward/threatens to self-harm if discharged?

Stay calm. Don't feel you have to be heroic by 'forcing her off the ward' – this is likely to backfire, e.g. escalating self-harm/rapid readmission out-of-hours.
- If Karen's very emotional, offer to talk once calmer
- Let her say what's upsetting her, e.g. feeling rejected/afraid
- Empathise, e.g. *It's scary, leaving the safety of the ward, and having to face problems at home*
- Emphasise that discharge *isn't* a rejection, but a positive step forward
- Remind her of the support arranged after discharge, and of her own resources.

If this doesn't help, or you feel Karen may be at high risk, discuss with your consultant. They may feel that Karen can take responsibility for the risk – or suggest a change of plan. Don't view the latter as a 'defeat'.

Take-home message

Working with people with EUPD is hard, and there are no easy answers or treatment templates. Plan for structure, but be flexible, and if you think you're getting into a 'battle of wills', step back and seek senior support.

Further reading

NICE (2009) CG78 Borderline personality disorder: Treatment and management.
Oldham J (2005) Guideline Watch: Practice Guideline for the Treatment of Patients With Borderline Personality Disorder. American Psychiatric Association.
http://psychiatryonline.org/pb/assets/raw/sitewide/practice_guidelines/guidelines/bpd-watch.pdf

CHAPTER 46

Older adults

Vivienne Mak[1] and Sean Lubbe[2]

[1] *South London & Maudsley NHS Foundation Trust, London, England*
[2] *UNSW Black Dog Institute, New South Wales, Australia*

RELATED CHAPTERS: CMHT older adults (30), delirium (55), treatment refusal (76)

Mr Delaney is 73 and was brought to hospital overnight by police under s136, after 'walking to work' along the motorway in pyjamas. He's now under s2, and you've been called to clerk him in.

With older adults, always consider the *Three Ds*: depression, dementia and delirium, but remember any diagnosis is possible (excepting puerperal psychosis). Older adults:
• More often show psychiatric symptoms of physical illness, and vice versa
• Have lowered alcohol tolerance (easier intoxication and side effects)
• Are never too old to misuse drugs
• May show more prominent or less flexible personality traits with age/changing circumstances
• May have sexual problems – often ignored by embarrassed younger staff (*ask!*).
Management is generally as for younger patients, but uses medication more cautiously, and recognises the greater role of physical health and disability.

Preparation

1. Notes and staff
• Admission circumstances, e.g. section papers, police s136 report
• Previous contact with psychiatric services
• Presentation on the ward, including evidence of memory/physical problems.

2. GP
• May know Mr Delaney well ± have relatives' contact details
• Confirm medications, PMHx
• Baseline MSE/cognitive testing/level of function
• Recent concerns/changes: physical, cognitive, psychiatric.

3. Social services
• Current care package, social situation
• Known housing/financial/safeguarding concerns.

Psychiatry: Breaking the ICE – Introductions, Common Tasks and Emergencies for Trainees, First Edition.
Edited by Sarah Stringer, Juliet Hurn and Anna M Burnside.
© 2016 John Wiley & Sons, Ltd. Published 2016 by John Wiley & Sons, Ltd.
Companion Website: www.psychiatryice.com

Assessment

1. Approach
Treat Mr Delaney the way you'd like doctors to treat your elderly relatives – with respect, interest and compassion. Try to understand his life: how the last 73 years make him the person he is now. This will help you make sense of his current behaviour and beliefs (even if he's very unwell), and personalise your plan to his needs.

2. Full history, remembering …
- *HPC*: does he remember what happened?
  - If not – cognitive impairment, delirium, substance misuse?
  - Triggers – life events, physical illness, recent medication changes
- *PPHx*: if an existing diagnosis, is this his usual relapse signature?
  - If not, think organic
- *PMHx* and DHx: organic causes, including polypharmacy
- *Substance misuse:* alcohol, illicit and prescribed drugs (e.g. benzodiazepines)
- *SHx*: functional assessment – ADLs, housing, finances
  - Ask: *What's a typical day like?*

3. MSE, remembering …
- Neglect
- Signs of depression (pseudodementia?)
- Cognition: use a standardised tool (Appendix D).

CARER VIEW:

They asked her, "Do you know the names of your children? Do you know how old they are? There's three things here, do you know what they are?" My mum was quite upset – she was insulted. But that's the standard procedure to assess whether she was becoming senile or whatever, but for my mum it was an invasion of privacy and also a disrespect.

'Carla'

---

4. Physical health assessment
A *full* physical examination is essential, remembering:
- Sensory deficits
- Pain, injuries
- Mobility
- Continence
- Nutritional status.

Ensure he has his glasses, hearing aids, dentures, mobility aids.

TIP: Relatives may facilitate physical examination, especially if he's agitated or frightened. However, maintain dignity – don't *expose* him in front of his children

5. Risk, remembering …
- Falls and physical health problems
- Neglect
- Suicide (old age increases risk).

Management

1. At admission
As part of the admission process, consider any:
• Advance Directive
• Lasting Power of Attorney (LPA): can be for property and financial affairs *and/or* health and welfare
• Deputyship: applies to finance and property.
Ask for copies of forms, rather than just taking the word of relatives.

Involve relatives/carers
Collateral histories are almost always informative and help *involve* carers. Find out:
• Timeline of problems
• Recent life events
• Concerns – memory, physical/mental health, functional changes
• Substance misuse.

Observation
Mr Delaney may be particularly vulnerable on a general adult ward. Have a lower threshold for 1:1 nursing if worried about:
• Disorientation/wandering
• Agitation (restraint and rapid tranquilisation are risky in elderly or frail patients)
• Harm from disturbed, strong, younger patients
• Self-harm.

Physical health
Proactive management is essential, not least because poor physical health can cause or worsen psychiatric illness.
• Exclude delirium and optimise physical health (Ch.55)
• Ensure investigations are reviewed promptly
• Liaise with geriatricians if complex physical problems.
Although Mr Delaney is detained, the MIIA doesn't cover physical treatments; the MCA may be needed if he refuses interventions and lacks capacity (p102–103).

Prescribing
Broadly speaking and wherever possible:
• Think holistically – minimise medications
• Start low, go slow ('homeopathic' doses may work; increase gradually)
• Choose medications with once-daily dosing where possible
• Reduce polypharmacy
  ◦ De-prescribe
  ◦ Don't treat side effects with more drugs; choose *better tolerated* medications
• Avoid drugs with …
  ◦ Alpha 1 blockade – hypotension, falls
  ◦ Sedation – falls, respiratory depression
  ◦ Long half-lives – harder to clear/stop if side effects; toxicity can build
  ◦ Anticholinergic side effects – confusion, constipation, urinary retention
  ◦ Potent liver enzyme inhibition – causes build up of other drugs
• Check renal, liver and cardiac function
• Avoid covert medication (hiding medications in food/drink). If essential, this must follow Trust guidelines and involve a best interests meeting (MDT plus carers).
Ask the pharmacist for advice, and check the latest Beers Criteria (see resources, p292) for the risks associated with different medications. Remember that *antipsychotics* carry greater risks of side effects in the elderly (especially if cognitively impaired):

- Heart attack, stroke
- Falls
- Cognitive impairment
- EPSEs/neuroleptic sensitivity reactions (especially in Dementia with Lewy Bodies or Parkinson's Disease).

Should rapid tranquilisation be required, see p447–8 and Table 74.3.

2. During admission
Hope and holism
Your default position is that Mr Delaney *will* go home. Are changes needed to enable this?
- Social services, e.g. care package, re-enablement services, respite
- Involve OT ± physiotherapy ±SALT ...
- Home adaptations
  ○ Falls prevention: rails, in-shower seats, removal of slippery rugs
  ○ Assistive technology and telecare, e.g. link alarms, medication reminders, wandering alarms
  ○ Other, e.g. switch gas cooker to electric/microwave to minimise explosions ...
- Geriatricians: refer for complex physical problems
- Psychological therapies may reduce disability or medication needs (don't assume he's 'too old' for them)
- Support with social issues, e.g.
  ○ Housing, finances, antisocial neighbours
  ○ Involve advocates early, e.g. IMHA.

Think about life
Especially if lonely or under-stimulated, link him in with old or new interests. Ask the community Mental Health of Older Adults (MHOA) team about local options, and check:
- Age UK: www.ageuk.org.uk/travel-lifestyle/hobbies/
- Local social services resources, e.g. day centres
- University of the Third Age: www.u3a.org.uk

Carers
Clarify their involvement and any stress. Do they need help?
- Practical, e.g. formal care package, respite
- Emotional, e.g. carer support groups
- Financial, e.g. attendance allowance (for patient); carer's allowance.

Older Adult referral?
Older Adult wards and MHOA teams have variable referral criteria – check whether he's eligible for specialist services. Criteria include:
- *New* patients meeting local age thresholds, e.g. over 65/75y
- *Known* patients who pass the age limit *and* develop older adult needs, e.g.
  ○ Frailty, e.g. falls, incontinence, blindness
  ○ Dependence, vulnerability, support needs, carer stress
- Cognitive impairment in general adult patients
- Older adult wards may accommodate particularly vulnerable older patients from general adult wards, though longer-term care remains with general adult services.

Memory Clinics manage uncomplicated cognitive impairment; they have a primarily diagnostic role. Referral criteria vary, but these clinics and MHOAs often pass referrals between each other to ensure patients get the most appropriate service.

Broach difficult issues

If Mr Delaney *can't* go home, or is likely to become more disabled, dependent or cognitively impaired, address this with him and carers, sooner rather than later, e.g. need for package of care.

If he needs a placement, social services will lead, but you'll complete medical parts of the Health-care Needs Assessment (HNA; 'banding') forms. Be accurate: they're part of a legal process to determine the correct care category and funding level, and will also influence how soon Mr Delaney will be discharged from your ward. You can also advocate for placements, balancing safety and support with his wishes about maximal independence, cultural or spiritual needs. The MHOA team can advise you on local service providers:

- Domiciliary services
- Day and outpatient care
- Sheltered housing < extra-care housing schemes < residential home ± dementia care < nursing home ± dementia care.

Highlight available legal options for planning future healthcare, welfare and finances (e.g. LPA, Advance Directive). If appropriate, broach end of life issues, such as palliative care, death, wills, funeral arrangements – but recognise when it's not appropriate to discuss these in front of him (e.g. lacks capacity, poor insight, stated wish not to be involved).

Risk management

As usual, but especially:

- Safeguarding (Ch.63) – report *any* suspected neglect or elder abuse
- Address risks at home, identified by Mr Delaney, carers, OT/staff on escorted leave.

3. At discharge

The usual principles apply, and discharge meetings may be very large if lots of agencies are involved, so send invitations well in advance. HTT may help, and some Trusts have an older adult specialist HTT.

Don't start or stop tablets just before discharge – any problems will be harder to monitor once home. If there's cognitive impairment or suicidality, decrease the risk of overdose with dosette box/carer dispensing. Ensure any hoarded/obsolete medications are removed from his home, e.g. during OT access visit.

What if ... ?

... He's informal or admitted under the MCA?

Ensure that his admission doesn't constitute a deprivation of liberty as this is subject to special provisions. The three key questions are:

- Does he lack capacity to consent to this admission?
  - *If yes ...*
- Is he subject to continuous supervision and control?
  - *If yes ...*
- Is he free to leave, should he wish to do so?
  - *If no ...* He may be being deprived of his liberty. Consider DoLS (p103) if the MHA isn't appropriate.

Take-home message

Use admissions to prevent admissions and always remember the medical aspects of care.

References

The American Geriatrics Society Beers Criteria Update Expert Panel (2012) American Geriatrics Society Updated Beers Criteria for Potentially Inappropriate Medication Use in Older Adults. American Geriatrics Society, New York.
  ○ http://www.americangeriatrics.org/files/documents/beers/2012BeersCriteria_JAGS.pdf

Further reading

Pinner, G., Hillam, J., Branton, T. and Ramakrishnan, A. (2011) Inpatient care for older people within adult mental health services. Faculty Report FR/OA/1. RCPsych, London.
  ○ www.rcpsych.ac.uk/pdf/FR_OA_1_forweb.pdf
  ○ Alzheimer's Society: support for patients and carers: www.alzheimers.org.uk

CHAPTER 47

Electroconvulsive therapy (ECT)

Sean Lubbe[1] and Vivienne Mak[2]

[1] UNSW Black Dog Institute, New South Wales, Australia
[2] South London & Maudsley NHS Foundation Trust, London, England

RELATED CHAPTERS: depression (21), mania (54), catatonia (68)

Mrs Smith, 63, was admitted 5 weeks ago with severe depression. She's failed to improve with medication, is barely eating or drinking, and her renal function is deteriorating. Your consultant asks you to prepare Mrs Smith for ECT.

ECT is a fast and effective treatment, typically used in severe depression, catatonia or mania. It's sometimes used in moderate depression where there's been a good prior response, and some argue for a role in treating clozapine-resistant schizophrenia. Early ECT *was* horrific and traumatic, and although it's very different now, many people still think it involves pain, screaming, smoke and sparks. Like many of the drugs used in psychiatry, we don't know exactly how it works. Your consultant is ultimately responsible for the decision to give ECT.

Preparation

1. Contact the local ECT lead (nurse coordinator/consultant)
- Where is the Trust ECT policy?
- Is there an ECT 'pack' to complete?
- When is ECT? (Usually 2 mornings a week)
- When should you refer? (E.g. >72 hours before the next session)
- How recent should blood tests (etc) be?
- How do you contact the anaesthetist?

2. Notes
- Is there an Advance Directive specifically refusing ECT?
- Is there a Lasting Power of Attorney or Court of Protection appointed Deputy with health-related powers? If so, involve them in discussions.
- Previous response to treatment, including medications and ECT
- PMHx, substance misuse, drug chart.

TIP: It's easier to explain ECT once you've seen it. Ask to observe an ECT list, and watch any Trust training films.

Psychiatry: Breaking the ICE – Introductions, Common Tasks and Emergencies for Trainees, First Edition.
Edited by Sarah Stringer, Juliet Hurn and Anna M Burnside.
© 2016 John Wiley & Sons, Ltd. Published 2016 by John Wiley & Sons, Ltd.
Companion Website: www.psychiatryice.com

Assessment

1. Indications
ECT is typically used for severe (life-threatening) or resistant:
- *Depression*
- *Catatonia*
- *Mania.*

ECT is occasionally used for moderate depression, or (not NICE-recommended) for 'maintenance' therapy. The decision to use ECT must weigh potential risks and benefits. Risks are higher for under-18s, pregnant women and older adults.

2. Consent
Ideally, a senior doctor should seek consent – try to observe. If possible, and with Mrs Smith's agreement, a relative or carer can attend, and provide written confirmation that you sought consent.
- Informed consent should cover the ECT *and* the anaesthetic though these don't need to be recorded separately
- Consent only covers one course of ECT. It *may* state a specific number of treatments – as agreed with Mrs Smith.
- Mrs Smith can consent to ECT if able to communicate her decision after understanding, retaining and weighing:
  - What ECT is, and what happens (including anaesthetic)
  - Purpose and likely benefits
  - Side effects/risks (general and specific to her)
  - Alternatives to ECT, e.g. medication, CBT
  - Consequences if no ECT.

Remind her that she can withdraw consent at any time. Give an ECT factsheet if possible (See Box 47.1). Document the consent discussion accurately in her notes.

Box 47.1 Key information for patients.

ECT:
- Can work faster than medications ± be life-saving
- Usually twice weekly, for 6–12 sessions
- An anaesthetist puts you to sleep under a general anaesthetic and gives muscle-relaxing medication. They closely monitor your heart, lungs and brainwaves
- A doctor passes a small electrical current across your brain for 2–3 seconds, causing a small fit
- Is not:
  - Like in *One Flew Over The Cuckoo's Nest*
  - Painful
  - Violent (no 'thrashing about' with the fit; toe-twitching or tensing are common).

Short-term side effects (settle within a few hours)
- Headache, muscle aches, nausea, tiredness
- Temporary memory problems, confusion, or distress on waking.

Longer-term memory problems:
- Can affect memories from *before* ECT: autobiographical (personal) memories and general memories
- Memories improve greatly after completing ECT, but some people have residual problems
- ECT technique can reduce the risk, e.g. unilateral electrode, lower dose
- The underlying illness may cause memory problems, so memory may *improve* with successful ECT.

Death:
- ~1 in 80,000 episodes (anaesthetic risk; similar to minor surgery risk)

3. Legal framework

See Table 47.1 for over 18s in England and Wales. Different legislation applies in Scotland and Northern Ireland but the principles are similar.

For under-18s, a formal second opinion (SOAD) is required, regardless of legal status.

4. Physical health assessment

Although you're responsible for the physical health work-up, the anaesthetist will also assess Mrs Smith and make a final decision about whether ECT is safe. Call them (or the ECT coordinator) regarding questions or concerns beforehand, e.g. whether to omit/delay regular medications on the morning of ECT.

History

- PMHx: particularly angina, MI, hypertension, CVA, asthma, diabetes, epilepsy, hepatitis. Note *any* current physical symptoms.
- Surgical history: previous anaesthetic (problems?)
- Substance misuse: smoking, alcohol, drugs
- DHx: full list
  - Remember that some medications raise or lower the seizure threshold, e.g. benzodiazepines, antipsychotics
- Allergies
- Pregnancy? (In women of child-bearing age.)

Examination

- Physical observations
- BMI ($\geq$32 = gross obesity)
- Cardiovascular, respiratory and neurological status
- Arthritis of neck/jaws
- Dentures/dental problems
- Cognition, as per Trust policy e.g. M-ACE/MMSE.

Investigations

- FBC, U&Es
- ECG

Table 47.1 ECT legal frameworks.

Legal Status	Capable of consenting?	Resisting or objecting?	Recommended action
Informal	Yes	No	Treat under normal rules of written consent
	Yes	Yes	Cannot use ECT
	No	No	Possible to treat under the MCA. Independent opinion advised
	No	Yes	Not appropriate to use MCA Consider using MHA for ECT
Detained under MHA	Yes	No	Treat with written consent and certificate of consent to treatment signed by RC
	Yes	Yes	Cannot treat with ECT except under criteria of s62 (emergency – see *What if … ?*)
	No	No	Treat if approved by SOAD
	No	Yes	Treat if approved by SOAD

- ± Glucose – if she has diabetes
- ± Sickle test (African/Caribbean/Eastern Mediterranean descent)
- ± CXR – if heart/lung disease
- ± Urine – pregnancy, UDS, dipstick as appropriate
- ± Other as needed, e.g. INR if on warfarin.

Other
- No absolute contraindications to ECT, but:
  - Risky if brain tumour or raised intracranial pressure
  - Defer if possible for three months after heart attack/stroke
  - Treat heart block, cardiac failure, hypertension or acute respiratory infection before starting ECT (unless emergency).

> **TIP:** Please never write, 'fit for anaesthetic' – it's ultimately the anaesthetist's call. I'm often asked to assess *notes* for fitness for anaesthesia and can't take the history from the patient myself. Suxamethonium is commonly used for ECT, but can trigger malignant hyperpyrexia. It's greatly reassuring if the SHO's asked, "Have any blood relatives had a problem with anaesthetic?" – and documented the answer in the notes.
>
> Alexander Scott, ST5 Anaesthetics

Management

1. Before ECT
- Check ECT has been prescribed (a set 'course' can't be prescribed beforehand, so one to two sessions are prescribed at a time)
- Book an interpreter if needed
- Nil by mouth for 6 h before ECT (including chewing gum/sweets); clear fluids allowed until 2 h beforehand
- Essential medications (e.g. antihypertensives) should be given with a sip of water
- The ECT pack, drug chart, obs chart and an RMN should accompany Mrs Smith to the ECT suite.

2. During
- Short-acting general anaesthetic and muscle relaxant; oxygen
- Seizure threshold is established during the first session. In subsequent sessions, a moderately suprathreshold stimulus is given (typically twice the seizure threshold for unilateral ECT).
- ECT can be administered by unilateral (non-dominant side) or bilateral electrode application
  - Unilateral reduces cognitive side effects but may be less effective.
- EEG is monitored throughout
- Durations of EEG seizure and convulsion are recorded
- She'll wake in the recovery room, and may feel briefly dizzy, confused, sick or achey. Painkillers are available if needed.
- She'll return to your ward and can eat and drink as usual.

3. After
- Assess for change in MSE *and* side effects after each dose
- Tell your consultant and stop ECT if …
  - Problems outweigh benefits
  - The psychiatric problem resolves

- ○ She withdraws consent (having previously consented to it)
- ○ The emergency has passed (if using s62)
- Clearly document reasons for discontinuing ECT
- If continuing ECT, capacity should be reviewed and documented before each treatment.

What if … ?

… It's an emergency?

Section 62 can be used to save life or prevent a serious deterioration in someone's condition if they're detained under the MHA (no matter what age). S62 applies either until the patient no longer meets the criteria or has received a second opinion (SOAD), but it's good practice to review it after every 2 treatments.

… ECT is being given in her best interests under the MCA?

This was commonplace, but is becoming more controversial. Seek legal advice if unsure, and consider whether Mrs Smith would be more appropriately treated under the MHA. If the MCA is being considered, hold a best interests meeting beforehand. It's good practice for another consultant to give an informal second opinion on medical necessity. Remember:
- The MCA can't override an advance decision refusing ECT
- Use the MHA if she is objecting or resistant (e.g. if restraint would be needed to facilitate ECT)
- Keep re-assessing capacity. The MCA doesn't apply if she regains capacity.

Take-home message

ECT works, but is only appropriate in specific situations. Clear explanations can decrease the fear about its use.

Further reading

Waite, J. and Easton, A. (2013) *The ECT Handbook*, 3rd edn, College Report CR176. The Royal College of Psychiatrists: London.
NICE (2003) *TA59 Guidance on the use of Electroconvulsive Therapy*. NICE, England.
  - ○ www.nice.org.uk/Guidance/TA59
ECT Patient information leaflet:
  - ○ www.rcpsych.ac.uk/expertadvice/treatments/ect.aspx

CHAPTER 48

Section 136 assessments

Anna M Burnside

East London NHS Foundation Trust, London, England

RELATED CHAPTERS: admission to discharge (34)

The unit coordinator bleeps you while on-call in the unit one weekend to assess Josh, 24. He was dancing naked in a shopping centre, so the police brought him to hospital under s136.

Section 136 is the police power to remove someone from a public place to a Place of Safety, to allow a full mental health assessment (Box 48.1). Trust protocols vary, so clarify your role beforehand, e.g.

- Contact the on-call senior/Approved Mental Health Professional (AMHP) to assess...
  - Immediately (you only clerk Josh if admitted)
  - After a brief interview and physical assessment
  - After a full clerking
- Full clerking + admit/discharge.

If the last option, your Trust's policy goes against guidance that the assessment should be completed by a s12 Approved Doctor ± AMHP (MHA Code of Practice). This isn't illegal, but we'd suggest you *never* discharge someone from s136 without full discussion with your registrar ± AMHP. It's also reasonable to ask your registrar to attend and help you, especially at first.

We'll assume you *are* expected to complete the assessment in order to explain the process.

Preparation

Josh has been detained by someone without mental health knowledge, so needs assessment by a mental health professional as soon as possible.

1. On the telephone
- Circumstances of detention
- Are police still present? Until when ... ?
- Physical concerns/substance misuse
- Alert and sober?
- Risks
- Agree when to attend (coincide with the AMHP if jointly assessing).

Psychiatry: Breaking the ICE – Introductions, Common Tasks and Emergencies for Trainees, First Edition.
Edited by Sarah Stringer, Juliet Hurn and Anna M Burnside.
© 2016 John Wiley & Sons, Ltd. Published 2016 by John Wiley & Sons, Ltd.
Companion Website: www.psychiatryice.com

Box 48.1 S136 key facts

Section 136
- The police power to remove someone from a public place to a Place of Safety if they seem:
  - Mentally disordered *and*
  - Posing a risk to self or others *and*
  - In immediate need of care or control
- It lasts *up to* 72 hours.

Place of Safety
- Is agreed by local services
- Usually a special assessment suite in a psychiatric unit
- Shouldn't be a police station or ED, but sometimes is.

Box 48.2 Tasers and tear-gas

- Police must *urgently* transfer anyone who's been 'tasered' to ED for medical assessment
- If tear-gas was used, Josh must be allowed to wash ± change clothing before the interview, especially if still symptomatic:
  - Tears, eye pain, blepharospasm
  - Burning throat, nose, skin
  - Rhinorrhoea, sneezing, coughing, retching
  - Most symptoms ease within 15–60 minutes
  - Breathing difficulties need ED.

2. On the ward
- *136 nursing coordinator:*
  - Josh's presentation since admission (± observe on CCTV if available)
  - Risks: do you need the ERT present to assess safely?
  - Ask to read police s136 papers
- *Police (if present):*
  - Handover – anything they haven't written down?
  - Use of taser/tear-gas (Box 48.2)
  - Agree how long they'll stay
  - Ask them to search Josh if it's possible he may have weapons
- *Check notes, particularly:*
  - PPHx, PMHx, substance history, risk history
  - Relapse signature – is this typical? If different, why?

TIP: The police may want to leave, but if you need them, give a clear, time-limited rationale *with* the lead nurse, e.g. *Based on the bruising, he may need transfer to casualty for medical assessment. Can you wait 20 minutes for me to check this?* Speak to their desk sergeant if required.

TIP: Check: does everyone feel comfortable interviewing in the room or should you initially speak via intercom?

Ruaidhri McCormack, ST5

Assessment

1. Approach
If assessing with the AMHP, ask how they'd like to run the interview – they're more experienced than you.

Josh may be frightened or angry. Explain he's not in any trouble, and hasn't been arrested – the police were simply worried about him.

If he's clearly intoxicated, you can't accurately assess him:
- Agree a sobering-up period (usually a few hours)
- Undertake a brief physical
- Ask staff to monitor and call you once sober.

2. Psychiatric history
Your focus is on *diagnosis* and *risk* assessment.
- Presenting complaint (why does he think the police picked him up?)
- PPHx
- PMHx
- Substance misuse
- Forensic history
- Past self-harm/violence.

The commonest diagnoses associated with s136 are schizophrenia, mania, drug-induced psychosis and personality disorder (Borschmann *et al.*, 2010).

3. MSE, especially ...
- Intoxication/withdrawal
- Mood
- Psychotic symptoms
- Thoughts of harm to self/others
- Disorientation/confusion/learning disability (LD)?
- Does he think he's unwell?
  - Would he accept help, e.g. admission; CMHT/HTT/GP follow-up?

4. Physical assessment, especially ...
- Physical examination (minimum = basic obs)
- Injuries, e.g. taser, handcuff bruising, fractures from any restraint
- Investigations, e.g. breathalyser, UDS, BM, paracetamol and salicylate levels.

5. Risk assessment, especially ...
- Suicide/self-harm
- Violence
- Other (related to admission), e.g. running in traffic, wandering.

6. Collateral history
It's essential to speak to a relative or close friend if considering discharge.
- Are they worried?
- Would discharge be safe?
- Can they offer support if Josh is discharged?

Management

If you've assessed with an AMHP, ask their opinion before making any decisions.

1. Manage physical illness
Treat minor problems on site. If Josh needs ED investigation or treatment, the police (or sometimes nurses) should transfer him there under s136; he can return once medical assessment is complete.

2. Consider specialist opinion
If Josh is under-18/possibly has an a learning disability, request assessment by someone with Child and Adolescent Mental Health Service (CAMHS) or LD expertise (AMHP *or* senior doctor).

3. Admit or discharge
You feel he requires admission; Josh is willing
Run your plan past your registrar (± HTT if required). Admit informally, as usual (p212–215). The Code of Practice states an AMHP should still review Josh and sign the papers to discharge the s136 (but local policies may differ).

> **TIP:** Re-consider the need for MHA assessment if admission involves transport to another unit and you're worried Josh might change his mind or become agitated en route.

You think he needs admission; he wants to go home
Contact your on-call senior (and AMHP) to undertake a MHA assessment. This is your default position for *any* concerns or uncertainty about Josh. Don't be pressurised to discharge him.

Discharge
If you're confident that Josh doesn't have a mental disorder, you may be able to discharge him. Always discuss first with your registrar and duty AMHP – especially if Josh *wants* admission. They may raise concerns you hadn't considered, or decide to assess him formally. If you suspect a mental disorder but still want to discharge, an AMHP *must* see the patient.
If discharging, consider aftercare, e.g.
- Seven-day follow-up by HTT/CMHT/GP
- Could a carer collect and support him?
- Make a crisis plan (p315)
- Give brief advice, e.g. about safe drinking if this is an alcohol-related presentation.

Officially, the AMHP should see him and rescind the s136, but local policy may let you sign the form. S136 ends once the assessment is complete, and Josh can't be held further.

> **TIPS:** Registrars are often responsible for s136 assessments. Try to attend, so you've seen a few before *you're* the registrar.

Take-home message

Have a low threshold for involving seniors.

Reference

Borschmann RD, Gillard S, Turner K, Chambers M and O'Brien K. (2010) Section 136 of the Mental Health Act: a new literature review. Medicine, Science and the Law **50** (1), 34–39.

Further reading

Department of Health (2015) The Mental Health Act 1983: Code of Practice. The Stationery Office, Norwich.

CHAPTER 49

Tribunals

Sarah Stringer

King's College London, London, England

RELATED CHAPTERS: admission to discharge (34)

Mrs Elaine Rice has paranoid schizophrenia and was placed on s3 MHA yesterday. She's very unhappy about it.

Most detained patients have a right to appeal their section in two ways:
- **Mental Health Tribunal**
  - Essentially a court hearing in the hospital, where an independent panel sits to hear the patient's appeal case
  - The panel consists of:
    - Chairperson ('president') – a lawyer
    - Medical member – usually a psychiatrist
    - Lay Person – often a social worker
- **Hospital Managers' Hearing**
  - Less formal
  - No medical or legal members
  - The panel *tends* to be less willing to discharge people.

In any case, it's the *team's* duty to prove the patient needs continued detention – not the patient's duty to disprove it.

Your role

1. Information

Encourage Elaine to appeal. This is her right if on s2 (within the first 14 days), s3 and some forensic sections (check before giving advice). She simply tells the nurses, who'll help her complete a form and find a *free* solicitor.

2. Report

Your seniors usually handle Tribunals, but may ask you to help write the medical report, based on the:
- Admission clerking
- Progress notes
- Risks
- Plan.

Psychiatry: Breaking the ICE – Introductions, Common Tasks and Emergencies for Trainees, First Edition.
Edited by Sarah Stringer, Juliet Hurn and Anna M Burnside.
© 2016 John Wiley & Sons, Ltd. Published 2016 by John Wiley & Sons, Ltd.
Companion Website: www.psychiatryice.com

Ask to see a good example from another patient's case, and expect your senior to tweak the legal wording at the beginning and end. Make sure you understand the criteria for detention (e.g. s2 or s3), including the risks (to Elaine's health/safety or others). For guidance on writing reports:

• www.judiciary.gov.uk/wp-content/uploads/JCO/Documents/Practice+Directions/Tribunals
  /statements-in-mental-health-cases-hesc-28102013.pdf

Other staff provide Nursing and Social Circumstances reports, and it's worth reading these, once they're available.

3. Attend tribunals

By observing a Tribunal, you'll know what to do once it's your turn, and find it easier to describe to patients.

You *don't* have to do Tribunals, and shouldn't feel pressurized over this. However, you may represent your team if feeling ready to do so – if so, the tips below will help.

Preparation

If representing your team at Tribunal:
• Dress formally
• Check your consultant's plan, should the Tribunal discharge Elaine
• Memorise the ICD criteria for Elaine's diagnosis (paranoid schizophrenia)
• Review:
  ○ Elaine's MSE on the morning of the Tribunal (working around the Tribunal doctor, who'll see her *alone* at some point).
  ○ The past week's events, particularly risks or medication issues
  ○ Your report (keep a copy with you)
  ○ The nursing and social circumstances reports (any mistakes/surprises?)
  ○ Drug chart: doses, adherence, PRN usage
• Set aside 2–4 hours. You should only be interrupted for *absolute* emergencies.
• Hand your bleep to another doctor and silence your mobile phone.

> **TIP:** Consider role-playing the Tribunal questions with your consultant beforehand in supervision, or asking them to observe you in the Tribunal and completing a WPBA.

During

1. Make a good first impression
• Outside the room, wait quietly until the Clerk invites you in
• If you can't stay for the whole Tribunal, ask the Clerk whether the Panel could let you leave to attend to clinical duties, once you've answered their questions
  ○ If they refuse, you *must* stay
• Sit where you're told to (often opposite the medic, and beside the patient's solicitor)
• Make eye contact with the Panel, and anyone speaking
• If Elaine interrupts, look to the Chairperson to intervene (don't step in)
• Listen to the Chairperson's introductions and their summary of the independent psychiatrist's meeting with Elaine.

2. Perform!

The Chairperson will address you, asking:

- If Elaine is suffering from a mental disorder of a nature or degree requiring involuntary treatment
  - Address them as Sir or Madam
  - State *yes* and whether nature and/or degree (don't justify yet)
- What the risks are if not detained
  - State whether these relate to Elaine's own health, safety *and/or* risk to others (don't justify).

The Medical Member will question you (usually 5–10 minutes)

- Talk about 'Mrs Rice', not 'the patient'
- Show empathy and compassion – don't be an automaton
  - Remember that Elaine is listening
- Be succinct but comprehensive
- They'll usually ask you to justify why you said nature/degree.
  - State that Mrs Rice is suffering with paranoid schizophrenia
  - To justify Nature, explain issues of insight, chronic/relapsing-remitting course without treatment, historic disengagement and relapse
  - To justify Degree: highlight key current symptoms demonstrating that she's unwell *now*
- When they ask for symptoms, you can and should:
  - Use formal terminology, with examples
  - Repeat things you wrote in the report
  - Mention today's positive MSE findings/recent symptoms on the ward
- Detail risks, when asked
- When asked about treatment:
  - Explain the current management plan, as a combination of psychopharmacological, psychological and social interventions
  - Start with medication details: drugs, doses, planned increases
  - Detail other management, e.g. 1:1 psychology sessions; OT groups; finding accommodation
- If they argue the diagnosis or management plan, calmly explain your team's reasoning.

The Chairperson and Layperson may then question you to:

- Clarify points
- Check concerns if Elaine is discharged today
  - State immediate risks
  - Explain contributing issues, e.g. ambivalence, recent problems, relatively recent mental state improvement, historic non-adherence, poor insight
- Ask what the plan would be if discharged today.

Finally, Elaine's solicitor will question you.

- Don't be intimidated: they've no psychiatric training and are often junior members of their firm, no matter how confident or sharply dressed they seem!
- Tilt your chair to face them (keeping yourself on view to the panel)
- Stay patient
- Be prepared for a grilling on the effects of detention on Elaine's human rights
  - Explain that her detention is the *least restrictive* option available now, and give reasons, e.g. won't stay informally; can't yet engage reliably with HTT due to limited insight
  - Explain how her detention *protects* her human rights, e.g. right to life, dignity, family life (p104)
  - State how immediate discharge would jeopardise these, e.g. suicide, sexual disinhibition, destabilizing her relationships.

You're done. Smile, thank the Panel and sit silently and attentively while colleagues are questioned.

After

Once finished, the Panel will meet privately to discuss their decision.
- They may call you back to hear the outcome, or deliver it by post a few days later
- Don't be upset if they discharge Elaine. This is exactly what they're set up to do, and an important safeguard for her human rights – not a sign that you've done anything wrong.
- Debrief with Elaine, *especially* if she's upset with you
- If discharged, put the plan into place as agreed with your consultant, e.g. TTOs, HTT/7-day follow-up with CC.

Take-home message

Tribunals can feel scary, but protect your patient's rights. Take opportunities to try them out *before* you're a registrar, if possible.

CHAPTER 50

Your first on-call shift

Rachel Thomasson[1], Sean Cross[2], and Anna M Burnside[3]

[1] *Manchester Royal Infirmary, Manchester, Lancashire, England*
[2] *South London & Maudsley NHS Foundation Trust, London, England*
[3] *East London NHS Foundation Trust, London, England*

You receive your oncall rota: you're on-call tomorrow night. A sense of dread descends …

With feet on both medical and psychiatric shores, you're the best person to assess:
- **Medical problems in 'psychiatric' patients**
- **Psychiatric problems in 'medical' patients.**

Of course, it's possible your foot isn't yet *firmly* on the psychiatric shore … Maybe the medical shore still feels slippery … OK, so you're waist-deep in water. Don't panic. This section ensures the practicalities don't increase your anxiety, and explains how to get help when out of your depth.

TIP: If you're feeling stressed, tired, or emotional from an incident, it's more important to take 10 minutes, have a cuppa and re-focus. It'll make you more able to deal with what's left, and in the long run, makes you more efficient.

Thom Proven, ST4

Preparation

Sort out the following things *before* your first on-call.

1. Where?
- Handover (e.g. if the liaison office is called *The Wellbeing Unit*, you'll never find it)
- Swipe-cards or keys – how do you get these?
- On-call room – how do you get in?
- Do you cover … ?
  - Psychiatric unit
  - General hospital and Emergency Department (ED)
  - Both.

Psychiatry: Breaking the ICE – Introductions, Common Tasks and Emergencies for Trainees, First Edition.
Edited by Sarah Stringer, Juliet Hurn and Anna M Burnside.
© 2016 John Wiley & Sons, Ltd. Published 2016 by John Wiley & Sons, Ltd.
Companion Website: www.psychiatryice.com

2. Contact numbers
- On-call seniors: general adult, Child and Adolescent Mental Health Service (CAMHS) ± other specialties
- Psychiatric Liaison Nurse (PLN)
- Duty Approved Mental Health Professional (AMHP)
- Bed manager
- On-call pharmacist
- Emergency Response Team (ERT) ± emergency medical team (if different)
- Yourself – bleep/mobile number; how to answer bleeps.

3. Equipment
In psychiatric units, you'll review medically unwell patients and complete a full physical for all new admissions. In ED, you'll sometimes see 'medically cleared' patients with worrying physical signs – a brief examination will either reassure you, or persuade medical colleagues to address concerns. Carry:
- Stethoscope (in a bag/pocket – not around your neck)
- Tendon hammer
- Pen torch
- ± Blood forms, urine drug screen (UDS), blood-taking kit.

Key protocols are usually available on the Trust intranet or in the liaison office – ask a PLN. Useful examples include:
- Rapid tranquilization (RT)
- Delirium management
- Alcohol detoxification ('detox').

> **TIP:** Collect a pack of useful forms and equipment. On-call, I carried phlebotomy equipment, drug charts, and blood forms round with me all the time. Saves having to leave a ward to go find them, especially when you've just persuaded someone to have their blood taken.
>
> Ben Spencer, ST6

4. Admissions
Check the admission procedure, including:
- Whether you need senior or HTT agreement before admitting someone
- Who finds the bed/organises transport, e.g. bed manager, PLN, you?
- What happens when there are *no* beds, e.g. private sector/inter-Trust agreements?

5. Referrals
Check how to refer to the Crisis/Home Treatment Team (HTT) and local Community Mental Health Teams (CMHTs).
- Referral forms? Letter/fax/email/telephone discussion?
- Mandatory referral information, e.g. risk assessment, full clerking
- Do you need to confirm receipt?

6. Emergencies
If covering a psychiatric unit, check the location and how to use emergency equipment, especially the ligature cutters, oxygen, suction and defibrillator. Don't assume you'll 'work out' how to use unfamiliar equipment in an emergency.

Table 50.1 On-call team-working.

Issue	Senior psychiatrist	Other
Psychiatric	✓	PLN
Aggression	✓	ERT
Medical/surgical	✓	Local medical/surgical registrar on-call
Medication	✓	On-call pharmacist
Protocols, admissions, nursing issues	✓	Unit holder/senior nurse/PLN
Mental Health Act (MHA)	✓	Duty AMHP
Safeguarding/child protection	✓	Duty AMHP/social worker

TIP: As far as possible, do the paperwork as you go along. Emergencies are rare in psychiatry and most things can wait. Otherwise, after 12 hours on-call you'll find you've created another 24 hours' paperwork to do.

On-call team

Don't struggle on alone – you're part of an experienced team (Table 50.1).

1. Psychiatrists

Senior doctors (consultant ±registrar) are usually on-call from home, covering ED, inpatients, police stations and community emergencies. They're contactable via the hospital switchboard, and sometimes have a bed management role, e.g. approving/reviewing admissions. You'll always have general adult and CAMHS seniors, and sometimes other specialists, e.g. older adults, forensics.

   Contact your senior at the start of your shift to introduce yourself and build a sense of teamwork. This also reminds them they're on call *before* they start an all-night party. Seniors *expect* you to contact them to discuss:
- Uncertainty, especially about admission/discharge decisions
- Tricky assessments
- Ethical/legal issues
- Prescribing
- Need for MHA assessments
- Feeling overwhelmed, e.g. urgent ED patients are piling up. Seniors may be able to attend and help clear the list, but if not, can help you prioritise and focus your assessments to speed things up.

Consultants have overall clinical responsibility and you should always feel able to contact them, especially if you have problems reaching the registrar.

TIP: You'll occasionally encounter a lazy registrar who refuses to help. Don't argue – just say you need senior support, so will contact the consultant if they can't help. This usually cures their lethargy.

Presenting patients over the telephone

Before calling your senior, plan the conversation, to sound competent and focused. They don't want an hour-long presentation, and can clarify extra points. Straightforward questions need short presentations (e.g. medication dose for a known patient); complex patients need lengthy discussions.

- Introduce yourself and say why you're calling, e.g.
  - *I'd like some prescribing advice*
  - *I'm not sure whether I should admit or discharge this patient*
  - *I think we need a Mental Health Act assessment*
- Patient details
  - Name, age, ethnicity, occupation, marital/housing status
  - Current location and MHA status
  - Whether known to psychiatric services; previous diagnoses
- Reason for presentation, triggers, duration of problems (or admission)
- Summarise current symptoms and problems
- Current medications and adherence
- *Relevant* background history – stick to issues affecting diagnosis or management:
  - Medical problems
  - Substance misuse
  - Social situation, e.g. lives with wife and baby
  - *Other* e.g. note a family history of schizophrenia in first episode psychosis
- Risks
- MSE – key points, e.g. chaotic, tearful, responding to hallucinations, refusing admission
- Physical findings/investigations
- Your plan
  - Offer this, however basic, to test out your ideas rather than simply being told what to do.

TIP: Before calling your senior for advice, make sure you've actually *seen* the patient. Disregarding this professional etiquette may leave you somewhat exposed.

Mark Tarn, Clinical Lead for Military Mental Health Scotland and Northern Ireland

2. PLNs

When covering ED, the PLN is an invaluable ally, who'll usually share your workload, or screen out patients who don't need to see you. PLNs provide:

- Expertise in assessing and managing self-harm risk
- In-depth knowledge of frequent attenders
- A sounding board to clarify your role/plans
- Chaperoning and support when seeing risky patients
- Logistical advice – referrals, MHA assessments, transfers.

They may ask your opinion, particularly if patients have complex medical problems, or may need a MHA assessment.

TIP: Spend time thinking about why you should see the patient, not why you shouldn't. If you're left in any doubt, just see the patient.

Angus Brown, Liaison Consultant

Placement specifics

1. Psychiatric units

This is just an extension of usual ward duties, the difference being that you're the only doctor on site, and most senior medical opinion in the unit. This can feel lonely, exciting, or a little scary – but again, don't be afraid to ask for help.

2. General hospital and ED

Psychiatric services are usually provided by separate mental health Trusts, so different record systems and protocols may make it harder to provide seamless care. You'll usually need to document in both medical and psychiatric notes, though it's often possible (and more useful to medics) to write briefly in the medical notes, while documenting the full history in the psychiatric notes.

The best EDs view you and the PLN as crucial teammates. Whether or not this is your hospital's culture, be helpful, proactive and keen to review patients: you'll improve working relationships and patient care, and generally find the medics reciprocate when *you* need *them*. Medical staff may know little about psychiatric care or facilities, so explain your decisions and plans in a non-defensive, non-patronising way, rather than expecting immediate agreement.

ED requires focused assessments and sound clinical decision-making in a time-pressured environment. However, psychiatric patients don't always fit into the ED's stringent time limits because:
- History and engagement replace quick diagnostic tests
- Patients may struggle to give a directly relevant history
- Intoxicated people need to sober up before you can reliably assess them
- Multiple assessments may be needed (e.g. MHA)
- It can take time to locate a psychiatric bed.

With experience, you'll get a better idea of how long things take. Try to manage expectations: if something's going to take a few hours, tell ED so they can plan around this.

PATIENT VIEW:

We were seen by a very nice casualty doctor. There just seemed to be gentleness and empathy. The way I was spoken with was respectful, non-judgemental. He had compassion for me. It was a just a case of, *this is another human being, who's going through a really bad time* and normalising it, you know? For him, it wasn't something frightening, annoying, overwhelming ... it was just, *'This person is another patient, clearly with difficulties other than physical manifestations.'* And yet I was being treated as a human being, a normal person. Which I really respected.

'Raphael'

The MHA in general hospitals

Use of the MHA can be trickier, so check how this works in your hospital. Chapter 15 gives an overview of the law; Table 50.2 provides key information in the on-call setting.

TIP: There can be pressure from all angles to *not* admit people ... However, there's nothing worse than laying your head on the pillow at night and finding you're deeply worried about the decision you've made. There are always seniors available to share the decision with, and at the end of the day, an unnecessary admission is better than an 'unnecessary' suicide.

Thom Proven, ST4

Table 50.2 MHA in general hospitals.

s5(2)	Only for *admitted* patients – excludes ED. Always check whether the patient has been *formally admitted* to the hospital.
	S5(2) papers must be received on behalf of the hospital managers before the section is complete. Find out who's responsible in the general hospital, e.g. site manager.
	Only the *Responsible Clinician* (RC; the doctor in charge of a patient's treatment) or their *nominated deputy* can authorize detention under s5(2)
	• There can only be one nominated deputy, so find out who that is, e.g. psychiatry SHO or medical registrar. If it's not you, you can't authorize s5(2)
	• Liaison psychiatry consultants can also detain, and then become the RC
	• There's no power to treat under s5(2), so the Mental Capacity Act (MCA) is used to justify treatment under *best interests* where someone lacks capacity. Common law is occasionally used to intervene and protect *other* peoples from the patient, or prevent immediate harm.
Transferring detained patients from a psychiatric unit	Detained patients are transferred from psychiatric units either under s17 leave, or s19 (emergency) transfer – check which is being used.
	Ensure the s17 or s19 form travels with the patient, and the receiving ward knows who the RC is for psychiatric treatment:
	• s17: the patient's inpatient psychiatry consultant
	• s19: the liaison psychiatry consultant
Patients brought in by police	When police bring someone to ED, check whether the person is voluntary, or under arrest/s136/the MCA. For s136 or MCA, the police should complete and give you a copy of the relevant forms.
	If s136, swiftly clarify whether the police expect:
	• Physical treatment before transfer to a psychiatric unit for further assessment
	• Assessment under s136 in the ED

Handovers

Your colleague should handover a list of jobs at the start of your shift. It's easy to forget things, so the essentials are listed below. Always check patients' exact locations and how urgently they need review.

1. New patients awaiting assessment
• ED
• General hospital
• Psychiatric unit admissions

2. Ongoing issues: psychiatric unit
• Medical reviews
• Investigations to chase, e.g. blood results
• New admissions clerked but with outstanding tasks or ongoing concerns
• Psychiatric problems needing review
• Seclusion reviews (Ch.39)
• Patients expected/admitted under s136 (Ch.48).

3. Ongoing issues – ED/general hospital
Patients awaiting:
- Your review (history/MSE) to determine management
- Senior review – if so, why, and is the registrar aware?
- Admission
  - Have a bed and transport been organized?
  - Is there a contingency plan if they change their mind?
- MHA assessments organisation (you/PLN/bed manager/AMHP?)
  - Contact the registrar, AMHP and s12 doctor to assess
  - Locate a bed
  - Organize transport.

Prioritizing

Prioritize based on immediate risk and the skills of the involved team. There's only one of you, but respectful delegation is possible, e.g. the PLN might start assessing someone in ED, or the Unit Holder may review a situation on the unit. Remember:
- Physical health problems in psychiatric units can't be delegated, and may be more serious than they sound
- Psychiatric inpatients are essentially *already* in a safe place, though acute mental health deteriorations may be hard for staff to manage
- ED patients may walk out (you can't use s5(2) in ED), so should generally be prioritized above general hospital patients. Where several patients are awaiting assessment, prioritize clinical need, while staying mindful of breaching ED waiting times.
- General hospital patients should be prioritized if agitated, refusing essential treatment or trying to leave
  - However, medics *can* offer prn, assess capacity or use s5(2)
- Prioritise s136 suite patients over routine admissions. This ensures timely admission/discharge, which is better for patients, and the staff covering the 136 suite.
Consider calling ward staff to gain further information, advise on initial management and give them some idea of when you'll attend.

> **TIP:** Documentation: if called away, make sure you've covered the formulation, risk assessment and management plan; you can add the rest later in your shift.

> **TIP:** When there's time at the start of an oncall, briefly visit each psychiatric ward, introduce yourself and proactively sweep up jobs. This reassures nurses, cuts down time spent answering non-urgent calls, and transforms you into That Lovely Doctor Who Says Hello.

Transfers

Table 50.3 summarises the key points to check before transferring someone between sites. A few minutes now saves time and confusion later.

Table 50.3 Transfer checklists.

Situation	Checklist
From psychiatric unit to ED	• RMN to accompany the patient and stay with them until they return • Ask the RMN to photocopy the drug and obs charts • Write a cover letter (p51) • Handover to liaison/duty psychiatrist for next day review if not returning

From ED/ general hospital to psychiatric unit	• Is the patient medically fit for transfer? (Box 50.2)
	• Clear plan if ongoing medical concerns, e.g. management, investigations, follow up
	• Copies to travel with the patient:
	  ◦ ED notes/medical discharge summary
	  ◦ ECGs, imaging reports, blood results
	  ◦ Drug chart (photocopy)
	• Once a bed's identified, speak to the ward nurse in charge:
	  ◦ Confirm they *have* a bed and are expecting the patient
	  ◦ Summarise the case
	  ◦ Confirm medical "clearance" (p315)
	  ◦ Highlight risks and management e.g. PRN medication, obs level
	  ◦ Ensure they have a copy of your assessment
	• Ask the PLN to help you arrange transport ± escort
	• Ask if the patient wants anyone informed of their admission

From ED to medical ward (patient with mental *and* physical problems)	• Review ED and psychiatric notes
	  ◦ Past self-harm, aggression, absconding?
	• History
	  ◦ Explain you're seeing them briefly, and don't want to delay transfer; a detailed assessment will happen later
	  ◦ Explore the presenting complaint
	  ◦ Screen: current mental illness, substance misuse, forensic history
	• MSE, considering how symptoms may affect admission:
	  ◦ Agitation/irritability/impulsivity
	  ◦ Thoughts of self-harm, violence or absconding
	  ◦ Psychotic symptoms
	  ◦ Insight and willingness to follow medics' plan
	• Assess capacity if refusing investigations/treatment (Ch.76)
	• Assess risk: to self and others, including absconding
	• Document your findings and plan, advising as relevant:
	  ◦ Use of MCA/MHA
	  ◦ Risk management, e.g. RMN, PRN medication
	  ◦ Regular psychotropics
	  ◦ What to do if they try to leave
	  ◦ Monitoring and management of any substance withdrawal
	  ◦ Contact details for liaison/duty psychiatrist
	• Handover to liaison/duty psychiatrist for next day review

Transfers may be fretfully pushed by referrers, or anxiously resisted by the receiving team, whether medical or psychiatric. Don't get intimidated or annoyed – get diplomatic. You're the best person to:
• Assess where the patient can be most safely managed
• Communicate the challenges or limitations of care at either site
• Provide medical or psychiatric support to staff on either side.

Involve your registrar early if the situation's becoming heated: senior level communication can resolve issues quickly.

Medically cleared?

Medics may insist on transferring 'medically cleared' patients, without appreciating the limitations of medical care on psychiatric wards. A clear explanation is usually all that's needed, and a useful rule of thumb is that the patient must be medically fit for *discharge home*. Specifically, psychiatric wards *can't* usually manage:

- IV medication or fluids
- Parenteral feeding
- Sliding scales
- Unstable diabetes
- Hoisting for transfer.

You may need to manage the psychiatric team's anxieties about transfer:

- Consider assessing the patient yourself. Your team will relax if you're happy the transfer is appropriate.
- If transfer is *safe* but requires ongoing medical care, get a specific person's contact details to provide telephone advice to the psychiatric ward, e.g. medical registrar, modern matron
- Where available, involve clinical nurse specialists who can liaise with the ward or provide in-reach, e.g. diabetes, palliative care.

Discharges

1. Patient – crisis plans

If discharging, always write the person a simple summary of your management plan, so they know what they need to do, and what you'll do for them. Include a *crisis plan*, should they feel worse, or become more risky (e.g. considering self-harm), e.g.

- Agreed strategies to cope with problems, e.g. stress/suicidal thoughts
- Contact details
  - Carer
  - Daytime: GP ±CMHT
  - Out-of-hours:
    - Samaritans (UK: 08457 909090; ROI: 1850 609090)
    - Crisis help-lines
- Attend ED if feeling worse/risky.

2. GPs

GPs are a great central information reservoir: should someone present at the other end of the country, their records are more easily traced through their GP than a mental health Trust. However, GPs may see 40 patients on a busy day, so don't want to plough through a 6-page assessment! Compromise by sending the named/duty GP a copy of your full clerking with a succinct cover letter stating:

- Date, place and reason for presentation (triggers, key symptoms)
- Diagnosis ± comorbidity (e.g. drugs/alcohol)
- Risks
- Management plan:
  - Short, numbered points
  - *Highlight* anything the GP should do, e.g. *I would be grateful if you could review her mental state within a week, refer for Cognitive Behaviour Therapy (CBT) and consider starting an antidepressant, e.g. fluoxetine 20 mg PO mane*
- Contact details of any involved services, e.g. CMHT/Care Coordinator (CC)
- Crisis plan, e.g. attend ED; involve police if aggressive.

TIP: Unless you've good reason to withhold it, give the patient a copy of their assessment and letter. They can show these to the GP/CMHT, should your letter get lost in the post.

3. CMHTs

Different teams have their own referral routes (e-mail, fax, telephone) and expectations (structured proforma; full clerking plus cover letter). Always think: will this team have access to my notes system? If not, include a copy of your assessment, otherwise they'll have to repeat everything from scratch. Copy the GP into all correspondence.

TIP: Try to call the person providing follow-up, *before* discharging the patient. You can confirm they received your referral ± get an appointment or realistic sense of when they'll see the person. Out-of-hours, ask the next doctor to check your referral's been accepted.

4. HTT

HTTs provide home visits as an alternative to hospital admission (Box 50.1). Services vary widely: some provide 9–5 care, while others are 24/7, or may base a teammate in ED to assess possible referrals.

Box 50.1 Common HTT referral criteria

- Manageable risk
- Patient agrees to engage
- Someone to facilitate access, if needed
- ±Taking medication which needs monitoring
- Admission is the only alternative

You must usually discuss referrals with the duty person over the telephone, *before* the patient leaves hospital. This is because they may advise admission if the person is too complex, severe or risky, *or* a CMHT referral if HTT isn't required. HTTs generally need the same information as GPs, as well as:

- Patient ± carer contact details, e.g. mobile numbers
- Whether the patient:
  ○ Can guarantee their safety between visits
  ○ Is happy to be visited at home by HTT
- Any risks/practicalities for home visits, e.g. ease of access, floor of building, aggressive pets.

PATIENT VIEW:

Things have gotten better with home treatment, but there's a lot of isolation – I can't exactly turn round to you and say, "Well, I've made a very close friend when I was ill this time." Because I've been treated in my home ...

'Sarah'

TIP: Always check: is the patient a carer? Urgently contact the duty social worker about children or vulnerable adults. If admitting, organise a carer to take keys and deal with pets. Nobody wants a dead goldfish on their conscience.

TIP: When I'm halfway through a long and particularly trying shift, and want to chuck my bleep in the bin, go home and never come back, I have a cup of tea and a biscuit and take five minutes to remind myself: in a few hours, I'm going home to my girlfriend, my nice flat, my friends. Many patients have been here for months without going outside for more than an hour or so. Many have been totally abandoned by everybody who should have loved them, or have pasts full of admissions or abuse. Many live in hostels I wouldn't want my dog to live in. Most of their problems are caused by a crippling illness they didn't choose, and because of the nature of the illness, they don't even realise they're ill. So they have to trust the people who've deprived them of their liberty, injected them against their will and dictated how they must live their life ... They have to carry on taking tablets that make them fat and sleepy, for an illness they don't believe they have. That usually gives me enough compassion, patience and sympathy to get through (the energy is topped up by the biscuit and tea).

Sam Porter, CT2

CHAPTER 51

Self-harm

Rachel Thomasson[1], Jane Bunclark[2], Sean Cross[2], Rory Conn[3], and Christina Barras[4]

[1] Manchester Royal Infirmary, Manchester, Lancashire, England
[2] South London & Maudsley NHS Foundation Trust, London, England
[3] Tavistock and Portman NHS Foundation Trust, London, England
[4] South West London & St George's Mental Health NHS Trust, London, England

RELATED CHAPTERS: self-harm on wards (71), treatment refusal (76)

Ben, 21, cut his wrists and took an overdose after his girlfriend dumped him. He was brought to ED by ambulance. Though distressed and tearful, he's accepting N-acetylcysteine. You've been called to assess.

Everyone presenting with self-harm or suicidal thoughts needs a full psychiatric assessment, no matter how low risk they seem. Whether self-harm *functions* as a suicide attempt or not, *any* act increases the risk of suicide in the following year.

Self-harm *can* upset and frustrate staff – but don't ignore dismissive, rude or angry behaviour. Rather than psychoanalysing colleagues, try to:
- Help them empathise with Ben
- Role-model compassion
- Be pragmatic. Unprofessional responses may prolong your assessment, complicate his presentation and increase his risks.

Finally, remember, self-harm *isn't* synonymous with *personality disorder*.

> **TIP:** Don't label patients with personality disorder, without a proper assessment. Especially not when on-call, and especially not teenagers, many of whom appear personality disordered, but are just having a difficult adolescence. A diagnosis on their records will stick and put them at long-term risk of being stigmatised and written-off throughout their contact with services.
>
> Lucinda Richards, CT3

Preparation

> **TIP:** Don't *refuse* to assess if Ben hasn't completed treatment or been 'medically cleared'. Work in parallel with ED to manage risk.

Psychiatry: Breaking the ICE – Introductions, Common Tasks and Emergencies for Trainees, First Edition.
Edited by Sarah Stringer, Juliet Hurn and Anna M Burnside.
© 2016 John Wiley & Sons, Ltd. Published 2016 by John Wiley & Sons, Ltd.
Companion Website: www.psychiatryice.com

1. *Briefly* check Ben (you/PLN)
- Calm and willing to stay? If not, ask security/a Registered Mental Nurse (RMN) to stay with him
- Sober? Intoxication will postpone your assessment (see *What Ifs ... ?)*
- Note down his physical description – if he absconds, security + police need this.

2. Gather information – paramedic, ED, psychiatric notes
- Circumstances:
  - Who called the ambulance?
  - Where was he? E.g. home, railway tracks
  - Attended willingly?
- Triggers
- Medical
  - Injury severity, e.g. nerve/tendon/vessel damage
  - Overdose details: what, how much, when? Does his presentation *match* his story?
  - Clues to undisclosed self-harm, e.g. drowsy; abnormal obs/ECG/bloods
  - Treatment: received; refused/outstanding + urgency
- Psychiatric
  - Diagnosis
  - Risks, especially historic suicidality/self-harm. How dangerous? Triggers?
  - Engagement
- Crisis plan/what's helped previously? Have previous admissions been helpful?

PATIENT VIEW:

I used to hurt myself. When I was in hospital I'd try to put bandages around my arms and I'd put rubber gloves on, but in the morning they'd all be off and all the bed was full of blood ... They said it was attention seeking. Whilst I'm at work, when I go through these periods, I put gloves on – I don't want anyone to see what I've done to myself. I hide it. It's not attention seeking. Then I'd go to hospital asking for help and they would just leave me, and I'd be all leaking.

'Amaya'

Assessment

PATIENT VIEW:

It's hard for people to understand why you self-harm. If you cut yourself, you go to hospital ... And they're all, "Why don't you talk to someone?" Because there's nobody to talk to.

'Rob'

---

1. Approach
Do:
- Hold the position that Ben saw self-harm as his *best* way to cope at the time
- Stay calm, acknowledge distress and try to understand the causes. Engagement helps minimize risk, and the interview itself can be therapeutic.
  - Explain that you want to work *with* him to try and find ways to help (but manage expectations – you can't solve everything/provide formal therapy yourself)
  - Take his problems seriously – start with the *triggers* for today's self-harm
  - Positively reinforce *any* attempts to seek help or engage, e.g. note courage or clear thinking despite distress

- ◦ Consider Ben's strengths: coping strategies, dealing with past stress
- ◦ Nurture ambivalence, e.g.
  - *It sounds like a big part of you wanted to die, but maybe a smaller part wanted to survive? Is that possible?*
  - *Do you think there's any reason you survived?* (E.g. family, skills, things he's still 'meant' to do)
- Jointly assess with the PLN if concerned about strong dynamics.

Don't:

- Minimise problems, e.g. jumping to say everything will be OK. Any suggestion he's over-reacted may trigger shame/anger
- Undermine his story, e.g. if his stated overdose doesn't match blood levels. This may prompt a bigger attempt to 'prove' he's serious.
- Brush over trauma, e.g. sexual abuse. Bearing witness communicates that you and future professionals have the strength and ability to help Ben with this.

In patients who haven't yet self-harmed:

- Positively reinforce help-seeking
- Check what's prevented them acting on thoughts so far
- Ask if they've rehearsed self-harm.

TIP: The only way to have a sense of safety about whether they'll repeat self-harm is understanding why they did it and helping *them* understand why. Help them to tell you. For example, if someone's been cutting, but says they don't know why they did it, help them return to the state of mind when the act took place. Start concrete, e.g.

- *Where were you? What were you doing in the kitchen? What were you cooking?*
- *Who was there? What was your boyfriend doing?*

If their boyfriend was criticising their cooking, ask:

- *What was he saying? How did you feel about that?*
- *Why did you feel so [e.g. furious]?*
- *So what did you do when he was being so critical?* [self-harm]

You now know which affective state they can't handle, e.g. anger when self-esteem is threatened. By helping them give their narrative, you can then say:

- *So, when your boyfriend's critical in future, what could you do differently?*

If they say it'll never happen again, be gently sceptical, e.g.

- *Was that the first time he's been critical?*
- *What makes you think he'll never be critical ever again?*

You can summarise that they're sensitive to criticism and may be vulnerable to that in the future, and might benefit from counselling to think about that.

Duncan McLean, Consultant Psychiatrist and Psychotherapist

---

2. Full history

Try to understand Ben's story, from the first self-harm thought, to being in ED, to future plans. Collect and weigh risk and protective factors – alongside your gut feeling – to decide whether he's safe for discharge. Tables 1–3 summarise higher and lower risk indicators.

- *History of Presenting Complaint* (HPC: Table 51.1)
- *Context: past history and demographic* (Table 51.2)
- *Current presentation* (Table 51.3).

By the end of your conversation, you should understand:

- The function of any self-harm
- How likely:
  - ◦ …Thoughts will become acts
  - ◦ …Acts will cause severe injury/death
- How to work with Ben to prevent harm.

Table 51.1 Self-harm HPC: risk factors for completed suicide.

Questions to ask	Higher risk	Lower risk
Triggers/stressors • *When did you first start thinking about this?* • *What was happening around then?* • *Was there a final straw?*	• Insoluble problems • Bereavements • Mental illness	Triggers resolved

Thoughts and plans
• *What thoughts did you have about self-harm/ suicide?*
• *What were your plans?*
• *Did you do anything because you thought you wouldn't be alive to do it later?*
	• Lengthy/extensive planning
	  ○ Researched methods
	  ○ Scoped out a site
	  ○ Gathered the means
	  ○ Rehearsed the act
	• Last acts, e.g.
	  ○ Changed/made a will
	  ○ Organised child/pet care
	  ○ Paid debts
	  ○ Said goodbye
	  ○ Suicide note
		• Limited planning
		• No last acts

Act: details and function
• *Take me through exactly what you did*
• *What was going through your mind?*
• *How did you feel during …? And after?*
• *What did you hope would happen?*
• *Did it help in some way?*
• *Did you want to die, or something else?*
• *Did you do anything to ensure you'd die / survive?*
• *How did you end up in hospital?*
	• Function = death
	• Method = violent/risky, e.g.
	  ○ Hanging
	  ○ Shooting/stabbing
	  ○ Jumping from height/in front of vehicles
	  ○ Overdose: large, staggered or poisonous
	• Believed lethal
	• Alone at the time
	• Precautions against discovery
	• Substance misuse during act
	• Accidentally found
		• Function = not suicide, e.g.
		  ○ Survive – cope/'get through' difficult situations
		  ○ Regulating or relieving anger, distress
		  ○ Express feelings
		  ○ Block, escape or distract from feelings
		  ○ Feel *something*, especially when emotionally numb
		  ○ Self-punish
		  ○ Communicate with/influence others
		  ○ Make self unattractive
		• Method = less harmful, e.g.
		  ○ Superficial cuts
		  ○ Most overdoses
		  ○ Self-biting
		  ○ Wound-picking
		• Didn't believe lethal
		• Safety measures, e.g. cutting 'safer' body areas
		• Alerted others/called for help

3. MSE, remembering …
- Scars, neglect, agitation, tearfulness, guarding, intoxication/withdrawal
- Low, perplexed, irritable, suspicious, flat/unstable affect
- Hopeless, wants to die
  ○ Intent/plans to self-harm
- Delusions
- Hallucinations/pseudohallucinations (including commands to self-harm)
- Dissociation, flashbacks
- Poor concentration, learning difficulties
- Willing to work with a crisis plan? Help-seeking?

Table 51.2 Historic and demographic risk factors for completed suicide.

Questions to ask	Higher risk	Lower risk

Past history and demographic
 	
• *Have you ever felt like this before?*
• *What triggered that?*
• *What did you do then?*
• *Can I ask you a few more general questions now …?*
	• PPHx:
	  ○ Past self-harm, especially attempted suicide/serious harm
	  ○ *Any illness*, including personality disorder
	  ○ Non-engagement
	• PMHx: illnesses which are:
	  ○ Painful/chronic/terminal
	  ○ Neurological
	  ○ Stigmatising
	• FHx: suicide/mental illness
	• Substance misuse
	• Personal:
	  ○ Abuse/adverse events
	  ○ Impulsivity
	• Demographic/SHx:
	  ○ Male
	  ○ Young + male
	  ○ Elderly
	  ○ Widowed > separated > single
	  ○ Unemployed
	  ○ Isolated/living alone
	  ○ Abusive/unsupportive relationships
	  ○ Homeless
		• Female*
		• Younger
		• Well-supported; lets you contact supporters
		• Employed/studying
		• Caring for children
		• Historic:
		  ○ Good engagement
		  ○ Help-seeking
		  ○ Coping strategies

*Women have higher self-harm rates, but men more often complete suicide, due to more violent methods.

Table 51.3 Current presentation: risk factors for completed suicide.

Questions to ask	Higher risk	Lower risk
MSE • *How do you feel about [self-harm] now?* • *Do you regret it?* • *What do you regret?* • *How are you feeling?*	Regrets survival; wants to die Ongoing stressors Mental illness, especially depression/psychosis Agitation Impulsivity Hopelessness Insomnia	Regrets self-harm Stressors resolved No mental illness Calm Hope
Future plans • *What are your plans for tonight/next week?* • *Do you still want to hurt yourself?* • *Are you thinking of killing yourself?* ○ If 'no': *It seems like it was so desperate … What's changed?* • *Does anything stop you hurting yourself?* • *What will you do if [stressor] happens again/ gets worse?* • *What do you want to happen next?*	Self-harm plans No protective factors Poor coping strategies Refusing help	No intent to self-harm Reasons to live Solid protective factors Good coping strategies Help-seeking

4. Risk assessment (see also p38–41)

List risk and protective factors, considering immediate and longer-term risk. Don't assume someone's safe, because of a single factor, e.g. being female. *Anyone* can kill themselves.

* Self: self-harm *and* suicide
  * Details of any ongoing plans: method, access to means, *where* and *when*
  * Triggers: current/future
  * Behaviours increasing Ben's risk
  * Can he seek help pre-emptively, or only *after* crisis/self-harm?
  * Coping skills. What stops him using these?
  * Access to means (e.g. tablets/other) – can you negotiate removal?
* Self: neglect, vulnerability to exploitation
* To others: aggression; child risk?

5. Capacity assessment

If Ben needs ongoing tests or treatment, assess his capacity to make these decisions (Ch.76).

6. Collateral history

* Can be hard, out-of-hours, but always try; record contact details
* Have they been worried about Ben?
* Why do they think he self-harmed? Were they surprised?
* Can they support him? How?

Box 51.1 Don't be fooled!

Some people seem low risk, but pose high risks of suicide. Listen to your 'gut feeling' and look out for patients who have:

* *Started to recover from depression*
  * More energy to implement plans
* *Recovered from a first episode psychosis*
  * Insight into the illness and potential disability may prompt self-harm
* *Recently been discharged from hospital*
  * Suicide is highest in the week post-discharge (even if seniors thought they were OK)
* *Made a serious suicide attempt, but suddenly want to live*
  * If stressors are unchanged, are they lying?
* *Lost their faith*
  * Suggests deepened hopelessness; may alienate them from support network
* *Chosen to cope alone*
  * Prevents carer awareness/support
* *Acted dangerously but didn't believe in the lethality*
  * Underestimating risk can accidentally kill
* *Repeatedly self-harmed*
  * Don't be blasé: their long-term risk is very high
  * Worry more if the frequency/type of self-harm changes

Management

TIP: Manage your own anxiety – try and be in a calm and reflective state of mind, rather than anxiously wanting to make a decision or sort a problem. Your need to *do* something or get somewhere in a hurry will prevent you taking in *their* difficulties. Try to think – not about trying to get it over with and go back to bed as soon as possible – but of a need to tolerate.

Duncan McLean, Consultant Psychiatrist and Psychotherapist

Take a break to step back and reflect on Ben's risk and any strong reactions you've had to him or his story, e.g. anxiety, irritation, helplessness. Don't underestimate complexity: to begin with, discuss *all* presentations with the PLN or senior on-call. This helps you think through options and stops you missing anything important.

1. Ensure medical problems are addressed

If Ben refuses treatment, but lacks capacity, treat in his best interests under the MCA (Ch.76).

PATIENT VIEW:

I cut myself once and it was pretty deep. Normally I take care of it myself but I went to hospital, waited about five hours and finally got seen. They said, "My first year student will stitch you up." The job he'd done was absolutely diabolical. I could do a better job and I can't even sew. I was just so, so angry.

'Henry'

---

2. Address mental illness

All mental illnesses increase the risk of suicide, so should be *treated* – often needing HTT, CMHT or admission. Treat people *safely*, remembering that prescriptions may become overdoses, and often won't work immediately, e.g. antidepressants. Discuss medication with your senior.

3. Instil hope

Whilst recognizing Ben may feel hopeless or overwhelmed, *you* can still have hope. Feedback on his strengths (e.g. intelligence, resilience, skills) and your belief things can improve. Back off if he resists this.

Ask whether he's had times when life felt very difficult. This may help him recognise that he's going *through* a very bad time, but won't always feel this way, especially if he can stay safe while tackling key problems.

4. Problem-solve

You may decrease risk by tackling stressors. List problems with Ben and target the most troubling/easily solved:
* Practical advice, e.g. sleep hygiene (p72), alcohol use
* Sign-post to help, e.g. Citizens Advice Bureau, homeless day centres
* Break problems into simple steps, e.g.
  ○ Tomorrow = call work to say ill
  ○ By Friday = see GP
* Involve family and friends
* Consider *limited* medication for insomnia/anxiety, e.g. three days' promethazine 25 mg.

5. Harm minimization and coping strategies

Ben may already want to avoid self-harm or minimise the risks. If not, use a motivational interviewing (MI, p74) approach to try and increase motivation for survival or safety, e.g.
* *What are the most helpful things about [X] (e.g. cutting)?*
* *Is there anything about [X] you don't like/that worries you?*
* *If you could change anything about [X], what would it be?*
* *I've met some people who self-harm but have found ways to make it a bit safer. Would it be OK if I shared some of their ideas with you?*

Skip this if Ben's dismissive or finds it patronising. Otherwise, discuss how he can meet the function of self-harm without placing himself in such danger. Introduce options respectfully, e.g. *It doesn't work for everyone, but would any of the following work for you … ?* (Table 51.4)

Table 51.4 Harm minimization.

Aim	Ideas
Identify and avoid triggers	• Keep a diary of situations triggering urges • If possible, avoid triggers until stronger • Don't be alone: seek out friends/family • Avoid alcohol/drugs (decrease inhibitions) • Store blades (etc.) out of sight • Avoid unmonitored self-harm websites/chat rooms

Reinforce motivation to stay safe	• List negatives/worries about self-harm, e.g.
	  ◦ Scars/not wanting to explain injuries to people
	  ◦ Hospital admission
	• Consider the effect of his death on loved ones
	• List positive things about himself
	• Build a shoebox of reminders of achievements/good memories; view when overwhelmed

Distract from self-harm thoughts	• Do something enjoyable, e.g. exercise, music/films, walk the dog • Help someone • Relaxation exercises/yoga
Delay self-harm	• Remember urges come and go • Set targets for *not* self-harming, e.g. walk dog, *then* review urges • Have non-self-harming reward for each target achieved
Alternatives to dangerous self-harm	*If the function requires pain:* • Squeeze ice-cubes • Bite a chilli/lemon • Take a cold shower • Snap an elastic band around his wrist *If the function relates to symbolism, e.g. self-punishment, expressing inner pain, marking his body:* • Draw 'cuts' with a red marker • Put plasters/bandages where he wanted to cut • Draw/photograph himself and draw self-harm or write his feelings over it $\pm$ destroy it.
If urges are overwhelming	• Buy a first aid kit • Don't self-harm while drunk/high • Use clean equipment, e.g. sterilize razors • Cut more safely, e.g. fleshy areas, avoid vessels • Call 999 if overwhelmed/injured.
If feeling suicidal or worried he'll self-harm dangerously	• Remove the means, e.g. give tablets/knives to carers • Contact friends/family • Call Samaritans • Attend ED

6. Admit or discharge?

After the above discussions, you should feel clearer about Ben's immediate risks. Involve him in the decision: how safe does he now feel? Run all decisions past seniors at first, and *always* consult when unsure (Table 51.5). You can:

- Discharge with GP/CMHT follow-up within seven days
- Discharge with HTT (*if* they accept him)
- Admit (± MHA assessment if refused).

If discharging, write Ben a simple *crisis plan* (p315) for feeling overwhelmed or suicidal, including contact details of carers, his CMHT and any crisis lines (e.g. Samaritans 08457 909090). He should attend ED if worse – explain he'll be taken seriously, even without self-harming.

Table 51.5 Factors affecting admission/discharge.

Discharge more likely	Admission more likely
• Good home support (confirmed *with* carers)	• High risk of self-harm
• Actively help-seeking	• Formed lethal plan and intent
• Confident he'd return to ED if risks increased	• Multiple risk factors
	• No/weak protective factors
	• Unsupported/lives alone
	• Unsure if he could return to ED, should risks intensify
	• Current psychosis, mania, severe depression
	• Ongoing stressors – clearly in crisis
	• No plans, but extremely hopeless/unpredictable

If Ben repeatedly self-harms:

- Admission may be unhelpful, e.g. preventing use of support networks
- You can fully acknowledge his distress without admitting him
- GP/CMHT could refer for psychology
- Link back in with existing care plans/teams, highlighting current difficulties
- If high risk, discuss with a senior. Admission, while best avoided, is no failure.

PATIENT VIEW:

The Samaritans saved my life that night. She listened to me, she understood where I was coming from. It wasn't too much for her to handle. The thing that kept me alive was she said, "I'll call you at nine" – this was at six. And it was that feeling – if she phones and I'm not here, I don't pick up, how's she going to feel? A complete stranger I'd never met, but I'd feel I'd be letting her down.

'Felix'

---

7. Documentation

Record your assessment and plan, including how you made decisions and excluded alternatives. Be defensible rather than defensive.

- Copy to the GP and involved professionals
- If ongoing psychiatric support's needed in the general hospital, handover to liaison
- If the assessment crosses into office hours, call Ben's CMHT. They may speak to him ± arrange same-day contact.

TIP: During busy on-calls, it can feel like people with personality disorders have rocked up with self-harm just to annoy you. Remember that however bad your day or night is going, it probably isn't as bad as theirs. Furthermore, you only have occasional days or nights like this. They experience lows like this many times a month.

Lizzie Hunt, ST4

What if ... ?

... He's a child?
See Ch.52.

... He walks out, mid-assessment?
See Ch.76

... He's drunk?
Don't assess until sober:
- He can't have a meaningful intoxicated conversation
- Intoxication increases risks of assault
- Sobriety may 'cure' suicidal thoughts.

Negotiate a realistic timeframe for assessment with ED, e.g. several hours if very drunk.
- Ensure a *full* physical assessment. Slurred speech, vomiting and ataxia *may* be alcohol-related, or more serious, e.g. head injury.
- ED may admit him to a medical assessment unit, reducing 'breach' pressures
- While drunk, he's likely to lack capacity, so may be prevented from leaving (MCA).

Once sober, assess for ongoing suicidality, and treatable mental illnesses.
- HTTs may refuse your referral if he's alcohol-dependent; discuss with seniors
- Some hospitals have alcohol liaison workers who'll assess people with primary alcohol misuse problems and signpost to local alcohol services. If so, consider referral. If not, signpost as appropriate to local addictions services.

... He's actively receiving medical treatment or is physically unwell?
Never refuse to see someone until 'medically cleared'. You might delay a full assessment, but can briefly review, gather information and advise on intermediate risk management, e.g.
- Where Ben can be most safely treated
- Need for 1:1 RMN/security
- Response if he tries to leave

... You tell Ben you're discharging him, and he *then* makes serious self-harm threats?
Take Ben seriously, and try to understand why he feels he needs admission. Are there other ways to meet these needs? If he says things that make discharge impossible, discuss with seniors, who may review him in person or advise a *short* crisis admission.

... He's on Section 136?

See Ch.48. If medical treatment isn't needed, ask the police to convey Ben to the designated Place of Safety for assessment. If he needs medical treatment:
- Commence immediately if consenting. If not, assess capacity, with the medics (Ch.76).
- The police may want to leave, especially if treatment's time-consuming. Negotiate with them, your senior, the AMHP and ED. If Ben's fit to talk, the s136 assessment may occur alongside medical treatment – this varies across the country, so discuss with seniors.

... He presents at your CMHT?

Ask someone to sit with Ben, whilst quickly gathering information.
- If you think he'll need HTT or admission, ask the Duty Worker to contact HTT/bed manager
- Jointly assess with the duty worker/CC
- In case Ben walks out, focus on the current crisis, risk/protective factors and MSE
- Discuss with your consultant ($\pm$ use it as a WPBA).

If sending Ben home
- Discussing psychology referral or medication may instil hope
- Consider HTT, or offer a swift review with you/CC (e.g. in 1–2 days)
- Document everything immediately, in case he presents out-of-hours
- Place him in Red Zone (p41).

If Ben agrees to a voluntary admission
- Ask someone (friend, relative, staff member) to sit with him whilst you organise this

If he refuses admission
- If high risk and unsuitable for HTT, discuss with seniors whether to arrange a MHA assessment. This may take a few days, so offer ongoing support/contact in the meantime.
- If *immediate* risks, your team *may* arrange an urgent MHA assessment at the team base.

If Ben walks out:
- You can't physically stop him – try to persuade him to stay
- You can either ...
  - Call the police: welfare check; if appropriate, they may pick him up on s136
  - Organise a MHA assessment at home.

... He's drunk at the CMHT?

It may be feasible for him to stay at the CMHT whilst sobering up.
- If impossible (e.g. late afternoon/against team policy), consider directing him to ED for assessment when sober. Discuss with the PLN first.
- Call the police if he becomes more risky. They can arrest him if drunk and disorderly (allowing him to sober up in custody) or intervene as above.
- Follow up the next day (review his notes, contact liaison if still in hospital; call Ben if he went home).

... Instead of attending, he calls, states he's suicidal, then hangs up?

Don't panic! This happens a lot. Consider the role of counter-transference: Ben has successfully displaced his anxiety onto you – but *has* communicated for a reason. If risks seem immediate (e.g. about to hang himself), try calling back immediately (e.g. dial 1471 to get his number) and find out more, including:
- His location
- Actual self-harm, e.g. details of overdose, if he's been sick, physical symptoms.

If risks don't sound imminent, briefly gather background information, including crisis plan. Discuss with seniors and PLN/CC – they may know Ben well and suggest helpful strategies.
- Call Ben back: engage, gain further information

- Offer to call an ambulance/assess him where you are (at the CMHT or ED)
- If he refuses help, is known and it's in office hours, his CMHT may clarify his crisis plan, make a home visit or call him back – so get them involved!
- Contact police for a welfare check if risks seem high or you can't contact Ben
- Document fully, including a timeline of calls and your follow-up plan.

Take-home message

Take a calm and thorough approach to self-harm assessments. Share decisions with colleagues and patients, documenting discussions. Well thought-out plans are usually defensible, even when things go wrong.

Further reading

Nordentoft, M. (2007) Prevention of suicide and attempted suicide in Denmark. Epidemiological studies of suicide and intervention studies in selected risk groups. *Danish Medical Bulletin*, **54** (4), 306–369.

Chehil. S. and Kutcher, S.P. (2012) *Suicide Risk Management: A Manual for Health Professionals*, Wiley-Blackwell, Chichester.

Kapur, N., Murphy, E., Cooper, J. *et al.* (2008) Psycho-social assessment following self-harm: results from the Multi-Centre Self harm project. *Journal of Affective Disorders* **106** (3), 285–293.

Broadbent, M. and Gill, P. (2007) Repeated self-injury from a liaison psychiatry perspective. *Advances in Psychiatric Treatment* **13**, 228–235.

NICE (2004) *CG 16 Self-harm: The short-term physical and psychological management and secondary prevention of self-harm in primary and secondary care*. NICE, England.

BMJ Best Practice series: Suicide risk management:
  ○ http://bestpractice.bmj.com/best-practice/monograph/1016/diagnosis/step-by-step.html

TOXBASE ~ www.toxbase.org

For patients

National Self-Harm Network: includes a forum for support and advice from other people who self harm: www.nshn.co.uk

CHAPTER 52

Self-harm in young people

Peter Hindley and Matthew Fernando

South London & Maudsley NHS Foundation Trust, London, England

> **RELATED CHAPTERS:** self-harm (51), child protection (64), child with challenging behaviour (75)

Kelly's 13 and was brought to ED by her father, Nick, following an overdose. Staff inform you she's medically cleared.

Assessing children and adolescents feels daunting before you've done a CAMHS job. The principles are the same as for adult self-harm (Ch.51), so this chapter focuses on the differences. You *must* discuss *every* presentation with the CAMHS senior on-call, and admit all self-harming under-16s to a paediatric ward overnight.

Preparation

1. Notes
- Known to social services? May show as an alert on ED notes.
  - If she's a Child In Need or subject to a Child Protection Plan, contact the duty social worker and consider assessing jointly
- Comorbidity, e.g. Autistic spectrum disorder (ASD), psychosis
  - Discuss complex presentations with your CAMHS senior first, as they may assess personally – observe, if possible.

2. Discuss with the treating paediatrician
- Any concerns or insights from observing Kelly's presentation and interactions with her dad.

3. Call Kelly's parents/carers to attend if not present

PATIENT VIEW:

Being a young person, someone taking the time just to listen and reassure me that I wasn't crazy was perfect. That these feelings were real and it was an illness just like any other. I was terrified, and a smiling face of someone who actually cared made the world of difference.

'Jo'

Psychiatry: Breaking the ICE – Introductions, Common Tasks and Emergencies for Trainees, First Edition.
Edited by Sarah Stringer, Juliet Hurn and Anna M Burnside.
© 2016 John Wiley & Sons, Ltd. Published 2016 by John Wiley & Sons, Ltd.
Companion Website: www.psychiatryice.com

Assessment

1. Approach
Don't try to be 'cool' – you'll seem ridiculous as you're officially *ancient*. Instead, be *interested* and show Kelly you take her seriously. Normalise your involvement: everyone sees a psychiatrist after self-harm.

Explain confidentiality early on. Under-18s are subject to parental authority, and you must share things with Nick to keep Kelly safe. You don't have to pass on non-risk-related information.
- *What we talk about will be kept private, unless I'm worried there might be a risk to you or other people. I'd tell you before sharing anything with your Dad or anyone else.*

Always make time to see the child and parent alone, but start with both together. Separate early if problems, e.g. rows/Kelly won't speak openly while Dad's present. The more collaborative your relationship with Nick, the safer Kelly will be at home. His importance is three-fold:
- Collateral historian
- His behaviour offers insights into family dynamics
- He may provide support and help with future therapy.

Judge whether to start with:
- The self-harm – best if Kelly may dismiss general conversation as pointless/ patronising
- Getting to know Kelly first – best if Kelly is shy or anxious, e.g. interests, friends and school. This can build rapport and highlights possible stressors, protective factors and resources.

> **TIP:** Be flexible, rather than following a rigid plan. This helps you come across as a person, rather than an intimidating doctor.
>
> **Lucy Wilford, ST3**

2. Full history, remembering...
- *Triggers:* bullying (including online), academic problems, relationship conflicts
- *Detailed self-harm history* (p319–322)
  - Check lethality – young people often greatly over- or underestimate this
- *SHx*
  - Resources: supportive friends, teachers, relatives; social media contacts
  - Current family functioning. Who's at home? Where are they now?
  - Tensions, conflict, domestic violence
- *Comorbidity*: screen for underlying problems, e.g. depression, psychosis
- *PPHx*: CAMHS, school counsellors, educational psychologists
- *Brief personal and developmental history*
  - Struggling or needing extra help at school; specific/general learning difficulties
  - ASD (p277)
- *FHx*: depression, suicide, substance misuse.

3. See Kelly alone (take a female chaperone if you're male)
- Explore areas where she's become quiet, guarded or embarrassed
- *Substance misuse*
- *Sexual history:* current sexual relationships? Consenting and age-appropriate?
- *Screen for abuse* – all types increase self-harm/suicide risk. Start open, becoming more specific, e.g.
  - *Has anything frightening or upsetting happened to you?*
  - *Has anyone done anything to you that you didn't want? ... Touched you in a way you didn't like? ... Made you do anything sexual against your will?*

TIP: Gay, lesbian, bisexual or sexually uncertain teens have higher risks of self-harm. If their sexuality hasn't yet coalesced into an identity, avoid labels and ask *who* they're attracted to, e.g. *Some teenagers have problems or worries about* who *they find attractive. Do you worry about that?*

Justin Wakefield, CAMHS Consultant

TIP: Do a 'digital MSE' – ask Who, What, Where, When and How about online activities and mobile 'app' use. Check both the support/benefits they get, as well any use linked to increasing risk or signs of ill-health. Be 'e-curious'! Build digital use into relapse signs and safety plans.

James Woollard, ST6 CAMHS

4. MSE, remembering ...
- Rapport
- Interaction between Kelly and Nick, e.g. supportive, over-involved, hostile? (Box 52.1)
- Self-harm scars
- Signs of abuse or neglect (Table 64.1, p395)
- Depression, e.g. self-neglect, tearfulness. Teens may show more overt irritability than sadness.

5. Risks, including ...
- Immediate self-harm/suicide
- Safeguarding – including siblings.

TIP: Kelly may be new to self-harm, and scared it's really weird. Reassure her and let her know it's a common problem. Conversely, she may have friends who self-harm or swap techniques. Find out where she's learnt things, and encourage her to suggest friends seek help too.

Matthew Fernando, ST5 CAMHS

Management

1. Discuss with the CAMHS senior
Trusts usually insist a CAMHS expert reviews all self-harming under-18s. If so, you'll usually explain what'll happen next, and document everything clearly.

2. Admit or discharge?
It's occasionally safe to send someone home with next day CAMHS follow-up, but the CAMHS senior makes *all* decisions.

Paediatric medical admission
All self-harming under-16s should be admitted overnight to allow a specialist CAMHS assessment the next day (NICE guidelines).
- Paediatrics know this, so you'll rarely have problems getting a bed, but if so, ask your senior to speak with the paediatric registrar
- Discuss supervision overnight with paediatrics, Kelly and Nick, e.g. 1:1 if very distressed.

Psychiatric adolescent unit admission

Kelly may need this if her risks can't be managed on a paediatric ward, e.g. actively self-harming; severe depression with pervasive suicidal thoughts; underlying psychosis.
• Your CAMHS senior must attend and assess *now*.

3. Instill hope and start problem-solving

Try to give hope by explaining:
• Self-harm can be frightening for all involved, but this is an opportunity to understand and tackle underlying problems
• Many young people self-harm, but most stop and find other ways to deal with stress; CAMHS will help with this.
Where appropriate, discuss basic, practical steps to resolve problems, e.g. bullying, conflicts.

4. Harm minimization and coping strategies

Start to develop a Crisis Plan (p315) with Kelly, including:
• Alternative strategies for coping with distress (Table 51.4, p325). Leave *safer* forms of self-harm to CAMHS, or Nick may think you're *teaching* Kelly to self-harm!
• Who to contact if distressed/irresistible urges (on the ward *or* at home)
   ○ ± Childline 0800 1111.

Box 52.1 Advice to carers

Nick may feel angry, overwhelmed, guilty or anxious. Explain self-harm isn't his fault (unless it is, e.g. child abuse). Offer him advice:
• Learn about self-harm, e.g. www.nshn.co.uk
• Be available to talk – neither avoiding nor forcing conversations
• Ask whether …
   ○ Kelly wants to talk about anything triggering self-harm
   ○ He can do anything to help
• Don't enforce 'help' – this removes Kelly's (probably limited) sense of control
• Stay calm and show concern but not shock, disgust or anger in response to self-harm
   ○ Strong emotions make everything worse
• Tell her he cares, and try to share enjoyable activities.

Nick should seek professional help when feeling out of his depth, and may need to talk things over with CAMHS.

5. Address mental illness

All under-18s presenting with self-harm need a CAMHS referral for follow-up within seven days. Explain to Kelly and Nick what to expect, e.g.
• *Reaction to social stressor but no psychiatric diagnosis* or *adjustment disorder*
   ○ Most presentations
   ○ CAMHS will focus on problem-solving and coping skills
• *Depression*
   ○ Primarily managed with talking treatments (CBT, interpersonal or family therapy, p68)
   ○ Medication may be used for moderate to severe depression, but psychotropic-use in under-18s is a specialist decision
• *Oppositional defiant disorder*
   ○ CAMHS will organise support, particularly helping Nick manage conflict and boundaries

- *Drug or alcohol misuse*
  ○ A substance misuse worker will work with Kelly
  ○ If Kelly doesn't want you to share this problem with Dad, ask your senior how much to share
- *Psychosis*
  ○ This uncommon presentation usually needs inpatient admission
  ○ Management combines talking treatments and medications (Ch.23).

6. Documentation

Clearly document your risk assessment and plan in the ED and psychiatric notes, handing over to ED, paediatrics and the incoming psychiatrist.

- Ensure a full CAMHS assessment happens tomorrow (you/CAMHS senior to refer)
- ± Refer to CAMHS for seven-day follow-up (check if the CAMHS registrar will do this)
- ± Refer to social services
  ○ Alert paediatrics and the duty social worker to suspected abuse or neglect
  ○ Paediatrics usually make the safeguarding referral
  ○ Self-harm may warrant a safeguarding referral in its own right – discuss with your senior. If referring, ensure Kelly and Nick understand this is to offer further support, otherwise it will come as a shock.

What if ... ?

... Kelly doesn't want you to tell her parents?

Balancing engagement and confidentiality can be tricky, but risk trumps everything. At the end of the interview, explain you'd like to tell Dad what Kelly's told you, but ask if there's anything she doesn't want you to share. Negotiate with her, but be clear you can't make a safe plan if the people she lives with don't understand the risks.

If there's something you think Dad should know, but isn't enough to break confidentiality (e.g. occasional drug use), it may be possible to get *Kelly* to tell him, e.g.

- *How do you think he'll react?*
- *Would it be easier if I was there when you tell him? Would you like me to tell him?*

... She tries to leave?

Find out why she wants to leave and encourage her to stay. If she has Fraser/Gillick competence (p103–4) and insists on leaving, you may need to use the MHA – but discuss with your senior. It is sometimes OK for a young person to leave with a safety plan in place, but again, you absolutely must discuss first with your CAMHS senior.

... She's a child?

Younger children may somatise depression, e.g. tummy aches/headaches. Ensure paediatrics exclude organic causes, and involve CAMHS seniors early.

... She's 16–17?

16–17year olds are treated more like adults and not routinely admitted to paediatric wards. You must still discuss with the CAMHS senior, and it may be best to keep Kelly on an adult medical ward overnight to allow a face-to-face CAMHS assessment tomorrow. If discharging, she'll need a clear crisis plan (p315), including CAMHS referral.

... Dad refuses an essential social services referral?

Explain that you're legally required to make the referral, but try to identify any fears, e.g. that social services will remove Kelly. Reframe involvement as a positive means of supporting the whole family.

... Dad wants to take her home?

Find out why Nick's so keen to take Kelly home, explaining this may prevent expert input. If Kelly won't be safe at home, she may need to be kept in hospital, against Nick's wishes. If extreme risks, the MHA may be needed, or even emergency police protection: discuss with the duty social worker and your CAMHS senior.

Take-home message

Most of the assessment is the same as for adults, but you're expected to rely on CAMHS seniors for management planning and discharges.

Further reading

Department of Health (2015) The Mental Health Act 1983: Code of Practice. (chapter 19). The Stationery Office, Norwich.
Department for Education (2015) Working Together to Safeguard Children: a guide to inter-agency working to safeguard and promote the welfare of children. Department for Education.
   ○ www.gov.uk/government/publications/working together to safeguard children 2
General Medical Council (2007) 0–18 years: Guidance for all doctors. General Medical Council, England.
   ○ www.gmc-uk.org/guidance/ethical_guidance/children_guidance_index.asp

Resources for patients/families

Help, support and information, primarily aimed at girls and women up to age 24: www.selfinjurysupport.org.uk/tess-text-and-email-support-service
Help, support and information on a range of mental health problems for patients and carers, including self-help guidance: http://www.youngminds.org.uk/

CHAPTER 53

First episode psychosis (FEP)

Rachel Thomasson

Manchester Royal Infirmary, Manchester, Lancashire, England

RELATED CHAPTERS: FEP CMHT (23), Psychosis – longer term (24), mania (54), Videos (See website)

You're asked to review university student Alex, 20y. He was recently referred to the CMHT but didn't attend. His mother brought him in as he's been withdrawn, mumbling to himself and today said the Secret Service was monitoring him.

Alex and his mum are unlikely to have come across psychosis before, and may have all kinds of worries about what's happening, e.g. brain tumour, spiritual possession, actual Secret Service involvement. Make this first contact reassuring and helpful: you'll allay anxieties, and make it easier for them to seek help in future.

TIP: Humanity – that would be my biggest request. When things are really scary, when you're losing your mind and you don't know if you can get back – to know you're being dealt with by *humans*, who have lives, families and loved ones. That's really important. Not only have I lost my sanity, but I've lost my humanity. The system can be de-humanising to staff as well, and sets up this situation where patients display horrible behaviour towards staff because they start forgetting that they're human beings. We're all in it together.

'Johan'

Preparation

1. Manage agitation – *if acutely agitated and risky, see Ch.74.*

2. Exclude/treat physical problems
- Discuss appropriate investigations with ED (Appendix A3), working in parallel to minimize delays
- If Alex lacks capacity, see Ch.76
- Alex may need sedation if highly agitated and investigations can't wait. However, ED staff may confidently give high doses, leaving him too sedated to assess for hours. Offer assistance!
- If Alex is resistant, but there's nothing clearly indicating an organic cause, tests *can* be organised from the ward or CMHT – use your judgment.

Psychiatry: Breaking the ICE – Introductions, Common Tasks and Emergencies for Trainees, First Edition.
Edited by Sarah Stringer, Juliet Hurn and Anna M Burnside.
© 2016 John Wiley & Sons, Ltd. Published 2016 by John Wiley & Sons, Ltd.
Companion Website: www.psychiatryice.com

3. Gather information – ED and psychiatric notes, collateral
- PPHx, PMHx, risks, substance misuse
- Mother: be sensitive, as talking privately may exacerbate Alex's paranoia
  - Current concerns/risk
  - Timeframe and impact on studies/relationships
  - Support at home if discharged.

> **TIP:** Don't *fight* medics who don't take physical concerns seriously – politely involve seniors.

Assessment

1. Approach
Logical curiosity is your best approach; showing disbelief or robustly challenging Alex's story will lose rapport. Think: *if* this was true, how would *you* feel, e.g. disturbed, shocked, frightened? Reflect these feelings back to Alex, rather than seeming unbothered.
Try to cross smoothly between hallucinations and delusions, e.g.
- If Alex tells you about the Secret Service (delusions):
  - *Have you heard them talking?* (hallucinations)
- If he describes the Secret Service talking about him (hallucinations):
  - *What do you think's going on? Why are they doing this to you?* (delusions)
Gently challenge towards the end of the assessment, e.g.
- *Is there any possibility there could be another explanation?*
- *As a psychiatrist, I've met people with similar problems where it's been related to mental illness. Is that possible with you? If I'm right, there are many things I can do to help you. Would you be willing to test out my theory?*

> **TIP:** When assessing someone with delusions, always regard the experiences as absolutely true whilst you're with them. This is the easiest way to avoid betraying any cynicism, and will automatically be felt by the patient as empathetic and understanding. It's usually quite possible to do this without expressing actual agreement with the beliefs discussed. If you're challenged about whether you share the beliefs, it's usually quite easy to sidestep it with phrases like, "I haven't experienced the things you have, but I can see that you're finding it very worrying." Patients usually accept this, if you genuinely mean it.
>
> **Lizzie Hunt, ST4**

2. Full history, remembering ...
- *HPC* (Ch.23)
  - Triggers, e.g. stress, drugs, non-adherence
  - Effect on life, e.g. studies, relationships
- *PPHx:* prodrome (p147) / duration of untreated psychosis (DUP) (p148)
  - Previous psychotic/affective episodes (Box 53.1)
- *FHx:* psychosis
- *Substance misuse*, especially cannabis, stimulants, legal highs
- *SHx*
  - Are family, partner, flatmates, university aware and supportive?
  - Can anyone at home support him?

Box 53.1 Psychosis differentials

Confusion (e.g. disorientation, clouded consciousness) indicates an *organic* – not functional – psychosis. However, being alert and oriented doesn't exclude organic causes.
- Organic
  - Intoxication/withdrawal
  - Delirium – any cause
  - Intracranial, e.g. space occupying lesion, trauma, infection, inflammation, temporal lobe epilepsy
  - Metabolic, endocrine or autoimmune problems
  - Medication (e.g. steroids) recently started/changed
  - Dementia
- Functional
  - Primary psychotic disorder
  - Severe depression/mania

3. MSE, remembering …
- Agitation; intoxication/withdrawal
- Formal thought disorder
- Mania, depression, irritability
- Delusions. *What will you do if this goes on … ?* (risk)
- Hallucinations
- Confusion (delirium?)
- Willing to engage? Wants to leave? Capacity to accept/refuse.

4. Risks, including …
- Self-harm/suicide; chaotic accidents; self-neglect
- Worsening mental/physical health
- Aggression
- Retributive violence.

Management

For psychoeducation about psychosis, see p150.

1. Exclude and treat physical health concerns
The depth of investigation depends on your level of concern and Alex's willingness to allow medical input (Ch.76 if refusing). Although Appendix A3 outlines useful tests, there's no definitive list for every patient, and different EDs have varied facilities. If barriers, think:
- *Would I be comfortable managing him on my psychiatric ward without this test?*
- *Will this test change immediate management?*
- *Is this:*
  - *Easily checked now, but harder later?*
  - *Hard to check now, but easier later?*

If Alex needs further medical investigation or treatment, admit to a medical ward. Provide a written plan (p314) and ask liaison psychiatry to review tomorrow.

2. Admit or discharge?
Weigh the following factors to decide if Alex's safe to go home:
- Immediate risks
- Symptom severity/complexity (in-patient assessment may help if severe / complex)
- Insight and willingness to engage

- Capacity
- Support at home (check by telephone if carers aren't in ED).

Home

If there's good support, few risks, and he's keen to engage, he can probably go home ±HTT. Refer to the local Early Intervention Service (if available and he meets their criteria), otherwise, the local CMHT.

- Ensure Alex knows who'll contact him, and when
- Draw up a crisis plan (p315) with Alex and Mum, including community contact details
- It's generally preferable to let CMHTs start antipsychotics, but discuss with your senior if needed
- *Consider* short-term symptomatic relief, e.g. 3 days' night sedation (zopiclone 3.75–7.5 mg or promethazine 25 mg).

Psychiatric admission

If concerned about Alex's safety at home, arrange a psychiatric admission.

- If unwilling or lacking capacity to consent to admission, ask him to stay in ED and organize an urgent MHA assessment (contact registrar ±duty AMHP).

3. Handover

Inform ED, Alex and carers of your opinion and plan. Complete community team referrals as necessary.

If admitting, handover as usual, plus:

- Try to assess medication-free to establish diagnosis and baseline symptoms
- If medication's needed for agitation …
  - Recommend benzodiazepines or promethazine, as neuroleptic naive
  - If antipsychotics are unavoidable, use low-dose, e.g. olanzapine 2.5–5 mg, aripiprazole 5 mg, risperidone 0.5–1 mg.

Update the GP, whatever the plan.

> **TIP:** With patients, stick to non-technical language as much as possible. Acknowledging a *mental health difficulty* or *vulnerability* – rather than prematurely ICDing a patient into a corner – can help with patient engagement, self-esteem and recovery.
>
> John Joyce, EIS Consultant

What if … ?

… It's drug-related?

Always check substance misuse, physical symptoms and offer a UDS.

- Try to decide if intoxicated, withdrawing, or both (i.e. polysubstance misuse)
- Intoxication states subside as the drug clears
  - Psychotic symptoms usually resolve fairly quickly
- Some drugs *trigger* ongoing psychosis that doesn't disappear with excretion
- Either way, psychoeducation and safety are essential, and admission may be needed
- Allow intoxication states to resolve in ED if brief (e.g. alcohol), or transfer to a medical or psychiatric ward if longer (psychiatric: only if medically fit)
- Assess the need for further input e.g. EI/CMHT/addictions services
- Withdrawal states are invariably unpleasant, but rarely fatal
  - The exceptions are severe alcohol/GBL withdrawal (Ch.77) – needing emergency inpatient medical management.

... It's not his first episode?

Common reasons for relapse include:
- Stress
- Medication non-adherence
- Substance misuse, especially cannabis/stimulants.

Explore and document relapse triggers and signs, to aid future care planning. Once medically cleared, you'd usually offer to restart his usual antipsychotic, unless:
- Clozapine >48h missed doses (needs re-titration, Ch.37)
- High side effect load (needs decreased dose/different medication)
- High doses (may need to restart at lower dose).

HTT/usual CMHT can often follow-up, but admission is needed if risks are high or medication management impractical, e.g. too chaotic/complex for HTT.

... He tries to leave? (see also Ch.76)

His mother may be able to persuade him to stay, but take over if this is becoming distressing. You can't use s5(2) in ED, but should decide if the risks require MHA assessment. If so, ask ED to call security (or an RMN) while contacting your seniors to arrange assessment. Decide whether the risks are such that – should Alex actively try to leave or behave dangerously – security should physically prevent this, using the least force possible. Document the framework:
- MCA – if lacks capacity
- Common law – if risks to others, or need to prevent immediate harm.

Security may have limitations, e.g. not trained in therapeutic restraint, policies they must follow; a face-to-face conversation is always more effective than asking staff to 'tell security to sit with him'.

Tell security that Alex is awaiting MHA assessment, and needs to stay in hospital:
- Ideally, provide them with written relevant ('need to know') information
- Cover: risks; legal framework being used; what to do if he tries to leave (e.g. physically prevent versus follow him and contact police if he walks out)

Offer medication as for agitation (p442–444). If he does leave, contact the police, explaining the circumstances, and need for MHA assessment – they may be able to find him and return him to hospital under s136 (Ch.48).

Take-home message

Always rule out organic illness in first episode psychosis. If not *now*, be clear *when* this will happen.

Further reading

Berger, G., Fraser, R., Carbone, S., *et al.* (2006) Emerging psychosis in young people – Part 1 – key issues for detection and assessment. *Australian Family Physician*, **35**, 315–321.

Compton, M. and Broussard, B. (2009) *The First Episode of Psychosis: A Guide for Patients and Their Families*. Oxford University Press, New York.

NICE CG 178 Psychosis and schizophrenia in adults: treatment and management (2014).

CHAPTER 54

Mania

Rachel Thomasson

Manchester Royal Infirmary, Manchester, Lancashire, England

RELATED CHAPTERS: bipolar affective disorder (BPAD, 25), first episode psychosis (53)

Police brought Josie to ED after she smashed a window. She's tachycardic, hypotensive and has a swollen hand. She hugged a nurse and shouted, "I'm living on light and sips of rainwater! Food's for lesser mortals!"

Manic patients can be humorous, provocative, intimidating and fun – sometimes simultaneously. Dramas can unfold quickly, so don't keep Josie waiting, and have a low threshold for a chaperone and senior support. You may also need to protect Josie's dignity and safety while she's too busy to think about such things.

Preparation

1. Manage agitation – if acute risks, see Ch.74.
2. Ensure ED address physical health
- Immediate problems, e.g. broken hand, dehydration?
- Organic causes, e.g. delirium, head injury
- If a first episode of psychosis, discuss the need for baseline tests (Appendix A3&4)
- UDS + pregnancy test, if possible
  - Sexual disinhibition raises the risk of unplanned pregnancy
  - Pregnancy affects prescribing and restraint decisions (p267)
- If refusing medical interventions, see Ch.76.

3. Gather information – police, notes ± collateral
- PPHx: diagnosis, usual relapse signature, effective treatments (Table 54.1)
- Risks
- Duration of carers' concerns? Can they support Josie if discharged?

Assessment

1. Approach
Don't mirror mania – you'll exacerbate it, e.g. by talking quickly and loudly, or playfully responding to flirting. Stay calm and set clear boundaries, e.g. *I want to help you, but we'll have to finish if you touch me again.*

Table 54.1 Differential diagnoses: high or unstable mood.

Differential	Subtype	Presentation
Single episode	*Depression*	See Ch.21
	Hypomania	Milder manic symptoms; social function intact
	Mania	Severe manic symptoms; loss of social function
	Mania with psychotic symptoms	Severe mania + psychosis
	Mixed affective	Simultaneous (or very rapidly alternating) manic and depressive symptoms
BPAD	*Bipolar I*	≥2 major mood episodes (at least one mania/mixed affective)
	Bipolar II	≥2 mood episodes (at least one hypomania; *never* mania).
	Rapid cycling disorder	≥4 affective episodes in one year
Cyclothymia		>2 years' mood instability. Neither depressive nor hypomanic symptoms are severe/enduring enough to diagnose BPAD II
Schizoaffective disorder		Psychotic and affective symptoms are equally weighted and arise together as schizomanic or schizodepressive episodes.
Emotionally unstable personality disorder (EUPD)		Chronic mood instability: 'mood swings' occur within the space of hours. Other EUPD symptoms are present (Ch.26)

Josie's poor concentration, pressured speech and flight of ideas may scupper a structured history, so:
- Keep questions succinct
- Interrupt politely when necessary
- Redirect the focus onto Josie (also deflects personal questions)
  ○ *I'd much rather hear about your rainwater diet. Tell me about that.*
- If a history's impossible, focus on the MSE.

2. Full history, remembering …
- *Key symptoms:*
  ○ Mood – elation, irritability; lability
  ○ ↑ – energy, interests, libido, ideas/creativity, confidence, optimism, impulsivity
  ○ ↓ – sleep, concentration, inhibitions
- *Triggers:* insomnia, stress, drugs, medications, non-adherence
- *SHx:* impact on work, finances, relationships
  ○ Who's at home? Can they support her?
- *PPHx*: previous affective episodes change diagnosis from a manic episode to BPAD
- *Substance misuse.*

3. MSE, remembering …
- Self-neglect, inappropriately dressed, overfamiliar, agitated
- Loud, pressured speech; flight of ideas, clang associations, puns
- Elation, irritability, lability
- Delusions, especially grandiose (talents, purpose) or persecutory
- Hallucinations
- Does she think she's unwell; does she want help?

> **TIP:** Flight of ideas and pressured speech can make it hard to follow manic conversations. If Josie's irritated by your inability to keep up, try appealing to her grandiosity, e.g. *I think I'm a little slow, compared with you!/I'm a bit out of my depth here. Could you explain that again, slowly?*

4. Risk assessment, including…
- Self-neglect, dehydration, exhaustion
- Self-harm – impulsive, planned, accidental
- Risky/unprotected sex
- Overspending
- Retributive violence
- Sexual/financial exploitation
- Aggression
- Driving
- Child risks?

Management

1. Admit or discharge?
Based on Josie's diagnosis, symptom severity and risks, decide whether she can be managed at home. As a rule of thumb, mania usually needs admission; hypomania *may* be treated assertively at home to prevent a full-blown manic episode (Table 54.2).

HTT ± Josie's regular CMHT must monitor closely for risk, treatment response, and need for admission. This will be more successful if they/you can:
- Offer practical support around psychosocial stressors
- Enlist carer support.

2. Medication
Discuss medication with your registrar and Josie.
- Stop any antidepressant
- Add night sedation, as insomnia worsens hypo-/mania, e.g. zopiclone 7.5 mg PO nocte
- Consider regular benzodiazepines if very agitated, e.g.
  - Clonazepam 0.5–2 mg PO qds *or*
  - Lorazepam 0.5 mg PO qds
- If relevant (and not pregnant), restart Josie's regular mood stabiliser/antipsychotic
  - Check if unsure whether to prescribe: usual dose/retitration/higher dose
  - Check mood stabiliser levels if possible
  - Advise team taking over to consider increasing dose to optimise response, if tolerance and levels allow, e.g. lithium aim for drug levels of 1.0–1.2 mmol/L
- If an antipsychotic is needed, start low dose, e.g. olanzapine 5 mg, aripiprazole 5 mg, *or* risperidone 0.5–1 mg
  - Take extra care if neuroleptic naive (risk of neuroleptic malignant syndrome, NMS, Ch.67) or you suspect an organic cause.

3. Handover
Document and inform everyone of the plan:
- If police want to press charges, take their details for follow-up
- Handover to the team taking over (HTT/ward/liaison)
- Share your plan with her GP
- If Josie's going home, give her a clear crisis plan (p315).

Table 54.2 Admission/discharge.

Home with HTT if …	Psychiatric admission	Medical admission
• Insightful and help-seeking, e.g. early relapse/hypomania • Capable carers at home (confirmed by telephone) • ±Known to services *Risky* if current substance misuse or historic disengagement	• High risks/chaotic/poor insight • No acute medical problems Arrange informal admission if willing and able to consent. Otherwise, organize urgent MHA assessment.	• Physical treatment needed (MCA) • ±MHA may be needed if refusing psychiatric treatment • Advise on medication + 1:1 RMN • Handover to liaison psychiatry – next day review

What if … ?

… It's a mixed picture?

Consider a mixed affective state (Table 54.1) if depression or mania *don't quite fit*, due to a mix of mood, drive and behavioural problems, e.g. depression with over-activity or sexual disinhibition.

• Differential includes rapid cycling (p164); mixed anxiety and depression, and mood lability in EUPD
• Explore depressive, manic, anxiety and psychotic symptoms
• Suicide risk is high
• Stop antidepressants
• Have a low threshold for admission. Patients may need intensive support and complex treatment regimes.

Take-home message

Support ED to investigate more thoroughly in first presentations or when an organic cause is *suspected*, e.g. history of cerebral SLE. Don't *over*-investigate patients with established BPAD, presenting with their typical relapse signature after a period of non-adherence.

Further reading

Bassett, D.L. (2010) Risk assessment and management in bipolar disorders. *Medical Journal of Australia*, **193** (suppl), S21–23.
Fountoulakis, K.N., Kontis, D., Gonda, X., Siamouli, M. and Yatham, L.N. (2012) Treatment of mixed bipolar states. *International Journal of Neuropsychopharmacology*, **15** (7), 1015–1026.
NICE CG185 Bipolar disorder: the assessment and management of bipolar disorder in adults, children and young people in primary and secondary care (2014).

Resources for patients/carers:

MIND booklet on bipolar affective disorder: includes self-help advice and guidance for family and friends: http://www.mind.org.uk/information-support/types-of-mental-health-problems/bipolar-disorder/#.VChEDRY1DXM.

CHAPTER 55

Delirium

Vivienne Mak[1], Sean Lubbe[2], and Sean Cross[1]

[1] *South London & Maudsley NHS Foundation Trust, London, England*
[2] *UNSW Black Dog Institute, New South Wales, Australia*

RELATED CHAPTERS: drugs (41), older adults (30, 46), safeguarding (63), treatment refusal (76), delirium tremens (77)

Mrs Black is 86 and lives with her daughter, Suki. The memory clinic recently diagnosed mild cognitive impairment. She was admitted to hospital three days ago with a fractured hip, and is now confused and trying to leave.

Delirium (acute confusional state) is a neuropsychiatric syndrome and medical emergency, with high mortality and morbidity rates. It's a *clinical* diagnosis, which should trigger a thorough investigation, rather than a shoulder shrug (Table 55.1). Remember:
- 'Confusion' is often used inaccurately, e.g. any unusual behaviour
- True confusion indicates an organic state, i.e. disorientation, clouded consciousness, muddled thinking, inattention
- Older adults don't always raise a fever or inflammatory markers, so normal results *don't* exclude delirium
- Top delirium risk factors are:
  - ≥ 65y
  - Pre-existing cognitive impairment
  - Current hip fracture
  - Severe illness.

Cases are often complex, and your role is supporting the medics, not taking over management. When unsure, encourage them to investigate as they would a *new* patient, and treat for delirium first.

TIP: Don't overlook *hypoactive* delirium: lethargy and psychomotor retardation. The 'well-behaved' patient, sitting quietly and fully compliant may be extremely unwell. These patients are often referred for 'depression' or poor engagement with rehabilitation.

Preparation

If Mrs Black *is* delirious, you'll probably need to gather information from other sources (Table 55.2).

Psychiatry: Breaking the ICE – Introductions, Common Tasks and Emergencies for Trainees, First Edition.
Edited by Sarah Stringer, Juliet Hurn and Anna M Burnside.
© 2016 John Wiley & Sons, Ltd. Published 2016 by John Wiley & Sons, Ltd.
Companion Website: www.psychiatryice.com

Table 55.1 Delirium signs and symptoms.

Onset	Acute change
Course	Fluctuating
Cause	**D**rugs / **D**rink / **D**ehydration
	Electrolyte disturbance
	Lots of pain
	Infection / **I**nflammation
	Respiratory failure (hypoxia/hypercapnia)
	Impaction (Faecal / constipation)
	Urine retention
	Metabolic disorder (liver/renal failure, hypoglycaemia) / **M**alnutrition
	Sensory impairment / **S**leep problems
Cognitive symptoms	Inattention/distractibility
	Altered conscious level: fluctuating, hyper-alert, drowsy
	Disorganised thinking
	Disorientation
	Poor short-term memory
Other Symptoms	Hallucinations or illusions – especially visual
	Labile mood
	Delusions – commonly persecutory
	Psychomotor agitation or retardation
	Disturbed sleep/wake cycle

NB: Mnemonic DELIRIUMS used with permission of Guy's and St Thomas' Hospital NHS Foundation Trust.

Assessment

1. Approach
If Mrs Black is confused, frightened or potentially aggressive, a friendly but polite approach can be disarming, e.g.
- *Hello, Mrs Black. I'm sorry to see you in hospital. I was talking to your daughter Suki, and she said you were unwell.*

Introduce yourself and explain why you're seeing her. Simple, clear communication is key (p276). Where able:
- Ensure she has her glasses/hearing aids
- Minimise distractions and background noise
- Reassure her she's safe and you want to help
- Re-orientate – remind her where she is and who you are
- Read behaviour as a form of communication, especially if she can't express herself verbally, e.g. if wandering, is she searching for something, escaping a persecutor, or desperate for the toilet?

If she rambles off topic, acknowledge *feelings* (even if the content's confusing) and gently refocus. Closed questions may help if very thought disordered.

> **TIP:** *Consider* gently holding her hands if she allows. This may reassure, help maintain attention, and give you an early warning if she tries to lash out.

2. Focused history, remembering …
- *HPC:*
  - Check for the common worries of psychosis and confusion, e.g. theft, people trying to harm her, poisoned food; seeing strange/frightening things; being lost
  - Systems review, especially pain, thirst, constipation, urinary symptoms

Table 55.2 Information-gathering in delirium.

Information needed	Source				
	N	I	DC	S	C
Carers' contact details	✓				✓
Cause(s) of delirium	✓	✓	✓	✓	✓
Delirium signs and symptoms	✓			✓	✓
Baseline cognitive function, ± historic test, e.g. MMSE / Abbreviated Mental Test (AMT) / M-ACE	✓				
Baseline function/ADLs + chronology of any deterioration	✓			✓	✓
Sensory impairment ± usual aids • Hearing aids, glasses; dentures, mobility aids	✓			✓	✓
PMHx, especially … • Chronic disease making delirium harder to clear • Affecting medication choice	✓				✓
PPHx, including … • Usual relapse signature • Pre-existing cognitive impairment	✓				✓
Medications • Delirogenic, especially opiates, steroids, benzodiazepines, TCAs, anticholinergics • Omission of usual medications, e.g. benzodiazepines, steroids • Delirium treatments: appropriate choice and dose? (p350) • Adherence • Drug levels	✓	✓	✓	✓	✓
Substance misuse, especially alcohol, benzodiazepines/sleeping tablets	✓	✓	✓		✓
Challenging or risky behaviour (home/ward)? • Wandering, falls, absconding • Aggression • Vulnerability to neglect/exploitation/abuse • Resisting essential medical/nursing care	✓			✓	✓
Current sleep pattern ± reversed sleep-wake cycle	✓			✓	✓
Eating and drinking	✓			✓	✓

Key: N = notes; I = Investigations; DC = Drug Chart; S = Staff; C = Carers

- As able, check:
  - PMHx – especially recent changes
  - PPHx
  - Substance misuse.

3. MSE, remembering ...
- Agitation/retardation, aggression, self-neglect. Packed and ready to leave?
- Rambling, repetitive speech. Formally thought disordered/mute.
- Labile/flattened affect
- Delusions, commonly persecutory; often ill-formed, changeable
- Visual hallucinations/illusions are typical; any modality is possible
- Fluctuating consciousness/hyper-alert/drowsy
  - Poor orientation, attention, short-term memory and ability to follow instructions
  - Easily distracted by other things going on
  - If well enough, MMSE/M-ACE and compare with baseline; if not, check orientation to time and place + attention with serial 7s/WORLD backwards
- Insight is usually limited.

> **TIP:** An AMT ≤7, or MMSE ≤24 *or* a new drop from usual performance – all increase the suspicion of dementia/delirium. *But* don't be a slave to numbers. A good score may reflect a lucid moment ...

4. Assess capacity
If Mrs Black wants to refuse care or leave, assess her capacity to make these decisions (Ch. 76).

5. Diagnosis
Delirium is the most likely diagnosis, but differentials are:
- *Dementia* (Ch.30)
  - A new stroke can cause a sudden step-down in cognition *or* delirium
  - Dementia with Lewy Bodies (DLB) typically fluctuates ± visual hallucinations
  - NB Treat a fluctuating picture as delirium first
- *Functional psychosis* – may cause thought disorder ± poor concentration
  - *Can* present late
  - If there's a history of psychosis, assume delirium unless this is the usual relapse signature, with clear consciousness and minimal cognitive change from baseline (Box 55.1).

Box 55.1 Short Confusion Assessment Method (CAM). (*Source:* Adapted from Inouye et al. 1990.)

Diagnosis of delirium = CAM Positive, i.e. 1+2 + (3 or 4)
1 Acute onset, fluctuating course
2 Inattention
3 Disorganised thinking (illogical/rambling)
4 Altered consciousness (drowsy or hyper-alert)
However:
- *Any* of these signs raises the possibility of delirium
- Being *CAM negative* doesn't *exclude* delirium (may indicate a lucid moment)

Management

1. Nursing

Good nursing care is essential. Be respectful and avoid patronising nurses when offering advice. They may more willingly accept tips from a PLN than you. Key points are:

- *Reassurance and reorientation* – as often as necessary
  - Good lighting in the day so she can see clearly
  - Low-level night lighting to help orientate if she wakes, but not prevent sleep
  - Avoid changing beds, bays and staff. Allocate one nurse per shift and consider a *single* move, closer to the nursing station or into a quieter bay.
- *Maintaining safety* – consider a 1:1 RMN while Mrs Black's a risk to herself/others
- *Good food and fluid intake* – assist/ensure sufficient time
  - ± Dietician review
- *Regular toileting* – monitor bowel movements
  - Treat constipation/UTIs
  - Don't catheterise unless essential
- *Pain monitoring* – staff may need to use pain scales adapted for cognitive impairment
  - ± Regular paracetamol to prevent discomfort
- *Mobilisation* – as soon as possible
  - Older adults decondition rapidly – a few unnecessary bedbound days may make the difference between her going home or into care
- *Sleep hygiene* (p72) – try to keep her awake all day; consider night sedation.
  - Melatonin may be worth a try

2. Medical

Delirium is a medical problem, with a medical cause. Work closely with medical colleagues to ensure a full delirium work-up (Appendix A2).

- Delirium can be caused by almost anything, especially in cognitively impaired patients. Don't be put off by, *"But she doesn't have an infection"*.
- There's often a delay between the underlying problem resolving and a delirium clearing (e.g. in some cases it can take months).

- Ensure they don't only look for one cause. Encourage them to keep looking and optimize physical health. This includes:
  - Removing unnecessary catheters/lines
  - Treating constipation
  - Treating pain
  - Checking the drug chart with a pharmacist for delirium-exacerbating drugs.

3. Psychiatric

Psychiatrists are often involved in diagnosing and managing delirium, particularly where it causes risky or challenging behaviour – though many hospitals now have a delirium service, which may take over care. Follow Trust guidelines and don't prescribe medication unless Mrs Black is:
- Posing risks to herself or others
- Very distressed, particularly by delusions or hallucinations (Box 55.2).

Remember that all sedatives can cause delirium. The key principles are:
- Use a single drug
  - Usually haloperidol 0.5 mg (maximum 5 mg/24 h in elderly)
  - Sometimes olanzapine 2.5 mg (maximum 7.5 mg/24h in elderly)
- Start prn: lowest dose, repeated as necessary 1–2 hourly
- Be prepared to go straight to regular medication if someone's very disturbed
- Clearly document the maximum 24h dose
- Review daily
- Tailor to age, body size and degree of agitation
- Titrate up as needed
- Use oral rather than IM, whenever possible
- Monitor physical obs closely after IM medications.

Use benzodiazepines *(e.g. lorazepam 0.5–1 mg max 2 mg/24 hrs)* instead if:
- Parkinsonism, suspected DLB
- Prolonged QTc (>440 ms in men; >470 ms in women)
- No ECG *or* there is history of arrhythmia
- Seizures
- Alcohol or drug misuse (see Ch. 77).

Medication is short-term (usually <1 week), and should be continued for a week after delirium has apparently resolved.

Box 55.2 Legal frameworks

You may also be asked to assist with capacity assessment (Ch. 76) or even to 'section' Mrs Black if she's trying to leave. There's often a question of whether DoLS or the MHA should be used.
- *Medical Treatment*
  - As a general rule, given under the MCA. The treating team should assess capacity and make a best interests decision for each treatment.
- *Confining a patient to a ward*
  - If it's felt to be in her best interests to stay on the ward, this may come under a different legal framework
  - DoLS vs MHA is a common area of conflict and confusion
  - Where there's deprivation of liberty and the person would be detainable under the MHA, this should be used if there is no less restrictive option
  - As the law around DoLS is changing rapidly, discuss individual cases with an AMPH/oncall senior

4. Talk to carers

Involve the family in management. This may comfort Mrs Black, reduce carers' anxiety and helplessness, and assist the medical team in providing the best possible care. Suki may be distressed by her mother's confusion, and fear the change is permanent – take time to explain delirium, and that it usually remits over time. Find a hospital leaflet on delirium (or download from the Alzheimer's Society).

Encourage her family to visit often, and:
- Reassure
- Reorientate
- Reminisce
- Bring personal items and family photos
- Offer favourite drinks and snacks at each visit
- Help with personal care if this is difficult, e.g. dressing, combing hair
- Avoid arguments; don't be frustrated by repetition.

5. Follow-up

Handover to liaison psychiatry to follow-up, especially ensuring antipsychotics/ benzodiazepines are stopped.

Delirium often resolves completely, but can also herald dementia – or uncover it. If Mrs Black wasn't known to any services, you'd ask her GP to formally test cognition, three months post-discharge and refer any concerns to the Memory Clinic.

As the Memory Clinic already know Mrs Black, write to them to update them and ensure they can review and monitor progress. The more complex her social or psychiatric history, the more appropriate a referral to the Mental Health of Older Adults (MHOA) service.

What if ... ?

... It's a young person?

Have a lower threshold for considering substance misuse as a cause. Drugs and alcohol can cause, mask or mimic a range of psychiatric symptoms, and multiple drugs may cause simultaneous intoxication or withdrawal (Appendix C6). Gain a UDS if possible.

Intoxication states subside as the drug is cleared, but the patient's risk and safety may need to be managed until then. Withdrawal may need to be managed assertively (Ch. 77).

Higher medication doses can often be used in fit younger adults, e.g. haloperidol 5 mg, olanzapine 5 mg, lorazepam 1–2 mg. Take extra care with antipsychotics if you suspect a post-ictal state, or alcohol withdrawal, as they lower the seizure threshold.

... Staff say she needs placement ('banding')?

Although delirious patients are likely to improve and go home, there's sometimes pressure to 'band' them for residential/nursing homes. Notice any talk of 'bed-blocking' and resist inappropriate placement, as this can cause them to irreversibly lose their home.
- Nobody should be permanently placed in a care home due to delirium alone
- Temporary transfer to a more appropriate environment may be needed if acute medical problems have resolved but there's ongoing challenging behaviour or need for supportive care, e.g. psychiatric ward, respite/rehabilitation placement. This may reduce the risk of iatrogenic infections, e.g. *C.difficile*. Involve MHOA psychiatrists.

In patients with underlying dementia, the admission may uncover an unsafe home situation.
- Once the delirium resolves, the MDT should assess the ongoing level of function and need
- A package of care should always be considered – and preferably tried – before placement
- Whilst someone lacks capacity, any important or irrevocable decisions should either be delayed or made via a *best interests meeting*, involving the MDT and family/IMCA.

Should a decision be taken that someone requires institutional care, conveying isn't generally viewed as a deprivation of liberty, so is done under the MCA. The nursing home can apply for DoLS in advance or upon the person's arrival.

Take-home message

Delirium is a medical emergency, but psychiatry often has a supportive role in diagnosis and behavioural management. Delirium's often multifactorial – so once you've found the cause of the delirium, keep looking. And remember, one third of cases are preventable …

Reference

Inouye, S., van Dyck, C. *et al.* (1990) Clarifying confusion: the confusion assessment method. *Annals of Internal Medicine*, **113** (12), 941–948.

Further reading

NICE (2010) CG103 Delirium: Diagnosis, prevention and management. NICE, England.
Potter, J. and George, J. (2006) The prevention, diagnosis and management of delirium in older people in hospital: concise guidelines. *Clinical Medicine*, **6** (3), 303–308.
Witlox, J., Eurelings, L.S.M., de Jonghe, J.F.M. *et al.* (2010) Delirium in elderly patients and the risk of postdischarge mortality, institutionalization, and dementia: A meta-analysis. *Journal of the American Medical Association* **304** (4), 443–451.

Patient/family resource:

http://www.rcpsych.ac.uk/healthadvice/problemsdisorders/delirium.aspx.

Video: *Barbara's story*

http://www.guysandstthomas.nhs.uk/education-and-training/staff-training/Barbaras-story.aspx.

CHAPTER 56

Obsessive compulsive disorder (OCD)

Natasha Liu-Thwaites[1] and Rachel Thomasson[2]

[1] *South London & Maudsley NHS Foundation Trust, London, England*
[2] *Manchester Royal Infirmary, Manchester, Lancashire, England*

RELATED CHAPTERS: anxiety (22), trauma (31), panic attacks (57)

Kwame, 23, was sent to ED by his GP after reporting he might sexually assault a woman. Staff report he's been tearful, refused to see the female doctor, and repeatedly asked if he's accidentally touched anyone. Kwame keeps checking his body for signs of arousal, and mentally 'retracing his steps' in case he's assaulted someone.

Distress is key here, suggesting Kwame's thoughts are egodystonic: going against what he values about himself. This chapter addresses sexual thoughts in OCD – if you can handle these, you can handle any OCD presentation. A good knowledge of symptomatology separates a high-risk sex offender from an extremely low-risk OCD sufferer, or someone with delusions of guilt. For *actual* sex offending, see Table 56.2, p355, p425–427.

Preparation

1. Gather information – collateral, GP, psychiatric notes
- PPHx: suggestion of OCD, depression or psychosis?
  - Usual presentation and treatment?
- Concerns when last seen?
- Risk history.

2. Review OCD symptomatology (Table 56.1)

Assessment

1. Approach
Keep calm and non-judgmental: empathise with how upsetting the thoughts feel. Kwame may be too ashamed to say what's wrong. Without putting words into his mouth, try suggesting areas, e.g.
- *Some patients I see have thoughts that really disturb them. Some might worry they're gay when they don't want to be. Others worry they're paedophiles, rapists or murderers. Do you worry about anything like that?*
If he's worried about you involving police or social services, explain:
- *I'd only break confidentiality if I thought there was a serious risk of harm to you or someone else. I'd tell you beforehand if I felt I needed to do that.*

Psychiatry: Breaking the ICE – Introductions, Common Tasks and Emergencies for Trainees, First Edition.
Edited by Sarah Stringer, Juliet Hurn and Anna M Burnside.
© 2016 John Wiley & Sons, Ltd. Published 2016 by John Wiley & Sons, Ltd.
Companion Website: www.psychiatryice.com

Table 56.1 OCD Symptoms.

Symptom	Description	Examples
Obsessions	Thoughts, images, impulses or doubts	Contamination
		Violence
	Recurrent, intrusive, distressing, egodystonic	Sex
		Religion
	Seen as illogical (at some level, when not acutely distressed)	Immorality
	Recognised as person's own thoughts	
Compulsions	Repeated rituals to 'undo' obsession and decrease anxiety	Cleaning
		Checking
	Can be overt (actions) or covert (thoughts)	Counting
		Ordering
		Silently repeating a prayer/phrase
Safety-seeking behaviour	Other means to neutralize or lower anxiety	*Avoidance* of triggers, e.g. children, if paedophilic obsessions
		Seeking reassurance
		Strict routines
		Being extra careful or slow to prevent mistakes

2. Full history, remembering…
- *HPC*: OCD symptoms and effect on life
- *Comorbidity*, e.g. depression, other anxiety disorders, substance misuse
- Exclude psychosis.

3. MSE, remembering…
- Compulsions, safety-seeking behaviours
- Anxiety ± depression
- Obsessions, covert compulsions
- Delusions/thought insertion = psychosis
- Suicide/self-harm.

4. Risk
- *To* others – likely to be extremely low if OCD (Table 56.2)
- *From* others if he's disclosed thoughts
- Suicide/punitive self-harm
- Neglect/unintentional harm e.g. of childcare responsibilities

Management (OCD)

If depression, see Ch.21; psychosis, Ch.53.

1. Psychoeducation
Be very clear that this is OCD, and there are effective treatments.

Everyone experiences intrusive thoughts, e.g. urges to jump in front of trains; images of sexually inappropriate behaviour. Most people just shrug their shoulders and move on. People with OCD:
- Try to block these thoughts, making them worse because their brain has to *think* about the thing to remember to block it out
- Tend to believe the experience is evidence that they're *bad* (or risky, abnormal, perverse)
  - It's not – it's *normal!*
  - Also, 'bad' people wouldn't worry like this!

TIP: Demonstrate intrusive thoughts
- Say: *Don't think about purple penguins for one minute*
- After a minute's silence, ask:
  - *What happened?*
  - *What do you make of that?*

Table 56.2 OCD or potential sexual offender?.

	OCD	Sex offending (p425–427)
Thoughts	Egodystonic → anxiety, distress, guilt	Egosyntonic →pleasure, excitement
	Resisted	Actively summons thoughts
Behaviours	Avoids triggers and potential 'victims'	Seeks out opportunities to see/contact possible victims
	Won't act on/masturbate to thoughts	Acts on/masturbates to thoughts
Other	Discloses irrelevant past sexual history	Hides/minimizes/normalizes/lies about sexual history
	Help-seeking	Avoids help/authorities
	Other OCD symptoms	No OCD picture

2. Admit or discharge?

Emergency admission is rarely needed, unless Kwame's at high risk of self-harm. Involve HTT if the risk is moderate, otherwise, refer for follow-up by the GP, or CMHT if more complex.

3. Treatment

Give information on the options.
- *Self-help*, e.g. see resources; mindfulness (Box 56.1), relaxation (p72)
- *CBT* – first choice treatment in OCD
  - Explain (p68) and suggest a referral, e.g. via GP
- *Medication:* SSRIs or clomipramine, preferably *with* CBT
  - Give information, but ask his GP/CMHT to start and monitor
  - A low-dose antipsychotic may be added later if poor response.

Box 56.1 Mindfulness approach

Help Kwame distance himself from his thoughts. Ask him to imagine he's on a bench by a road; the passing cars are his thoughts. It's stressful and pointless to:
- Try stopping all the cars or shout at them to go away
- Scrutinize each car intensely, searching for hidden danger.
Thoughts, like cars, come and go – try to just *notice* them, rather than judging, resisting or getting caught up in them. It's hard at first, but easier with practice – mindfulness (p68) may help.

> **PATIENT VIEW:**
> They tell you that you need to relax. They don't tell you about alternative therapies like yoga that tell you *how* to de-stress.
>
> 'Helena'

Take-home message

Phenomenology is key. Don't drag an OCD patient through an excessive risk assessment, which may be harmful, e.g. confirming their worry that they're dangerous.

What if ... ?

... You're asked to assess a sex offender?
See p425–427.

Further reading

NICE (2005) CG31 Obsessive-compulsive disorder and body dysmorphic disorder. NICE, England.
Veale, D., Freeston, M., Krebs, G., Heyman, I. and Salkovskis, P (2009) Risk assessment and management in obsessive-compulsive disorder. *Advances in Psychiatric Treatment*, **15** (5), 332–343.

Patient resources

Challacombe, F., Oldfield, V. and Salkovskis P. (2011) *Break Free From OCD: Overcoming Obsessive Compulsive Disorder with CBT*. Vermilion: London.
OCD-UK. Support and resources including a telephone advice line: www.ocduk.org
OCD Action. Support and resources including local support groups and advocacy: www.ocdaction.org.uk
Mindfulness resources:
  ○ www.headspace.com
  ○ www.bemindful.co.uk

CHAPTER 57
Panic attacks

Natasha Liu-Thwaites

South London & Maudsley NHS Foundation Trust, London, England

RELATED CHAPTERS: anxiety (22), trauma (31), panic attacks (57), somatisation (61)

Linda, 36, has been 'blue-lighted' to ED three times this week with palpitations, chest pain, breathlessness and dizziness. Each time, she thought it was a heart attack. The ED registrar has fully assessed Linda, excluded a medical cause, and requests your review.

Panic attacks are terrifying, and often mistaken for medical emergencies. Once medical causes are excluded, your role is to contain Linda's anxiety and offer psychoeducation. Panic attacks can be one-off events, recurrent (panic *disorder*), *or* denote severity in another anxiety disorder (Ch.22).

PATIENT VIEW:

It was clear from the way she spoke to me that I was being troublesome because I'd come out-of-hours. And that surely I could have managed my anxiety at home if I'd just tried to rest and quietened myself down. The way she spoke to me was with utter disrespect and a kind of patronising manner, that I was causing a considerable amount of trouble. I felt utterly patronised, undermined … humiliated. All the efforts I'd made to stay well had been impeded by the system and now that system was blaming me for where I sat.

'Jenny'

Preparation

1. Gather information – collateral, ED and psychiatric notes
- Have medical diagnoses been excluded? E.g. asthma, cardiac, hyperthyroidism
- Check for a normal, recent ECG and relevant bloods (FBC, TFTs, glucose)
- PPHx, including treatments.

2. Take
- Investigation results
- Information leaflets on panic attacks/anxiety.

Psychiatry: Breaking the ICE – Introductions, Common Tasks and Emergencies for Trainees, First Edition.
Edited by Sarah Stringer, Juliet Hurn and Anna M Burnside.
© 2016 John Wiley & Sons, Ltd. Published 2016 by John Wiley & Sons, Ltd.
Companion Website: www.psychiatryice.com

Assessment

1. Approach
Stay calm, kind and reassuring. Initially reflect Linda's words (e.g. 'heart attacks', 'funny turns') – rather than labelling the problem *panic attacks*, which may feel dismissive.
Aim to understand her:
- Interpretation of symptoms
  - *What do you think's happening when you get these feelings?*
  - *What thoughts go through your head at these times?*
- Feared outcome
  - *What's the worst thing you think could happen?*
  - *… And what's the scariest part for you about that?*
  - If not forthcoming: *Some people might worry they'll faint, lose control, go mad, have a stroke, or even die. Do you worry about anything like that?*

2. Full history, remembering …
- *HPC*: detailed description of panic attacks
  - Suffocating feelings, chest tightness, can't 'catch' breath (hyperventilation)
  - Paraesthesiae: lips, fingers, toes; digit cramp/spasms
  - Depersonalization/derealization
  - Intense fear/discomfort
- *Triggers*
  - Out of the blue, or clear trigger?
  - Stressors *before* attacks started, e.g. family heart attack
- *Safety-seeking behaviours:* avoidance, escape, taking aspirin, calling 999 … ?
- *Comorbid*
  - Anxiety disorder, especially agoraphobia
  - Substance misuse: drugs, alcohol, caffeine
  - Depression (*Would you still be depressed if the attacks ended?*).

3. MSE, remembering …
- Reassurance-seeking
- Hyperthyroid signs?
- Anxiety, panic, depression.

4. Risk, remembering …
- Suicide/self-harm
- Iatrogenic.

5. Physical assessment
Go through Linda's test results with her, but don't reinforce anxiety by repeating investigations or examination – they'll temporarily allay fears, but are never enough!

Management (Panic disorder)

See Ch.22 for other anxiety disorders

1. Psychoeducation

After a full history, introduce the idea of panic attacks. Linda may be relieved *or* find it hard to accept, especially if still frightened something bad will happen. Stay patient and empathic – the more she understands, the more likely she'll accept therapy.

- Panic attacks are the most extreme version of the 'fight or flight' response (p144)
  - They *feel* terrifying but are harmless
- People commonly misinterpret the symptoms as a sign of catastrophe
  - In her case, heart attacks
  - This misunderstanding worsens panic and makes attacks more likely
  - It's completely understandable that she seeks medical help …
  - … But other treatments are essential to get better (below).

2. Admit or discharge?

Emergency admission or HTT are rarely needed, unless there's a risk of suicide. Refer to the GP for follow-up, or CMHT if more complex, e.g. severe agoraphobia.

3. Treatment

Give information on the options.

- *Self-help*, e.g. information leaflet; see Resources
  - Relaxation (p71), sleep hygiene (p72)
  - Reduce/stop: caffeine, drugs, alcohol
- *CBT:* the first choice treatment for panic disorder
  - Explain (p68) and suggest a referral, e.g. via GP
- *Medication*
  - SSRIs (preferably *with* CBT)
  - Give information, but ask her GP/CMHT to start and monitor.

Don't prescribe benzodiazepines in the ED, and educate your colleagues about this! Though effective short-term, they're highly addictive and may worsen Linda's longer-term prognosis. If she's using benzodiazepines or other sedatives, she and her GP should withdraw these gently.

TIP: Remember the patients are at the core of all we do. Our job is a privilege; we ask a lot of our patients, so it's important we give back to them.

Sam Gray, PLN

What if … ?

… It's her first panic attack?

It may be the only one she ever has. Explain, advise, and inform the GP. Formal therapy isn't needed unless it becomes a recurrent problem.

… The panic attacks are part of another anxiety disorder?

Treat the underlying anxiety disorder with CBT ± medication (usually SSRIs). See Ch.22.

… She suffers a panic attack during the assessment?

Stay calm. Linda will be very distressed, and may think she's dying. Panic usually peaks within 10 minutes and passes in 30–40 minutes. Don't explain a complex CBT model! Say:

- *Linda, this is another panic attack. It feels frightening, but I promise you it's harmless and will pass. Nothing bad is going to happen to you.*

Just sit with her, doing *nothing* but soothing and encouraging.

- If she *demands* an intervention, she can breathe into her hands, cupped over her nose and mouth. This rebalances carbon dioxide levels, decreasing symptoms. It's discouraged longer-term (a safety-seeking behaviour), but can be usefully contrasted with heart attack/stroke treatment.

Afterwards, debrief and explore her understanding, e.g.

- *You did really well there*
- *It passed without any medical help. What do you make of that?*

Take-home message

Help people understand panic without minimizing how terrifying panic attacks feel.

Further reading

NICE (2011) CG 113 Guidelines for the management of anxiety (panic disorder, with or without agoraphobia, and generalised anxiety disorder) in adults in primary, secondary and community care.

CBT based self help manual: Shafran, R., Brosan, L. and Cooper, P. (2013) *The Complete CBT Guide for Anxiety (Overcoming Series)*, Constable and Robinson, London.

NHS Choices patient information, including self help advice around exercise, breathing, relaxation etc. Available at: www.nhs.uk/Conditions/Panic-disorder/Pages/self%20help.aspx

CHAPTER 58

Drug-seeking

Isabel McMullen and Lisa Conlan

South London & Maudsley NHS Foundation Trust, London, England

> **RELATED CHAPTERS:** alcohol (40), illicit drugs (41), opiate overdose (66), aggression (74)

Eddie, 28, attended ED after his methadone prescription was stolen. Staff report he's angry, abusive and demanding methadone.

The bottom-line is this: we rarely dispense addictive medications from ED, since it reinforces drug-seeking behaviour and can kill people – whether the patient or their customers (many drugs are sold on). Don't be pressured into prescribing: methadone withdrawal is unpleasant but not life-threatening. Methadone overdose kills.

Preparation

1. Gather information – notes and professionals
- Alerts for drug-seeking/violence
- Known to addictions services?
  - In office hours, contact them to discuss
- If 'out-of-area', contact his local ED/psychiatric service for information.

2. Safety
- Take a chaperone and interview where staff can easily observe you
- See Ch.74 if aggressive.

Assessment

> **TIP:** It's often better to think more and do less. It's always better to listen at least as much as you talk.
>
> **Elizabeth Venables, Consultant**

Psychiatry: Breaking the ICE – Introductions, Common Tasks and Emergencies for Trainees, First Edition.
Edited by Sarah Stringer, Juliet Hurn and Anna M Burnside.
© 2016 John Wiley & Sons, Ltd. Published 2016 by John Wiley & Sons, Ltd.
Companion Website: www.psychiatryice.com

1. Approach
Be kind but firm. Explain that you want to help, and can see he's upset, however he:
- Must be patient and answer important questions
- Will have to leave if he shouts or threatens you.

Eddie's wish to get methadone may occasionally override his honesty. Be alert to inconsistencies in his history but don't challenge them – you'll only inflame the situation.

2. Focused history, remembering...
- *HPC:* explore – this will help Eddie feel understood
  - Has he reported the theft to police and got a crime reference number?
- *Substance misuse* (p34 for detail)
  - Clarify current methadone dose and prescriber's contact details
  - Previous and current drug use
- *Recent 'discharge' from prison, hospital, residential detox placement?*
  - Opiate tolerance is lost quickly, so there's a high risk of fatal overdose if Eddie plans to try his 'usual' dose of heroin/methadone.

3. MSE, remembering...
- Opiate intoxication/withdrawal (p261)
- Suicidal/violent thoughts (check *before* refusing to prescribe!)
- Psychotic symptoms (suggest other drug use/underlying psychosis).

4. Physical assessment
- Full examination – drug users often have poor physical health
- If *overdue* methadone, Eddie should show *some* signs of withdrawal (p261).

5. Risk, remembering...
- Self-harm
- Violence
- Accidental overdose.

Management

1. Explain your role
Set boundaries around your role in ED: you *can't* prescribe methadone.

Be helpless
Explain you have no choice in this situation. It's harder for Eddie to be angry if you're helpless, than if you seem to be willfully withholding help.

Be helpful
- You *can* help him access the local addictions team who *can* prescribe methadone. If he wants to go, provide details *and* ensure they're expecting him in the morning.
- Consider stat symptomatic relief for active diarrhoea or vomiting, e.g. loperamide 4 mg or metoclopramide 10 mg, but don't give TTOs.
- Help Eddie reflect on how he's coped with past withdrawal. Would these options work now?

2. Psychoeducation

The key points are:

- Withdrawal is unpleasant but not fatal
- There are high risks of death through overdose if using opiates:
  - 'On top' of methadone
  - After a period of abstinence
  - With alcohol/benzodiazepines
- He's responsible for his actions – especially important if threatening violence/crime.

3. Handover

Document your assessment. Fax/e-mail a copy to the GP and addictions team. Add drug-seeking ±
aggression alerts to his notes, as relevant.

What if ... ?

...Eddie threatens to use drugs overnight?

That's his choice. Empathise with his distress but hold firm.

...He storms out, shouting he'll kill himself or mug someone for drug money?

If he wasn't suicidal *before* you refused methadone, this is a rather hollow threat. He wants opiates,
and will most likely approach another ED or a dealer as his next move. Try to remind him he's
responsible for his actions before he leaves and document clearly. Contact the police if he's targeting
a specific person or carrying weapons.

...He threatens suicide unless admitted?

Explore his plans. Explain that methadone won't be prescribed until the next ward round; visiting
the addictions service will provide swifter relief. This often resolves suicidality.

...He's lost a benzodiazepine prescription?

The same principles apply. Withdrawal is more dangerous (e.g. fits) but most people will
self-medicate with alcohol or street benzodiazepines. Giving a prescription interferes with any
addictions team treatment plan. *Never* prescribe benzodiazepines to heavy alcohol users, except as a
formal alcohol detox.

...There's a good reason to prescribe methadone?

Occasionally, you may decide to prescribe, e.g. a pregnant methadone-user in clear withdrawal.
Always discuss with specialists before prescribing. The UDS should be positive for methadone but
otherwise negative. See Ch.41+42.

...He demands an alcohol detox?

Praise Eddie for wanting to stop drinking – it's a big decision, and he should be proud of himself for
taking this first step. In office hours, consider redirecting swiftly to addictions services.

Assess for:

- Intoxication/withdrawal (postpone interview if drunk)
- Reasons for wanting a detox *now*

- Motivation to change
- Past and current alcohol usage
  - Other drugs, especially benzodiazepines
- Previous attempts at abstinence (assisted or not)
  - Fits or delirium tremens (DTs)?
  - Reasons for relapse
- Comorbid mental and physical illness.

Admit and organise a detox (p254) if:

- Current withdrawal fits or DTs (Ch.77) *or* seriously ill, e.g. decompensated liver disease, severe malnutrition
  - Medical ward
- High suicide risk *or* serious psychiatric comorbidity
  - Psychiatric ward.

Otherwise, alcohol detox isn't usually possible via ED.

Recognise any frustration and explain Eddie should self-refer to the local addictions service. They'll organise a planned (elective) detox, and:

- Provide support before and after, e.g. MI (p74), rehabilitation, keyworker
- Assess whether a home detox is possible, e.g. if good social support; no comorbid medical conditions, previous DTs or withdrawal seizures.

This is much more likely to succeed than a sudden admission.

Before discharging:

- *Explain he mustn't stop drinking completely, due to risk of death from fits or DTs*
  - He *can* try cutting down gently and 'topping up' with alcohol when shaky
- Give details of the addictions service, e.g. print off a map and opening times
- Fax or e-mail your assessment to the team to ensure they're expecting Eddie. This may make your assessment feel more useful for him.
- Consider dietary advice ± prescribing B vitamins (p256)
- Alcoholics Anonymous (AA) may help. If Eddie's found AA helpful before, or never tried them, encourage him to attend.
  - Find local meetings via www.alcoholics-anonymous.org.uk
  - He only needs a *desire* to stop drinking – he shouldn't turn up drunk, but doesn't have to be abstinent to attend

Take-home message

Don't be pressured to prescribe methadone (or organise non-urgent alcohol detoxes) in ED – signpost to specialist services.

CHAPTER 59

Learning disability (LD) and behavioural change

Rory Sheehan

North London Training Scheme for Psychiatry of Intellectual Disability, London, England

---

RELATED CHAPTERS: inpatients with LD (44), delirium (55), safeguarding (63), treatment refusal (76)

Rufus is 23, lives in a residential home and has a severe LD. Over the past week, he's become increasingly agitated and aggressive. Staff called an ambulance as they could no longer manage his behaviour. Rufus hasn't co-operated with the ED doctor, who requests your assistance.

Be aware of *diagnostic overshadowing* – the tendency to assume the presentation is due to the LD, rather than looking for another cause. This issue prevents people with LD receiving the care they need. Although Rufus is likely to have very limited speech (Table 44.1, p275), this doesn't mean he *can't* communicate – just that you must work more flexibly. With his carers, try to understand what the changed behaviour communicates – whether a biological, psychological or social change (Table 59.1).

Preparation

1. Gather information – notes, obs chart, prescriptions/medication boxes
- Current physical health concerns
- PMHx, PPHx ± diagnosed genetic syndrome?
- Regular medication. Changes? Adherence?

2. Collateral history – carers, family ± GP
- Usual level of function/ADLs
- Health passport (p278)/communication method ± sensory deficits
- Recent GP involvement?
- Recent behaviour
  - Gradual or sudden change?
  - Possible triggers (Table 59.1)
  - Staff response (any inadvertent reinforcement?)
- Previous similar episodes?
  - Triggers? Management?
- Risks to Rufus, residents, staff.

3. Try to find a quiet side room for the interview

Psychiatry: Breaking the ICE – Introductions, Common Tasks and Emergencies for Trainees, First Edition.
Edited by Sarah Stringer, Juliet Hurn and Anna M Burnside.

Table 59.1 Causes of behavioural change.

	Possibilities
Biological	Delirium (Ch.55)
	Dementia (early onset risk in Down syndrome)
	Pain, especially toothache, constipation, ear infection
	Epilepsy
	Medication, e.g. side effects, withdrawal
Psychological	Stress, sadness, frustration
	Adjustment disorder
	Depression (screen changes in sleep, appetite, interest, enjoyment)
	Psychosis
	Abnormal perceptual experiences
Social/	Changed accommodation, routine, carers or residents
environmental	New communication difficultly, e.g. wax blocking ears, lost sensory aid
	Stress
	Boredom / lack of sensory stimulation
	Abuse

Assessment

1. Approach
Discuss Rufus' preferred communication method with his carer beforehand, e.g.
- Makaton (language programme using signing and symbols with speech; Figure 59.1)
- Picture books
- Computer.

Check if Rufus has interests you can use to engage or relax him. The carer may support communication between you, but you should speak to Rufus directly, using simple, clear communication (p276). Even if Rufus can't communicate verbally, introduce yourself and say why you're there.
- Be reassuring – the new environment and people may frighten him
- Keep speech simple and slow, using his name at the start of sentences
- Make eye contact and smile
- Use facial expressions or simple drawings to help communicate
- Sentences should convey one message/action at a time
- Give Rufus time and encouragement to respond
- Keep a safe distance if he's been aggressive.

2. History and MSE ...
- Focus on MSE if unable to gain a history
- Evidence of distress/pain, e.g. sweating, grimacing, holding part of the body, limited movement
  - Use pain face scales if helpful
- Evidence of psychosis or depression (when unsure what a behaviour means, ask the carer if it's normal for Rufus)
- Capacity to make decisions about investigations and treatment.

3. Risks, remembering ...
- Worsening physical/mental health
- Self-harm
- Neglect/abuse
- Aggression.

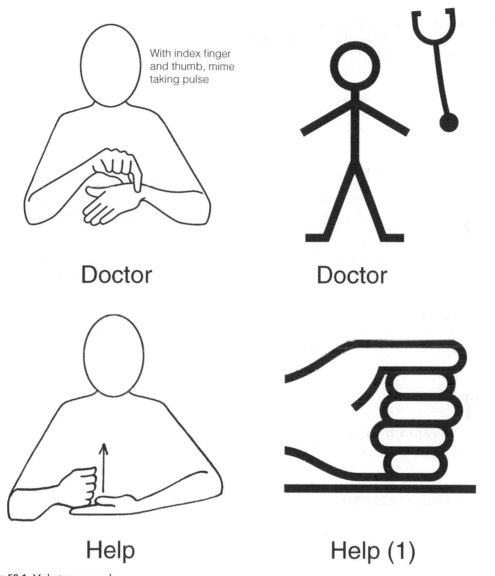

Doctor

Doctor

Help

Help (1)

Figure 59.1 Makaton examples.
British English version of Makaton, used with kind permission of The Makaton Charity. For further training or resources, see www.makaton.org

Management

1. Investigate and treat physical illness

ED *must* rule out physical causes, and will appreciate your support. If Rufus lacks capacity to make decisions about his physical health, investigate and treat in his best interests under the MCA (Ch.76). In order to examine and conduct tests, consider using:
- Proportionate restraint
- Simple analgesia, e.g. paracetamol
- Low dose anxiolytic, e.g. lorazepam 0.5 – 1 mg PO (only IM if refused and *essential*).

> **TIP:** People with LD, *don't* have higher pain thresholds, but may respond to *much* smaller drug doses than usual. They're more sensitive to paradoxical reactions with benzodiazepines, so use when necessary, but monitor closely.

If Rufus needs a medical admission, liaise early with the ward and consider the need for DoLS (p103). Request a 1:1 RMN with LD experience, and handover the information you've gathered on Rufus' communication needs.

2. Admit or discharge?

Once you've addressed medical causes ask the residential home whether they feel able to look after him. (If Rufus was living with family, discuss emergency respite care with carers and social services.)

If Rufus' symptoms are ongoing or severe, he may need psychiatric admission, but a general adult ward could be very frightening.

- Discuss with your on-call senior (LD registrar if available)
- Consider waiting until morning to discuss with his community LD service ±letting them review. They're better able to diagnose underlying psychiatric problems, and start/monitor psychotropics.

3. Handover

Document clearly – including Rufus' communication needs. If he's staying in hospital, handover to liaison psychiatry for follow-up. Copy notes to his GP and LD team.

What if … ?

He needs rapid tranquilisation?

Be cautious and use old age guidelines (Table 74.3, p448).

Take-home message

Consider a wide differential in people with LD presenting with acute behavioural change. Work closely with carers to understand the problem.

Reference

Mencap:
  ○ www.mencap.org.uk/about-learning-disability/information-professionals.

Further reading

NHS Lanarkshire Adult Learning Disability Communication guide:
  ○ www.healthelanarkshire.co.uk/assets/files/TGD.COMAID.71078.P-1.pdf.
Royal College of Psychiatrists 'Challenging Behaviour' easy-read leaflet:
  ○ www.healthelanarkshire.co.uk/assets/files/TGD.COMAID.71078.P-1.pdf.

CHAPTER 60

'Social' presentations

Sean Cross[1] and Rachel Thomasson[2]

[1] South London & Maudsley NHS Foundation Trust, London, England
[2] Manchester Royal Infirmary, Manchester, Lancashire, England

RELATED CHAPTERS: psychosis – long term (24), safeguarding (63)

James, 48, has had intermittent contact with psychiatric services and numerous diagnoses over the years, including schizophrenia, borderline LD, and dependent personality disorder. He's presented to ED for the third time this week, seeking help – but is vague about his needs and doesn't appear suicidal, depressed or psychotic.

Try to think beyond the labels of well/unwell (Table 60.1). Social problems may:

- Trigger or exacerbate mental illness
- Indicate underlying mental illness, e.g. through functional impact
- Be the most acceptable way of seeking help for mental illness.

It's an old maxim in medicine that if someone returns for the third time with the same problem, it's time to look again – consider whether something's been missed.

> **TIP:** Patients often communicate distress by making various demands: to change their medication, sort their complex housing problem, find them a job, make a difficult situation better, etc. Often you won't be able to resolve the problem quickly, but what's more important in the first instance is that you listen to the demand and try to understand the anxiety behind it. If you can respond to the anxiety you may find the demand itself goes away.
>
> Marcella Fok, ST5

Preparation

Gather further information – notes (including old discharge summaries), staff
- Current supports, e.g. GP, CMHT
- Is he entitled to s117 aftercare (p99)?
- What's been tried on previous presentations?
  - Why didn't this work?
  - What hasn't been addressed?
- Check basic obs have been completed.

Psychiatry: Breaking the ICE – Introductions, Common Tasks and Emergencies for Trainees, First Edition.
Edited by Sarah Stringer, Juliet Hurn and Anna M Burnside.
© 2016 John Wiley & Sons, Ltd. Published 2016 by John Wiley & Sons, Ltd.
Companion Website: www.psychiatryice.com

Table 60.1 Vague presentations – differential.

Problem	Examples	Notes and tips
Organic	Delirium, non-convulsive status, brain tumours, encephalitis, endocrine disturbance	• PMHx and full physical assessment • May present with subtle disturbance in conscious level, disorientation, ↓attention
Cognitive impairment	Learning disability/difficulties	• Often undiagnosed in older people • Check schooling and employment history
	Delirium Dementia	• Vague changes in older adults may signal an impending acute illness
Psychosis	Prodrome (no previous psychosis diagnosis)	• ↓Concentration, apathy, sleep disturbance, • Low, perplexed, blunted, anxious, irritable, suspicious • Social withdrawal and ↓function
	Negative symptoms (previous psychosis, often chronic – see Ch.24)	• Psychomotor retardation • Blunted affect • Apathy/poor motivation • Anhedonia • Self-neglect • Social withdrawal/loss of function • Poverty of thought • Poor concentration
Depression		• Look for negative cognitions
Stress reactions	Adjustment disorders Acute stress reaction Post-traumatic stress disorder (PTSD) Fugue/dissociative states	• Establish history of stressor(s) and timeline
Language and cultural barriers	Limited English Different service expectation Sensory impairments	• Use interpreters • Collateral to establish if *changed* behaviour
Malingering	Factitious medical/psychiatric disorder	• Inconsistent or overinclusive presentations • It's hard to fake thought disorder • Consider 'gain' (Box 60.1) • Obstructing collateral history-taking • See *What ifs … ?*

Box 60.1 Gain – an underused concept

Gain describes the different motivating factors associated with help-seeking, whether for diagnosis, treatment or admission.
• May be conscious or unconscious
• *Primary gain* includes psychological motivators, e.g. *If I'm admitted to hospital I'll feel less stressed.* Includes somatisation presentations (Ch.61).

> • *Secondary gain* tends to be associated with external advantage, e.g. financial support, housing; avoiding work or criminal charges
> • Staff responses may provide gain and reinforce helpful/unhelpful behaviour.

Assessment

1. Approach

If James is vague or rambling, try to add structure, e.g.

- Interrupt politely
  - *Sorry to interrupt. You mentioned problems sleeping. What time do you go to bed?*
- Reframe
  - *You've talked a lot about the difficulties with your neighbours. Is that why you're here today? How do you think we might help?*
- *Take me through what you did yesterday* (may offer important insights).

Collateral history is often very revealing – so get one! If James has 'nobody' you can talk to, he's either very isolated *or* worried what his contacts may say …

If you suspect malingering, be wary of asking leading questions. Be alert to James endorsing rare or unusually numerous symptoms (e.g. *all* first rank symptoms), especially where there's a subjective/objective mismatch.

2. Full history, remembering …

- *HPC:* why did he attend? How does coming to hospital help him?
  - *Think:* What's the 'gain' for repeated attendances? (Box 60.1)
  - New symptoms since last assessment?
  - Inconsistencies?
- *Problem areas/worries*
  - Finances
  - Housing
  - Work/studies
  - Relationships
  - Physical complaints
- *Screen for mental illness*
  - Depression
  - Psychosis, including disorganization and negative symptoms
  - Cognitive impairment
- *Screen for physical illness*
  - PMHx and systems review, particularly neurological symptoms
  - Current/recent medications; adherence
- *Substance misuse*

3. MSE, remembering …

- Self-neglect
- Intoxication/withdrawal
- Physical illness
- Medication side effects
- Psychotic/affective symptoms
- Poor concentration or organisation
- Formal cognitive testing (Appendix D).

4. Risks, including …
- Self-neglect
- Deterioration of mental/physical health
- Self-harm
- Safeguarding issues; exploitation.

Management

If James is under a CMHT, you primarily need to pass concerns (his and yours) to the team. The less contact he has with formal services, the more there is to do.

> **TIP:** Have the confidence to give your formulations and suggestions. Sometimes you'll be more able to see the forest for the trees than a hassled, busy team.
>
> Greg Shields, ST4

1. Diagnostic review and follow-up options
Decide whether James' presentation *fits* with established or provisional diagnoses. Discuss uncertainty with your registrar, and consider the best next step for follow-up:
- *Medical* – refer acute concerns back to ED
  - Use unscheduled presentations for opportunistic healthcare. Alert his GP ($\pm$ CMHT) to concerns and encourage James to attend for follow-up.
- *Psychiatric* – consider further assessment if problems have deteriorated, changed or been overlooked. The CMHT is usually appropriate, unless risks require admission.
  - If known to a CMHT, agree with the CC that James will be redirected to the CMHT in future ED presentations (unless physically ill)
  - If he's under the Care Programme Approach (CPA) suggest a CPA review (Ch.19)
  - If James hasn't had recent CMHT contact but would benefit from this, discuss the reasons for discharge/disengagement. Social problems may now facilitate engagement.
- *Social* – if there are *no* psychiatric issues, focus on social interventions.

2. Social interventions
If social problems are driving James' presentation, try and intervene (Ch.13). The PLN/duty social worker will know how to access local options, so ask their advice and signpost as needed, e.g. Citizen's Advice Bureau. Address carers' needs where appropriate.

3. Handover
If ED *isn't* the best way for James to access support, gently but firmly make this clear, including advice on where he *should* go. This may help James *and* prevent repeated ED presentations.

Ensure that ED are aware of your plan, and copy this to the GP. If suggesting that a diagnosis may be wrong or overlooked, do so respectfully, e.g. *At interview he showed signs of X and Y, suggesting he may be suffering with Z. I would be grateful for your review.*

What if ... ?

... He's demanding?
If James makes inappropriate demands (e.g. *I'm not leaving until you give me housing!*) empathise with his distress, but calmly and firmly explain that you can't help in the way he wants. Give written advice on accessing help (e.g. attending the Homeless Persons Unit) but don't reinforce the behaviour by bending the rules to placate him – this will only encourage further attendances.

... He's malingering?
James needs to go home, but see p379 first.

Take-home message

Don't be helpless, just because you can't prescribe.

Further reading

http://www.mentalhealth.org.uk/our-work/policy/physical-health-and-mental-health/
http://www.poverty.ac.uk/

CHAPTER 61

Medically unexplained symptoms

John Moriarty

South London & Maudsley NHS Foundation Trust, London, England

RELATED CHAPTERS: anxiety (22), panic attacks (57)

You're on-call one Saturday. Pat Sykes is a 40-year old carer, admitted with leg paralysis. All tests are normal and the medics want to discharge her – but have requested you review first.

Frustration builds when people experience symptoms that can't be explained by physical causes (Table 61.1).

- Patients feel staff aren't taking them seriously, or think they're lying
- Staff may be dismissive, or order unnecessary tests, worried they're 'missing something'.

Tensions may rise further when Pat realises the medics have called a *psychiatrist*: surely proof they think it's 'all in her head'! Don't expect a warm welcome or a miraculous cure. Instead, try to:
- Validate the reality of her experience
- Prevent iatrogenic harm
- Help her *consider* the possibility of psychological support.

TIP: Use the label that helps Pat most – often *no* label.

Preparation

1. Gather information – medics + *all* notes
- *Why* does the team believe they've excluded a physical cause?
  - If unclear, ask
- What's Pat been told about her condition and the purpose of your assessment?

2. Pause
- Ensure you've enough time and aren't feeling irritated/harassed
- Try to observe Pat before assessing her:
  - Presentation ± inconsistencies, e.g. unconscious leg movements
  - People's reactions to her, e.g. undermining/reinforcing the sick role.

Psychiatry: Breaking the ICE – Introductions, Common Tasks and Emergencies for Trainees, First Edition.
Edited by Sarah Stringer, Juliet Hurn and Anna M Burnside.
© 2016 John Wiley & Sons, Ltd. Published 2016 by John Wiley & Sons, Ltd.
Companion Website: www.psychiatryice.com

Table 61.1 Medically unexplained symptoms.

Terminology	Explanation	Examples

Dissociative disorders	• Loss of integration between sensation, consciousness and bodily control
	 • Onset often sudden, after trauma/life event
	 • Usually remits within weeks/months
		• Dissociative fugue, amnesia, seizures
		 • Conversion disorders
		   ○ Sudden loss of specific sensory/motor function
		   ○ E.g. paralysis, blindness
		   ○ Refers to psychodynamic idea that emotional pain is 'converted' to physical symptoms

Somatisation disorder	• Multiple, recurrent and frequently changing physical symptoms (≥ 2y) • Commonly present to many different specialists • High use of hospital care	• Briquet's disorder
Somatoform autonomic dysfunction	• Similar to somatisation disorder, but autonomic dysfunction • E.g. trembling, sweating, gastrointestinal symptoms, palpitations	• Irritable bowel syndrome • Hyperventilation syndrome
Persistent somatoform pain disorder	• Similar to somatisation disorder, but persistent, severe and distressing pain, occurring with psychosocial problems	• Back pain • Tension headache • Atypical facial pain
Hypochondriacal disorder	• Extreme, persistent physical concerns, with underlying fear of a specific illness, e.g. cancer	
Medically Unexplained Symptoms/ Functional symptoms or syndromes	• Umbrella terms for unexplained symptoms	• Globus hystericus • Fibromyalgia • Chronic fatigue syndrome • Repetitive strain injury

Assessment

> **PATIENT VIEW:**
>
> I suffer from non-epileptic attack disorder. It's linked with anxiety. When you're in there for something they think is possibly life-threatening, you actually feel believed. Then they come back and tell you, 'its psychological', and that sense that you're deserving of help is gone ... it feels like they're saying you're making it up, you're being manipulative. When you have no control over it, it's awful.
>
> 'Jax'

1. Approach

Imagine how it feels to *know* something's wrong, but feel no one believes you. Empathize, establish rapport and respect Pat's perspective.

- Acknowledge her reservations, e.g.
  - *What did you think when they said you'd see me?*
  - *Sometimes people are angry about seeing a psychiatrist. They might feel it means doctors don't really believe them …*
- Normalize your involvement, e.g.
  - *I'm asked to see lots of medical and surgical patients in this hospital. I'm yet to find an illness which isn't worse with stress and worry – whether appendicitis, heart attacks or even cancer. I've often helped these patients, so perhaps it's possible I can help you?*

Try the *BATHE Technique* (Lieberman and Stuart, 1999). This was designed to rapidly assess the impact of symptoms, and may help broaden your conversation to a psychosocial understanding of illness. Put questions into your own words.

- **B**ackground
  - *Tell me about what's been happening to you …*
  - *How does it affect your everyday life?*
- **A**ffect
  - *How do you feel about it?*
- **T**rouble:
  - *What troubles you the most about this?*
- **H**andle:
  - *What helps you handle that?*
- **E**mpathy:
  - *This sounds really difficult. I think anyone in your situation would feel frustrated/fed-up*

2. Full history, remembering …

- *HPC:* Try the BATHE approach
  - You don't need to take a standard history of each symptom – it's been done repeatedly
  - Summarise problems back or physically make a list to show you've understood
- *Illness behaviours*
  - Explore impact, duties and responsibilities (work, dependents, hobbies)
  - *What do you do in a typical day?*
  - *How do you relax?*
  - *Are there things you must avoid?*
  - *Do you feel self-conscious about your symptoms or disabilities?*
- *Illness beliefs*
  - *What's your greatest fear about what's going on here?*
  - Prompt if needed, e.g.
    - *Are you worried you'll never get better … ?*
    - *Have you read worrying things on the internet or in medical books?*
- Less inflammatory once you've gained rapport:
  - *Triggers:* recent and historic stress, including early illness experiences
  - *Comorbidity:* depression, anxiety disorders

TIP: Some people have simply been doing too much, for too long. *If so*, see how Pat responds to the idea of cutting down some duties.

3. MSE, remembering …

- Illness/safety-seeking behaviours, e.g. checking pulse, fixed posture, using medications
- Depression, anxiety
- Psychological mindedness.

4. Risk assessment, including ...
- Iatrogenic harm
- Suicide/self-harm.

Management

1. Psychoeducation
Diagnostic labels (Table 1) are fraught: though some people take comfort in knowing there's a recognised term for their condition, others will be offended. It's more important to keep Pat engaged and come to a shared understanding of the problem, than to inflict a diagnosis – if you simply discuss her 'leg problems', fine. 'Stress' can be a helpful term, but avoid it if she's adamant her problems are nothing to do with stress. Never say:
- *The tests are all negative. There's nothing wrong with you*
- *Fortunately, this is all in your head/psychosomatic ...*
Consider this approach (it won't work for everyone):
- *You're definitely experiencing problems*
- *Do you use a computer or smartphone ... ? [Use the most familiar example – not both]*
  - *What programs/apps do you use most?*
- You might then explain ... Computers/mobiles are made up of hardware and software
  - Hardware: physical parts, e.g. keyboard, screen, and bits you'd see if you opened it up
  - Software: programs/apps
- *The body's a bit like a computer/mobile ... In your case, the hardware's fine, but for some reason, the programs/apps aren't playing normally. That's why you're experiencing problems* (e.g. legs not working).
Medical tests simply can't pick up 'software' problems, e.g.
- *The approach of running tests doesn't seem to have helped, and might even have added to your worries and frustration*
- *The good news is that that your body itself is OK, even though it's not working properly just now.*
Let Pat ask questions before moving on.

PATIENT VIEW:

They said, "the hardware in your brain is working fine, but the software isn't". But there was no discussion about *how* the software interacts with the hardware. There's something that doctors either aren't explaining properly, or they literally don't know. And they're not going to tell *us* they don't know. Dr X was at least honest: he said, "We still don't know enough about how this impacts on how your body functions."

'Jax'

PATIENT VIEW:

Hardware! Software! I remember sitting in the hospital bed and I said to them, "I'm not a fucking computer!"

'Kelly'

---

2. Realistic hope
Be clear and confident about what will happen next, e.g.
- *Further tests won't find the cause of the problem*
- *We can help you ...*
  - *Train your body to work better and get back to ...* (nice things she misses)
  - *± Reduce any stress which makes it harder to deal with symptoms.*

Be optimistic about recent symptoms, e.g.
- *You've had a temporary block to the control of your leg. We're certain it's not a stroke. You're likely to make a full recovery, quite quickly.*

However, multiple complaints over many years are more resistant, and excessive optimism is often unhelpful/unrealistic. Focus on:
- Her regaining control of her body
- Decreasing disability/helping her live as normally as possible.

3. Involve family

Use discretion: some families will be invested in physical causes, while others will be helped by your explanation, and will reiterate key messages and encourage Pat with her treatment.

4. Treatment options

Treatment will target the problem(s) Pat recognises, e.g.
- Treat comorbid depression/anxiety (Ch.21 and 22)
- Rehabilitation, especially physiotherapy
- CBT
  - Your referral should state whether to focus on anxiety/mood or exploring (and challenging) illness beliefs and behaviours
- Liaison psychiatry outpatients (complex cases)
- Antidepressants (even if not depressed). Her GP/liaison psychiatrist might suggest these later.

Where possible, offer a second meeting – it's a lot to take on, all at once.

5. Handover

Feed back to the medics so they can reiterate the same messages supportively and compassionately. Ensure the hospital and GP know:
- *Not* to further investigate existing symptoms
- To *sensibly* investigate new symptoms (neither ignore nor over-investigate).

What if ... ?

... She refuses help?

Psychological treatment won't help if Pat doesn't want it. If she's sceptical of your advice but received a respectful and empathic assessment, she may accept *future* help, so don't feel you've wasted your time.

... She's malingering?

Malingering is a behaviour, not a diagnosis. It *can* cause unexplained physical/psychiatric symptoms... *or* simply reflect staff frustration or dislike of a patient. To be confident someone's malingering, you need strong evidence of:
- *Deliberate* and *conscious* feigning of symptoms
- Deliberately misleading professionals *and*
- Aiming to gain *something*, e.g. benefits, sick-leave, opiates.

It's often hard to prove, but when certain, discuss with seniors. Help the medics address their concerns directly with the patient, who's likely to be upset or angry, but then seek input at another hospital. Pass concerns and evidence to the GP to prevent unnecessary uptake of NHS resources and iatrogenic harm.

... This is a factitious disorder? (Munchausen Syndrome)

Unlike malingering, the gain here is usually formulated as an *unconscious* need to adopt the sick role. In reality, there's usually a mix of primary and secondary gain. Again, you need proof of deliberate feigning or production of symptoms. Specifically assess risks from iatrogenic/self-inflicted medical problems or suicide. Support the medical team to raise their concerns *with* the patient, explaining:

* Factitious disorder is a recognized illness
* Outpatient psychological treatment is available.

The person will usually walk out. They may threaten suicide; if so, and they weren't suicidal *before* the discussion, it's more likely they'll move to another hospital than self-harm. Discuss the case with seniors and the liaison psychiatry consultant – a senior medic or psychiatrist may raise a patient alert if there's *high* risk of iatrogenic harm.

Reference

Lieberman, J.A. and Stuart, M.R. (1999) The BATHE Method: Incorporating Counseling and Psychotherapy Into the Everyday Management of Patients. *The Primary Care Companion to the Journal of Clinical Psychiatry* **1** (2), 35–38.

Further reading

Stone, J., Carson, A., Sharpe, M. (2005) Functional symptoms and signs in neurology: Assessment and diagnosis. *Journal of Neurology, Neurosurgery and Psychiatry,* **76** (suppl 1), i2–i12.

Patient resource:

Information and advice (also useful clinician tips in the *In the mind?* section) www.neurosymptoms.org

PART III
Emergencies

CHAPTER 62

Acute relapse

Laurine Hanna
South London & Maudsley NHS Foundation Trust, London, England

RELATED CHAPTERS: bipolar affective disorder (BPAD, 25), disengagement (27), mania (54)

Jean, 45, has a history of BPAD. Her husband, Tom, called today because Jean drove dangerously fast to a hardware store and bought the entire stock of white spirit. She's carried a kitchen knife for protection when unwell previously.

Working with relapsing patients feels very different when they're in the community, rather than 'safe' in hospital. You can't constantly monitor Jean or restrict her movements, and it may take an uncomfortably long time to organise an admission or Mental Health Act (MHA) assessment. Meanwhile, your main challenge may be managing your own anxiety or uncertainty. Share these feelings with colleagues, who'll often be very experienced at 'holding' risk in the community, and containing the anxiety this creates.

Preparation

1. Gather information – Tom, Care Coordinator (CC), notes, General Practitioner (GP)
- Recent
  - Relapse indicators
  - Likely triggers
  - Medications ± non-adherence
  - Risky behaviours
  - Home situation: level of support, relationships, children?
- History: relapse signature, previous admissions, known triggers
  - Risks
  - Crisis plans
- Tom – call 999 if immediate danger. Otherwise, ensure he can call you for advice.
- What are Tom and Jean's views on HTT / admission?

Psychiatry: Breaking the ICE – Introductions, Common Tasks and Emergencies for Trainees, First Edition.
Edited by Sarah Stringer, Juliet Hurn and Anna M Burnside.
© 2016 John Wiley & Sons, Ltd. Published 2016 by John Wiley & Sons, Ltd.
Companion Website: www.psychiatryice.com

2. Team + consultant discussion
- Depending on urgency and risks:
  - Offer an appointment at team base
  - *Or* an urgent home visit (Ch.20)
  - *Or* a formal MHA assessment (police will attend)
- Check local Home Treatment Team (HTT) policy:
  - Referral criteria
  - Whether they need to 'gate-keep' (assess Jean / agree that HTT isn't appropriate) before admission is allowed
- Consider:
  - Asking HTT to attend
  - Senior doctor review – if they're 'Section 12 Approved', they can complete the first medical recommendation for a section, if detention is necessary
  - Contacting the bed manager regarding possible admission
- Safety: see with a colleague ± Jean's family
  - If high risks, involve police.

If the situation is more risky/chaotic
- Can Tom persuade Jean to visit the Emergency Department (ED)? If so:
  - Call the Psychiatric Liaison Nurse (PLN) ± fax over information
  - It may foster goodwill if you/CC meet Jean at ED to jointly assess
- If Jean isn't at home/is erratic/wandering the streets, call the police with a description and last known whereabouts. They might use s136 (p99; Ch48) if they see her.
- Consider circulating details to local EDs.

> **TIP:** Advance statements may help you select options Jean prefers, but shouldn't override risk considerations and clinical judgement.

Assessment

1. Approach
Emotions are likely to be running high: Tom will be stressed; Jean may be excited, angry, or frightened. Your calmness is essential to contain the situation. If Jean blames Tom for raising the alert, try to divert the blame onto you and the team, e.g. *Whatever Tom's worried about,* we're *concerned about you – Tom hasn't done anything wrong.*

2. Collateral
Full update from Tom, including:
- Recent behaviours
- Current views on admission versus Jean staying at home with extra support, e.g. HTT
- His stress, needs, safety.

3. Focused history, remembering ...
- *History of presenting complaint (HPC):*
  - Current symptoms/problems
  - Triggers e.g. stress, non-concordance
  - Impact on function and relationships
- *Substance misuse*
- *Past medical history (PMHx):* including systems review (physical illness/delirium?).

TIP: If too chaotic for even a basic history, focus on Mental State Examination (MSE)

4. MSE, remembering ...
- Agitation/retardation; aggression, disinhibition, impulsivity
- Intoxication/withdrawal; poor physical health
- Pressured/slowed speech; flight of ideas/poverty of thought
- Irritability, elation, depression
- Delusions, e.g. grandiose/nihilistic/persecutory
- Thoughts of harm to self/others
- Hallucinations, especially auditory commands
- Poor concentration/confusion; capacity?
- Views on HTT/medication/admission.

5. Risk assessment, remembering ...
- Self-harm, chaotic accident, spending, self-neglect
- Vulnerability from others, e.g. sexual
- Driving, aggression
- Child risks?

Management

Consider withdrawing to speak privately with your colleague ± call your consultant to share ideas. You can then return to Jean and Tom with a possible plan.

1. Admission
Consider admission when:
- Jean requests it
- Significant immediate risks
- Highly unpredictable/chaotic
- Treatment isn't feasible at home, e.g. poor insight, refusing HTT
- Physical complications
- Complex social circumstances, e.g. home alone; tense dynamics
- Carer(s) under great strain/can't cope.

Offer to phone HTT if they gate-keep admissions, but aren't yet involved.

If Jean agrees to voluntary admission and has capacity to consent to this:
- Your colleague(s) will arrange transport to hospital
- Reassure Jean and her family. Answer their questions.
- If at home, help Jean to collect personal belongings for hospital.

If Jean refuses voluntary admission (or agrees, but lacks capacity / is likely to change her mind):
- For extreme immediate risks, see *What ifs ... ?*
- MHA assessment may be needed: discuss with your team. You might help by discussing Jean's case with the Approved Mental Health Professional (AMHP)
- MHA assessments often take a few days to organise
  - Explain the process and probable timeframe to Tom. The AMHP will seek his views before proceeding.
  - Make sure he can contact the team quickly for support
  - He should call 999 if things deteriorate
- Meanwhile, ask Jean to consider CMHT/HTT contact ± medication
  - Advise her not to drive ± suggest Tom takes her car-keys (Ch.32)

- If children are at home, discuss childcare, e.g.
  - Can a relative look after them?
  - Should social services be involved? (Ch.64).

2. Treatment at home

Jean's relapse may be managed at home if:
- Risks aren't high or immediate
- She can consent to a treatment plan
- Family are willing and able to support her.

Care plan

Involve Jean and Tom in the plan, e.g. *We want to keep you out of hospital – how can we work with you to do this?* Discuss simple self-help, e.g. sleep hygiene (p72), distraction from voices, reducing alcohol. Write the plan down.

Increased support

Suggest HTT and make a referral if not yet done (your team may remain involved, depending on local protocol). Provide CMHT/HTT contact details and out-of-hours plan, e.g. attend ED/call 999. *Medication* (If your patient does not have BPAD, see relevant chapters for specific medications). Check for side effects, then:
- Improve adherence
  - Supervision, e.g. HTT/CMHT/Tom (if he's comfortable with this)
  - Aids, e.g. dosette box
- Restart or increase antipsychotic/mood stabiliser
- Sedation/night sedation, e.g. zopiclone 7.5 mg/promethazine 25 mg/regular benzodiazepines.

Reviews

- Frequent contact with HTT ± CMHT
- Offer to review personally over the coming days (unless HTT exclusively *takeover* her care)
  - Focus on risks, side effects and whether the plan's working
- Be ready to revise quickly if necessary, e.g. organise admission if deteriorating.

3. Documentation and handover

Communicate with the GP and other involved professionals, e.g. housing officer. See if they can offer support.

Document your assessment and plan, and place Jean in Red Zone (p42) for regular team discussion if remaining in the community. Don't see a subsequent admission as defeat.

4. After the crisis

With Jean, reflect on what helped. Include this in her relapse prevention / crisis plan. If HTT are handing back her care, ensure a formal handover and document and medication changes.

> **TIP:** If your anxiety is problematic, discuss it in supervision, but don't expect to banish it completely!

What If ... ?

... She refuses admission but is *extremely* risky?

There are two options:
- S4 MHA (p94) – this may allow a same-day admission, provided police/ambulance can attend quickly. You need to find a S.12 Approved Doctor and an AMHP, first.
- If she's showing risky behaviour in a public place (i.e. outside her home) *or* has broken the law, you can call the police. They could place her under S.136 (in a public place) or arrest her if she's committed a crime. Either way, you can then arrange a MHA assessment.

Take-home message

The earlier you spot relapse, the more easily you can manage it at home, so respond quickly to signs of relapse, and swiftly review patients who are starting to worry CCs. With experience you'll become more comfortable supporting unwell patients without admission.

CHAPTER 63

Adult safeguarding

Rory Conn[1], Vivienne Mak[2], and Sean Lubbe[3]

[1] Tavistock and Portman NHS Foundation Trust, London, England
[2] South London & Maudsley NHS Foundation Trust, London, England
[3] UNSW Black Dog Institute, New South Wales, Australia

RELATED CHAPTERS: learning disability (LD; 44, 59), child protection (64), alleged sexual assault (70)

Jeremy, 66, has an autistic spectrum disorder (ASD), mild LD, and depression; historically he's tied clothing around his neck as nooses, when distressed. He was discharged from hospital to supported accommodation several months ago. The care home manager has requested you review Jeremy's recent tearfulness. On arrival, you notice bruises on Jeremy's neck and wrists.

A *vulnerable adult* is anyone who may struggle to self-care or protect themselves from harm, abuse or exploitation – whether due to age, illness, or disability. They *don't* have to lack capacity, though this may be important. Remember that the ability to consent/make choices can also be impaired by duress or power imbalances.

Abuse is any violation of human or civil rights by someone else, including:
* **Physical, e.g. assault, unlawful restraint, rough handling**
* **Emotional**
* **Sexual**
* **Financial exploitation**
* **Neglect**
* **Discriminatory, e.g. treating someone differently due to race, sexuality**
* **Institutional – inadequate care/practice affecting a whole care setting, e.g. lack of choice, ignoring people's rights to privacy, dignity, respect.**

Raising safeguarding concerns can feel paternalistic or uncomfortable, especially where the patient doesn't believe they're vulnerable, or you get on well with their carers. These issues mustn't prevent thorough exploration of the cause of Jeremy's bruises (Box 63.1).

Box 63.1 Abuse risk factors

Patient:
* Isolated/living alone/homeless
* Elderly/frail
* Female
* Mental illness, especially depression, cognitive impairment
* Physical disability/illness
* Substance misuse

Psychiatry: Breaking the ICE – Introductions, Common Tasks and Emergencies for Trainees, First Edition.
Edited by Sarah Stringer, Juliet Hurn and Anna M Burnside.
© 2016 John Wiley & Sons, Ltd. Published 2016 by John Wiley & Sons, Ltd.
Companion Website: www.psychiatryice.com

Carer:
- Unpaid, stressed, tired
- Mental illness or LD
- Substance misuse

TIP: Read your Trust's safeguarding reporting procedures. Know how to contact the Safeguarding Lead and keep your Safeguarding Vulnerable Adults training up-to-date (often available online).

Preparation

1. Gather further information – CC, GP, notes, staff, family
- Jeremy's baseline: communication problems, level of function
- Recent changes, e.g. appetite, sleep, challenging behaviour
- Medication: concordance/supervision
- History:
  ○ Self-harm pattern/triggers
  ○ Challenging behaviour
  ○ Previous allegations of abuse/safeguarding concerns
- Environment:
  ○ Level of support. Are staff on or off site?
  ○ Relationships with other residents, e.g. conflict, bullying
- Is Jeremy known to social services?

2. Manager
- Ask questions *around* the subject – don't probe!
  ○ Concerns
  ○ Jeremy's cooperation with staff/how he's settling in …

TIP: Raise a safeguarding alert and remember it's for the Safeguarding Vulnerable Adults team to do the disclosure interview. Inexperienced interviewing changes evidence!

Viv Mak, Older Adults Liaison Consultant

Assessment

1. Approach
Remember general principles for assessing people with LD (p246). Jeremy may not disclose abuse for many reasons, e.g.
- Communication problems
- Confusion about what is happening
- Embarrassment
- Fear, blackmail, intimidation
- Loyalty to staff.

Be sensitive and kind.
- Start with broad, neutral questions, e.g.
  - *How are you getting on here?*
  - *What do you like doing?*
  - *What are the staff like?*
  - *What do staff help you with? Do you mind them helping with that?*
- Move to more focused questions, e.g.
  - *Is there anything worrying you at the moment?*
  - *How did you get these bruises?*
- Don't ask leading or closed questions, e.g. *Did someone hurt you?* This may alarm Jeremy, or 'con-taminate' evidence.
- Reassure him it's OK to tell you his worries.

If Jeremy voluntarily discloses abuse, explain:
- You *must* pass it on (you can't keep it a secret)
- You'll do your best to support and protect him.

If there's abuse in one modality, it may well be happening in another. Spot clues, e.g.
- Frequent accidents, falls, ED/hospital admissions
- STIs, genital itching/soreness
- Over-protectiveness of money/possessions
- Physical examination (below)
- Inappropriate/hostile environment (p391).

2. Focused history, remembering ...
- *Current circumstances/stressors*
  - New accommodation
  - Relationships with residents/staff
- *Evidence of depression or self-harm*
  - If bruises are self-inflicted, check triggers and function
  - New self-harm behaviours, e.g. overdose, cutting, burning
- *PMHx*, current concerns or injuries
- *Substance misuse*
- *Function:*
  - ADLs: what can he do himself? What do carers do for him?
  - Activities, social networks
  - Finances – awareness, arrangements, budgeting
- If Jeremy discloses abuse, write verbatim quotes
  - Has he told anyone, e.g. manager, other staff?
  - *Avoid detailed probing*

3. MSE, remembering ...
- Rapport. Oppositional/overly-compliant stance.
- Shabby, smelly, dirty
- Flinching, aggression, acting out, sexual disinhibition
- Oversedation
- Communication difficulties
- Depression, fear
- Thoughts of harm to self/others; immediate safety concerns
- Cognitive impairment
- Capacity to make decisions about safeguarding issues
- Does he want help?

4. Physical exam, remembering ...
- Pain/reluctance to be examined
- Pattern and age of bruising. Draw a body map of bruises.

- Other injuries, e.g. scars, cigarette burns, black eyes
- Malnourished, dehydrated, incontinent
- Mobility, hearing, visual problems
- Pressure sores.

5. Environment
- Accommodation: general atmosphere, cleanliness, organisation
- Room, e.g. squalor, hoarding, unchanged linen, cigarette butts, beer cans
- Access to appropriate aids, e.g. walking frame, rails
- Other residents' behaviour
- Interaction with carers
- Carers' attitude/remarks about Jeremy

6. Risk assessment, remembering ...
- Neglect/abuse/exploitation (Jeremy *and* other residents)
- Self-harm: accidental, deliberate
- Wandering or running away from the home
- Refusal of care, medication
- Deteriorating physical/mental health
- Home risks: fire, flooding, infestation
- Aggression

Management

This is a complex presentation and you might not be *sure* why Jeremy has bruises. Discuss with your consultant and team, recognising the situation and solutions may continue to evolve.

1. If you suspect significant injury
Arrange an urgent GP assessment or call an ambulance. If Jeremy refuses help, consider using the Mental Capacity Act to facilitate examination or admission to hospital. (MCA; Ch.76).

2. If the injuries are definitely self-harm
Treat the underlying illness (e.g. depression, Ch.21) and consider options:
- Psychiatric admission if high risk
- Extra support at accommodation, e.g. HTT, staff support/education

There may still be safeguarding issues if staff have ignored – or not taken steps to address – the self-harm; the manager didn't mention it to you, after all.

3. Safeguarding
You *must* report suspicions of abuse or neglect. Safeguarding procedures will guide your plan as Jeremy is a *vulnerable adult* and you have concerns about *significant harm or risk of harm*.

The safeguarding process (Table 63.1) is coordinated by local adult social services and aims to:
- Arrange multidisciplinary investigation
- Develop a *proportionate* support plan

Tell Jeremy you want to keep him safe and tell your colleagues about his situation. Explain the safeguarding process *simply*, and try to reassure him. Ask what he'd like to happen next and talk through ways to help. If he doesn't want you to disclose and is ...
- *Incapacitous* – discuss with your team and Safeguarding Lead
  - You may need to act in his best interests (Ch.76)

Table 63.1 Safeguarding process.

Step	Action	Time frame
Alert	Record suspicions of abuse	Immediately
	Deal with immediate safety	
Referral	Refer to safeguarding team	Same day
Decision to investigate	Social services/police decide whether case meets threshold for safeguarding	End of next working day
	Investigation lead identified	
Safeguarding assessment	Strategy meeting	Within 5 working days
	A multiagency plan is developed to assess risks and address immediate protection needs	
Safeguarding investigation	Information gathering, e.g. care records, interviewing staff ± disciplinary/criminal investigation	Within 4 weeks of referral
Safeguarding plan	Safeguarding plan implemented	Further 4 weeks, then regular reviews

- *Capacitous* – you *may* break confidentiality if you think a crime needs prosecuting *or* there's risk of harm to a third party
  - Discuss with your Safeguarding Lead

You won't lead the safeguarding investigation as a trainee, but should:
- Tell the manager you're worried about Jeremy and will discuss with your team. *Don't* interview staff or detail your concerns.
- Discuss with your team manager ± Safeguarding Lead as soon as you finish the assessment (out-of-hours, contact the duty social worker)
- Call the police if you suspect a prosecutable crime, e.g. assault or rape. Ask what steps you should take to record/preserve evidence (Ch.70).
- Make a safeguarding referral, following the steps in your Trust's *Safeguarding Vulnerable Adults Policy* (look on your intranet)
  - If Jeremy needs immediate protection, the safeguarding team/social services may urgently review the placement ± provide respite care (Table 63.1).

Other agencies may become involved:
- Care Quality Commission (CQC) – when allegations involve a care home
- Multiagency risk assessment conference (MARAC) – identifies people at risk of domestic violence and works to reduce risk
- Multi-agency Public Protection Arrangements (MAPPA; p42).

4. Documentation and follow-up
Document promptly, including your concerns and Jeremy's capacity and wishes.
- Write facts, *not* opinions
- You may need to complete an incident form
- Ensure ongoing plans are made to support Jeremy
- Inform the GP, your consultant and team manager.

What if … ?

… Jeremy lives with his brother and says his brother recently hit him. He doesn't want you to take action.
Ask Jeremy how he'd like to handle it, and explain how safeguarding or practical steps could help, e.g. information on domestic violence services, meeting the brother or offering carer support. Regularly review the situation and Jeremy's capacity.

If Jeremy is capacitous and nobody else is at risk, you *may not* have grounds to break confidentiality or override his wishes. Nonetheless, discuss (± anonymously) with the Safeguarding Lead.

... His family discover him living in squalor and bring him to ED?

Possible causes include:

- Physical, e.g. delirium, poor mobility/vision
- Psychiatric, e.g. dementia, depression, substance misuse, chronic personality or coping difficulties
- Social, e.g. decompensation following bereavement or loss of informal carers; poverty
- Neglect – if he has carers, why haven't they prevented this?

Interview Jeremy and his relatives together and separately. Check his baseline level of function, onset and triggers for change. Assess for the causes above. Check whether he has a Lasting Power of Attorney (LPA) or Advance Directive. Address safeguarding issues, following the procedure described above, and treat the underlying cause, e.g. delirium (Ch.55), depression (Ch.21).

If you suspect dementia and Jeremy's unsafe to return home, he should usually be admitted under the medics to establish the diagnosis and enable a full MDT assessment ± package of care. Alert liaison psychiatry to review, and only consider a psychiatric admission if he's physically fit, but can't be safely managed on a medical ward, e.g. due to challenging behaviour. Protect him on the ward, e.g. restrict access from suspected abusers. If available, emergency interim placement is another option (via social services) with psychiatric follow-up.

If discharging (e.g. to concerned and capable relatives), refer back to his existing team, or to the Mental Health of Older Adults (MHOA) if newly presenting and over 65. Include physical investigations and cognitive testing in your referral.

Take-home message

Have a low threshold for raising an alert. Discuss concerns with colleagues, clearly documenting reasons for action *or* inaction.

Further reading

Department of Health and Home Office (2000) No secrets: guidance on developing and implementing multi-agency policies and procedures to protect vulnerable adults from abuse. Department of Health, London.

Hodgson, R. and Rheade, J. (2013) Safeguarding vulnerable adults: The psychiatrist's roles and responsibilities. *Advances in Psychiatric Treatment* **19**, 437–445.

Social Care Policy, Department of Health (2011) Safeguarding adults: The role of health service practitioners. Department of Health, London.

Resources for patients

Victim Support: www.victimsupport.org.uk

CHAPTER 64

Child protection concerns

Peter Hindley[1], Juliet Hurn[1], and Sarah Stringer[2]

[1] *South London & Maudsley NHS Foundation Trust, London, England*
[2] *King's College London, London, England*

RELATED CHAPTERS: child self-harm (52), adult safeguarding (63), alleged sexual assault (70), aggressive children (75)

Daniel was admitted 2 days ago with a manic episode, exacerbated by cannabis use. He lives with his partner, Sam, and their children Phoebe (3) and Jack (5). During a visit to the ward, you notice the children have bruises to their faces and upper arms, some of which resemble finger marks. They seem wary of Daniel and hide behind Sam when he approaches.

Mental health problems *don't* mean someone can't be a good parent, though can sometimes make it harder. The risk of neglect or abuse increases with:
• Substance misuse, poverty, overcrowding, domestic violence
• Parental history of childhood abuse
• Children who have disabilities or were 'unwanted'
• Psychotic disorders where delusions are focused on the child
Although it's important not to jump to conclusions, any concerns should trigger a child safeguarding referral (Table 64.1, Box 64.1).

Box 64.1 The Children Act 1989.

- *Child:* anyone under 18
- *Children in need:* children needing service provision to reach a satisfactory level of health or development (includes disabled children)
- *Children at risk of significant harm:* a sub-set of children in need. Their risk of harm requires compulsory intervention in their best interests.
- *Maltreatment:* physical / sexual / emotional abuse, fabricated / induced illness; neglect
- *Section 47:* section dealing with enquiries into maltreatment/abuse
- *Child protection:* measures taken to protect children at risk of significant harm.

Psychiatry: Breaking the ICE – Introductions, Common Tasks and Emergencies for Trainees, First Edition.
Edited by Sarah Stringer, Juliet Hurn and Anna M Burnside.
© 2016 John Wiley & Sons, Ltd. Published 2016 by John Wiley & Sons, Ltd.
Companion Website: www.psychiatryice.com

Table 64.1 Signs of child neglect and abuse.

Signs or behaviours	Problem suggested			
	N	E	P	S
Weight loss/underweight/constantly hungry; stealing or scavenging food	✓			
Delayed development (physical, emotional, social)	✓	✓	✓	✓
Dirty, malodorous, head lice	✓			
Clothing: tatty, poorly fitting or inappropriate for the weather	✓			
Tired all the time/sleepy	✓	✓	✓	✓
Few friends (forbidden/not facilitated)	✓	✓	✓	✓
Excessive maturity, e.g. caring for younger siblings, taking a parental role	✓	✓	✓	✓
DNA healthcare appointments/untreated medical problems	✓		✓	
Frequently late or missing school/day care	✓	✓	✓	✓
Sudden or unexplained behavioural change, such as ...	✓	✓	✓	✓
• Withdrawal				
• Regressed behavior, e.g. rocking, sulking, return to bedwetting				
• Nervous behavior, e.g. hair twisting				
Emotional problems, e.g.	✓	✓	✓	✓
• Self-harm, aggression, distress, depression, anxiety, nightmares, eating disorders, substance misuse				
• NB Young children may present with vague 'tummy aches' or 'headaches', rather than saying they feel anxious or sad				
Flinching when touched or approached			✓	✓
Possessing unexplained money				✓
Reluctance to get changed, e.g. in sports			✓	✓
Running away / fear of going home	✓	✓	✓	✓
Reluctance to have their parents contacted		✓	✓	✓
Unusual deference to adults		✓	✓	✓
Precocious sexual knowledge/language; sexualized behavior				✓
Having 'secrets' they can't tell		✓	✓	✓
Excessive fear of making mistakes		✓	✓	
Low self-confidence	✓	✓	✓	✓
Excessive need for approval/affection/attention; overfamiliarity with strangers	✓	✓	✓	✓
Unable to cope with praise	✓	✓	✓	✓
Injuries:			✓	
• Unconvincingly explained				
• Covered with clothing – even in hot weather				
• Untreated				
• Bruising – especially where injuries through play are unlikely (e.g. face, chest, thighs)				
• Fractures – especially in under 2s				
• Bite marks				
• Burns, especially circular (cigarettes) or clearly demarcated				
• Scalds, especially:				
○ 'Tide marks' – child forced to stand/sit in hot water				
○ Upward splash marks – water deliberately thrown over them				
Evidence of sexual contact:				✓
• Genital/anal itching, bruising, bleeding or discharge				
• Incontinence				
• Stomach pains				
• Discomfort when sitting or walking				
• Unexplained, recurrent urinary tract infections (UTIs)				
• Sexually transmitted infections				
• Pregnancy				

Key: N = neglect, E = emotional abuse; P = physical abuse; S = sexual abuse

Preparation

Though preparation is important, don't delay in dealing with the problem. If you've immediate concerns about Daniel's MSE and risks, send a colleague to chaperone or separate him and the children *now*.

1. Gather information – notes, staff, GP
- Previous child safeguarding concerns
- Child risk screen
- GP: repeat presentations at surgery/ED for 'accidents'
  - Concerns about weight or development
- If a Children and Families social worker is already involved, speak to them.
  - Concerns from school//nursery?

2. Involve senior colleagues
- Tell your consultant – they may want to take the lead
- Ask Daniel's named nurse/ward manager to join you for the assessment

Assessment

1. Approach
Your role is clarifying and communicating concerns, *not* investigating the problem. Don't interview the children, as you're not trained to do this, may distress them, and could contaminate the evidence by putting words into their mouths.

See the family together
- Don't blame or appear disapproving of either parent
- Observe the family's interactions
  - Do parents respond to children's needs: interested, affectionate, appropriate (e.g. picking up if crying, setting boundaries)?
  - Are parents rejecting, unresponsive, critical or heavy-handed?
  - Are the children afraid of Sam? Is she afraid of Daniel?
- Acknowledge strengths
- Explain that time in hospital/coping with illness is stressful, and you want to check how you can support the family

Then interview Daniel and Sam separately, taking care not to increase Daniel's suspiciousness or irritability. A colleague should stay with the children and other parent.

2. Focused history, remembering …
- *Any worries about the children?*
  - Health/behaviour/development
  - School, including bullying
  - Involvement of health visitor, school counsellor, educational psychologist or Child and Adolescent Mental Health Service (CAMHS)
- *Have they noticed the bruises?*
  - What are their explanations? (Plausible? Appropriate?)
  - Cultural practices are *not* acceptable reasons for abuse, e.g. female genital mutilation
- *Explore parenting knowledge and style*
  - Practical care, e.g. *Are you managing to get them up? Make meals? Get them to school/crèche?*
  - Home environment, e.g. *How do you keep them safe around the house?* (Medications/sharp objects out of reach, sockets guarded)

- ○ Problems:
  - *Do you ever feel you can't cope?*
  - *How do you deal with naughtiness?*
  - *Have either of you ever lost your temper with them? What happened?*
  - ○ How does Daniel's illness affect him/the children?
    - Irritability, risk-taking
    - 'Protection' from harm, e.g. seeking repeated medical attention, keeping them indoors
  - ○ Own experience of being parented, including childhood abuse or adversity
- *Support*
  - ○ *Would you like more help at the moment?*
  - ○ Did/do they have a social worker? What was that to help with?
  - ○ Help with childcare, parenting groups, activities outside the house
- *Substance misuse*
- *Other household members/contacts, including babysitters*
  - ○ Relationship with children and parents
  - ○ Any concerns?
- *Sam:* does she fear for her own safety?

3. MSE (both parents), remembering ...
- Intoxication/withdrawal, self-care
- Elated/low, irritable
- Look specifically for thoughts or delusions incorporating the children, e.g.
  - ○ *They have no future ...*
  - ○ *I must protect them*
  - ○ *They're up to something ...*
- Hallucinations, including commands
- Poor problem-solving/understanding of children's needs; learning disability (LD)
- Do they think there's a problem with the children's safety or care?
  - ○ What and why?
  - ○ What would help?

4. Risk assessment – other issues
Include things the children *witness*, as these are also damaging, e.g. adult self-harm, domestic violence, pornography.

Management

1. Discuss with seniors
There are multiple indicators that Jack and Phoebe are at risk, and Child Safeguarding protocols must be followed.
- Urgently contact your Trust's Child Safeguarding Lead who will advise on next steps, including whether the children can safely go home with Sam today
- Involve your consultant and ward manager.

> **TIP:** Making decisions ... if you've got the first bit right (e.g. listening, considering people's views) you'll be better placed to get the second part right, i.e. to make the decision. Be prepared to change your view. This doesn't mean you got it wrong – it's a sign that you've listened, synthesised what colleagues are saying, and made a different decision at the end. Not many people do that, but it's to be respected.
>
> **Christopher Wheeler, Approved Mental Health Professional (AMHP)**

2. Tell the parents you're making a referral to social services

See Sam and Daniel with a senior colleague to explain the need to refer to Social Services *before* making the referral, *unless* this will increase the risk to the children.
- Sensitively explain your concerns
- Emphasise your legal duty to report any concerns about children, take action to keep children safe, and share information with social services
  - Stress that the aim is to offer more support at this stage
  - Say that you'd like the parents' consent … but must break confidentiality if refused
- Explain that social services will investigate, but always try to keep families together and offer extra parenting support
- Empathise with upset
- Apologise for causing distress

3. Make the safeguarding referral

Immediate concerns (or suspicions) of significant harm, must trigger a safeguarding referral to the social services Child Protection Team, following local protocols.
- Fax/email your report, then telephone to check it's been received
- If the family's known to social services, speak to the named social worker or their manager – otherwise the duty social worker (also available out-of-hours).

For extremely urgent concerns, where you can't/don't have time to contact social services, call the police. Social workers, the police, or the National Society for the Prevention of Cruelty to Children (NSPCC) can urgently remove a child from the home after seeking an Emergency Protection Order (EPO) from the court. In exceptional circumstances, they may remove the child without an EPO, though this would be in a case of dire emergency.

4. Document

Document your concerns and actions clearly.
- Focus on facts and write statements verbatim
- Avoid interpretation/value judgments
- Place an alert on Daniel's notes
- Update his child risk screen.

5. Follow-up

Check the progress of the referral daily. If you *can't* follow up the referral, ensure a specific colleague takes responsibility and give social services their contact details. Ensure all colleagues are aware of the safeguarding referral and are updated with progress, including the GP.

Working with the family

Children of people with mental illness – even if they're not *harmed* – may take on adult carer duties, or feel worried, confused, ashamed, or guilty. Discuss their needs with your team, e.g. education about parental illness, input from local young carers services, support by another caring adult.

Parents – especially those who lose custody of their children – are likely to experience strong emotions: anger, anxiety, guilt or despair. Your ongoing relationship with Daniel and Sam will be easier if you stay calm, viewing the problems as symptoms of wider difficulties within the family, rather than proof that one or both parents are 'bad'.
- Be alert to thoughts of suicide/self-harm, or a worsening of mental illness
- Ensure they each have support
- Explain that adherence to treatment plans for mental illness or substance misuse will be crucial in the eyes of social services (Box 64.2).

Box 64.2 What happens after referring to social services?

Within 24 hours, the social worker decides on the response and feeds back to the referrer, e.g.
- *No further action needed*
  - Signposting or request completion of a Common Assessment Framework (CAF) form to identify needs and support for the child/family
- *Child in need* but not likely to suffer significant harm. Results in a Child In Need Plan which will:
  - Provide services to the family
  - Define expectations for parents
  - Define measurable outcomes for the children
- *Child at risk of significant harm*: further assessment under Section 47. This may include:
  - Paediatric assessment of children's current functioning and evidence of abuse
  - Foster placement if unsafe to stay with either parent. Social Services will try to place children with a relative or family friend.
  - Parenting assessment
  - Child Protection conference and plan
  - Family Court proceedings
  - Ongoing reviews; meetings chaired by an allocated social worker.

If you're asked to attend a conference or write a report, discuss this with your consultant. Most psychiatrists have the expertise to comment on parental mental illness, but *not* parenting skills.

What if ... ?

... A child discloses abuse directly to you?

It's upsetting to hear allegations of abuse. Stay calm.
- Don't make negative comments about the alleged abuser
- Don't show disgust or shock
- Don't promise: *'everything will be alright'*/to keep secrets
- Listen without interrupting
- Only ask questions to clarify what's been said, not to dig deeper
- Take everything they say seriously, making verbatim notes
- Say that you're sorry this has happened to them
- Reassure them:
  - They've done the right and brave thing by telling you
  - It's not their fault
  - They won't be in any trouble
  - You'll ensure they're protected and supported
- Explain that you'll need to tell certain people who will know what to do.

Follow safeguarding protocols, as above.

... Your concerns are more vague?

Maybe you suspect emotional neglect, or just have a *feeling* things aren't quite right. You may follow steps as above, however:
- Discuss with your Child Safeguarding Lead before making the referral
- Your team may arrange further assessment/collateral, e.g. GP, paediatrician
- You'll have more time to discuss with the family and gain consent for any referrals
- Your team may complete a CAF *with* the parent(s) to structure the initial needs assessment and decide whether to proceed with the safeguarding referral
- Try to increase the family's support through links with relevant services e.g. parenting groups
- Review regularly

Take-home message

Mental illness doesn't mean people can't parent. However, if you're concerned that a child faces imminent risks of harm you must act immediately to ensure their safety. Always discuss concerns with the Trust's Safeguarding Lead and senior colleagues.

Further reading

Department for Education (2015) *Working Together to Safeguard Children: A guide to inter-agency working to safeguard and promote the welfare of children.* Department for Education, London.
Cleaver, H., Unell, I.and Aldgate, J. (2011) *Children's Needs – Parental Capacity. Child Abuse: Parental Mental Illness, learning disability, substance misuse and domestic violence, 2nd Edition.* The Stationery Office, Norwich UK
Department for Education (2015) *What to do if a child is being abused: Advice for practitioners.* Department for Education, London.
NICE (2009) Clinical Guideline CG89 When to suspect child maltreatment. NICE, England.

Resources for families

Children's Society young carer information: www.youngcarer.com

CHAPTER 65

Medical emergencies

Katherine Beck and Abigail Steenstra

South London & Maudsley NHS Foundation Trust, London, England

---

RELATED CHAPTERS: delirium (55), opiate overdose (66), stiff, feverish patients (67), catatonia (68), lithium toxicity (69), self-harm on ward (71), hanging (72), death (73)

While on-call, you're contacted about an inpatient named Roy. He's 48 and has schizophrenia, but appears physically unwell: short of breath, pale and sweaty. The nurse requests your urgent review.

Assessing and managing physical illness on a psychiatric ward can be stressful and challenging. You'll usually be the medical expert in the unit, but shouldn't let this stop you from seeking help from the local medics.

Preparation

1. On the telephone
- Roy's full name, age, MHA status and ward
- *SBAR:*
  - *Situation* – symptoms/signs, main concerns
  - *Background* – psychiatric and medical diagnoses, medications, MSE changes, previous similar episodes
  - *Assessment* – obs, Early Warning Scoring (EWS), blood sugar
    - Request now if missing
  - *Response* – what's their question? What do they want you to do?
- *Immediate response:*
  - *Advise* – of *your* working diagnosis, plan and timeframe
    - E.g. *This may be a heart attack. I'll be there in 5 minutes.*
  - *Instruct* – on immediate management
    - E.g. *Call 999 and the Emergency Response Team (ERT). Get the resus bag, ECG machine, drug chart, obs chart and notes. Start 100% oxygen and repeat physical obs and blood sugar.*

2. On the ward
- Get a clinical update and risk assessment
- Briefly view Roy, to check he isn't *in extremis*
- Read relevant notes
- Take a nurse with you to chaperone, reassure and assist/gain help if Roy deteriorates

---

Psychiatry: Breaking the ICE – Introductions, Common Tasks and Emergencies for Trainees, First Edition.
Edited by Sarah Stringer, Juliet Hurn and Anna M Burnside.
© 2016 John Wiley & Sons, Ltd. Published 2016 by John Wiley & Sons, Ltd.
Companion Website: www.psychiatryice.com

Assessment

1. Focused history and examination

Assess as you would on any medical ward, including ABCDE approach and checking allergies. Remember additional problems for psychiatric patients (Box 65.1). Involve the nurse if Roy's uncooperative, e.g. to demonstrate the examination or help him keep still.

Box 65.1 Additional problems for psychiatric inpatients

- *Medication side effects*
  - ○ Acute e.g. extrapyramidal side effects (EPSE), sedation
  - ○ Chronic e.g. metabolic syndrome
- *Behavioural factors*
  - ○ Intoxication/withdrawal
  - ○ Self-harm, including overdose
  - ○ Neglect of physical health conditions (not help-seeking)
  - ○ Dehydration/malnutrition (poor oral intake)
- *Specific conditions*
  - ○ Acute dystonias (Table 36.1, p226)
  - ○ Lithium toxicity (Ch.69)
  - ○ Neuroleptic Malignant Syndrome (NMS) / serotonin syndrome (Ch.67)
- *Psychosomatic symptoms*

TIP: Always, always, always think, *Is this person taking clozapine?* That boring cough/cold or constipation suddenly become a big issue.

Ben Spencer, ST6

2. MSE, especially symptoms complicating assessment and management …

- Intoxication/withdrawal
- Agitation/resistance
- Thought disorder/mutism
- Suicidal/violent thoughts
- Psychotic symptoms
- Confusion
- Poor insight.

Think: are symptoms part of Roy's usual presentation, or new and related to physical illness?

3. Investigations

Tests are limited and may take longer to process, compared with the general hospital, e.g. sending blood samples to lab by taxi!
- Usually possible: blood tests, ECG, urine drug screen (UDS)/urine dip
If more complex/rapid tests are needed to exclude a serious diagnosis, transfer to ED.

Management

1. Decide where to treat (psychiatric unit versus ED)
Can you safely manage Roy on the unit?
- Discuss with the nurses – they'll know local systems better than you
- IVIs can't be given on the unit
- Limited physical medications (check): usually glyceryl trinitrate (GTN), aspirin, glucagon IM, flumazenil IM, naloxone IM/IV
  - Follow algorithms for emergency drugs
- If unsure whether there's a *medical* indication to transfer, call the local medical registrar and gain parameters for transfer, e.g.
  - Pulse above X
  - 'Red flag' symptoms such as chest pain
- What are the risks of transfer, e.g. absconding, violence?
Discuss options with Roy.

2. If transferring to ED
- *MHA considerations*
  - Detained patients *don't* need section 17 leave for emergency transfer
  - For non-emergencies, the RC should write up s.17 leave, e.g. routine GUM appointment
  - If unsure, discuss with a senior.
- *Nurses*
  - Arrange transport, specifying urgency, e.g. *blue light* ambulance / ambulance / taxi
  - Photocopy drug and obs chart
  - An RMN should escort and stay with Roy. Staff shortages must be escalated to the unit manager or hospital manager. You'll occasionally need 2:1 or police escort.
- *Cover letter for the medics* (p51) including:
  - What to do if Roy tries to leave, e.g. hold under MCA/MHA
  - Symptoms which may make him hard to assess/treat (give advice if so)
  - Symptoms which look 'psychiatric' but are new or suggest organic illness
  - Ward and duty doctor contact details
  - Specify who should be contacted before transfer back to your unit

3. Handover and follow-up
- If Roy stays on your ward, ensure staff know *what* to do and *when* to call you back (specific parameters, EWS, 'red flags')
- Handover to the regular ward doctor(s)/next duty doctor
- Consider asking Liaison Psychiatry to review if Roy's admitted under the medics

TIP: Most ward nurses know the patients very well. We may not always go on medical jargon or scientific facts but sometimes we just have intuition, hunches – we are a bit witchy! Sometimes we just know when something's not right.

Sam Gray, RMN

What if ... ?

... Roy refuses to comply with the plan

The MHA can't be used to treat physical conditions against a patient's will. If Roy lacks capacity with respect to the intervention, treat in his best interests under the MCA (Ch.76). Consider the practicalities of enforcing necessary management, and where/how this is best done. Discuss with your senior if needed, and *always* discuss if medical treatment would be serious or irreversible. In an emergency, you can act quickly without consulting seniors/family, if a delay could be fatal.

Take-home message

Teams differ in their ability to manage acute illness on a psychiatric ward, depending on the ward facilities, staff training and even time of day. Take guidance from the team when making transfer decisions, but never let insufficient resources trump urgent medical care.

Further reading

Resuscitation Council (2011) *Immediate Life Support*, 3rd edn, Resuscitation Council UK, London.
Royal College of Physicians (2012) National Early Warning Score (NEWS): Standardising the assessment of acute-illness severity in the NHS. Report of a working party. RCP, London.

CHAPTER 66

Opiate overdose

Isabel McMullen and Lisa Conlan

South London & Maudsley NHS Foundation Trust, London, England

---

RELATED CHAPTERS: illicit drugs (41), death (73)

You're urgently bleeped. Chrissie, 35, has collapsed, following unescorted leave. She has a history of drug misuse. A used needle was found beside her.

Opiate overdose is a medical emergency. *Always* **transfer to ED.**

Preparation

1. On the telephone – request
- Ambulance (999) and someone to meet paramedics
- ERT (2222)
- Resuscitation trolley/bag
- Drug and obs charts

2. Run to the ward – go straight to Chrissie

3. Brief summary from senior nurse
- Diagnosis
- Substance misuse
- Medications
- Recent presentation

Assessment and management

1. Assess ABCDE
- Safety, e.g. remove used needles
- *Airway*
  - Head-tilt, chin-lift
  - Remove obstructions, e.g. food/gum/vomit; suction if trained
- *Breathing and Circulation – 10 second check*
  - Breath: look, listen, feel
  - Pulse: feel

Psychiatry: Breaking the ICE – Introductions, Common Tasks and Emergencies for Trainees, First Edition.
Edited by Sarah Stringer, Juliet Hurn and Anna M Burnside.
© 2016 John Wiley & Sons, Ltd. Published 2016 by John Wiley & Sons, Ltd.
Companion Website: www.psychiatryice.com

- *Disability: AVPU*
  - Alert
  - Voice responsive
  - Pain responsive
  - Unresponsive
- *Exposure:* expose and briefly look for cause, e.g. bleeding needle marks

2. Immediate life support (ILS)

- *Not breathing / no pulse*
  - Fit airway if trained
  - Ventilate via bag-valve-mask (attached to O_2 at 15L/min)
  - CPR – 30 chest compressions:2 breaths
  - Defibrillator: attach pads, turn on, follow voice prompts
  - Attempt IV access
- *Pulse, but Respiratory Rate (RR)<8*
  - Fit airway if trained
  - Ventilate via bag-valve-mask, 1 squeeze every 6 seconds
- *Breathing normally*
  - Place in recovery position and monitor RR

3. Opiate overdose (OD) specific

- *Assess for opiate OD*
  - Unconscious
  - Respiratory depression (RR<8)
  - Pin-point pupils
  - Signs of recent drug use, e.g. needles
  - Blue lips, cold skin
  - Drug chart: recent methadone/other opiates?
- *If you suspect opiate OD, give naloxone 0.4–2 mg IV (IM if no IV access)*
  - If no response, repeat every 2–3 minutes (max 10 mg)
  - Ask one nurse to record doses and timings

4. Ongoing management

- *No improvement: check blue light ambulance coming*
  - Continue CPR $\pm$ defibrillation
  - Reassess ABCDE, consider other causes
    - Check blood sugar
    - Benzodiazepine OD? (Consider flumazenil, p491)
    - IV access and take bloods if possible
    - Consider fluid resuscitation
- *If she improves:*
  - Continue high flow oxygen
  - Explain to Chrissie what's just happened
  - Find out what drugs she's taken
  - If OD – accidental or deliberate (is she suicidal?)
- *Await paramedics*

5. Handover

- Paramedics – summarise the history, your assessment and management
- *Transfer to ED for medical monitoring, no matter how well she looks now*
  - Naloxone's half life is shorter than most opiates, wearing off in 20–60 minutes

- Send an RMN with her (1:1) – be explicit about any risk of absconding/suicide
- Handover to ED doctor, including contact details (ward + your bleep number)
- Document clearly and strike off opiates (including methadone) until further review
- Help staff complete critical incident reports
- Verbal handover to ward doctor

TIP: Practice cases like this in your yearly Immediate Life Support (ILS) training, preferably as a ward team

Take-home message

Check for signs of opiate overdose, and if unsure, administer a trial of naloxone.

Further reading

Resuscitation Council (2011) *Immediate Life Support*, 3rd edn, Resuscitation Council UK, London.

CHAPTER 67

Stiff, feverish patients

Anna M Burnside

East London NHS Foundation Trust, London, England

RELATED CHAPTERS: common side effects (36), medical emergencies (65)

You're called to review Niruban Gunawardena, a 22-year old Sri Lankan student, admitted with psychosis 1 week ago. He's required rapid tranquilisation (RT), and is now drowsy, stiff, confused and feverish.

Neuroleptic Malignant Syndrome (NMS) is a life-threatening syndrome associated with dopamine antagonism; Serotonin Syndrome (SS) looks similar, but results from excessive serotonin. Both can kill, and mild presentations can precede full-blown syndromes. Think NMS or SS with *any* combination of HARD symptoms:

    H yperthermia
    A utonomic instability
    R igidity
    D rowsy/delirious

The differential includes lethal catatonia, malignant hyperthermia, alcohol withdrawal, infection (encephalitis / meningitis / sepsis) and drug toxicity. SS often presents with low-level discomfort, and may resemble opiate withdrawal, hypomania or antidepressant side effects.

    Attend immediately, and have a low threshold for transfer to ED.

Preparation

1. On the telephone – request
- Repeat physical obs, blood sugar
- Resus bag, drug and obs charts, notes.

2. On the ward
- *Quick look:* Airway, Breathing, Circulation
  - Looks very sick – call 999 now?
- *Notes*
  - Background information
  - Medication on admission
  - PMHx, baseline physical exam, obs, investigations + *current obs*
    - Underlying physical cause, e.g. infectious, metabolic, neurological, toxic?
  - NMS risk factors:
    - Neuroleptic naïve/history of NMS

Psychiatry: Breaking the ICE – Introductions, Common Tasks and Emergencies for Trainees, First Edition.
Edited by Sarah Stringer, Juliet Hurn and Anna M Burnside.
© 2016 John Wiley & Sons, Ltd. Published 2016 by John Wiley & Sons, Ltd.
Companion Website: www.psychiatryice.com

Table 67.1 Causes of NMS and SS.

Syndrome	Usual culprits	Other prescribed medications	Other causes
NMS	**Antipsychotics** especially • New • Increased • High dose • First generation antipsychotics (FGAs) **Antiparkinsonian drugs** withdrawn	Antidepressants Promethazine Metoclopramide Lithium Cholinesterase inhibitors	Illicit drugs, especially amphetamines
SS	**Antidepressants** especially • Selective serotonin reuptake inhibitors (SSRIs) • Combined with other serotonergic medications	Second generation antipsychotics (SGAs) Lithium Valproate Opiates, especially methadone and tramadol Ondansetron Metoclopramide Selegiline Linezolid Sumatriptan and other 'triptans'	Illicit drugs, especially LSD, ecstasy, amphetamine, cocaine, opiates Over the counter (OTC) medicines: dextromethorphan (cough syrups) St. John's wort, tryptophan NB: rare case reports of SS with Electroconvulsive therapy (ECT) in combination with antidepressants

- Substance misuse and UDS (especially amphetamines)
- Recent dehydration
- *Drug chart* (see Table 67.1)
  - Recent medication changes
  - Allergies/past drug reactions.

Assessment

Take an experienced nurse, in case of agitation/deterioration.

1. Physical assessment
- *Check*
  - Airway, Breathing, Circulation (call 999 if needed)
  - Glasgow Coma Scale (GCS)
  - Confusion: check orientation. Fluctuating attention?
- *Physical examination*
  - Table 67.2 for signs
  - Full neurological exam essential

2. Focused history, remembering ...
- *Medications:*
  - Changes – prescribed or over-the-counter (OTC)
  - Adherence
  - Overdose – accidental or deliberate (causes many cases of SS)
- *Substance misuse*
  - Illicit drugs
  - Alcohol

Table 67.2 Comparison of NMS, SS and lethal catatonia.

Factor	NMS	Serotonin syndrome	Lethal catatonia (Ch.68)
Medication	Recent (past 72h) exposure to dopamine antagonist or withdrawal of dopamine agonist	Serotonergic addition /↑ coinciding temporally with symptoms Neuroleptic *not* recently added or increased	May have been non-concordant with antipsychotics
Onset	Days-weeks	Hours-days	Varies
Progression	24–72h	Hours	Varies
Hyperthermia	>38°C on at least 2 occasions	Fever	Fever (NB: non-lethal catatonia - hot only during excitation phases)
Autonomic signs	↑BP (systolic or diastolic ≥ 25% above baseline) BP fluctuation (change within 24h of ≥20mmHg diastolic or ≥25mmHg systolic) ↑HR (≥25% above baseline) *and* ↑RR increase (≥50% above baseline) Sweating (often profuse)	↑HR ↑/↓BP Sweating	↑HR ↑/↓BP Sweating
Rigidity + other neurological findings	Lead-pipe rigidity ±Tremor	Rigidity Hyper-reflexia Myoclonus Tremor Ataxia Clonus Fits	Rigidity Posturing
Drowsy/ delirious	✓	✓	Usually alert, but unresponsive
Other physical signs	Bradykinesia *or* agitation Urinary incontinence Drooling Pallor	Hyperkinesia/agitation Diarrhoea Shivering Dilated pupils, Nausea ↑bowel sounds	Stupor/excitation (may alternate)
Bloods	↑Creatinine kinase (CK) (≥4x the upper limit of normal) ↑WCC ±Renal failure (if rhabdomyolysis)	CK may ↑ WCC may ↑ ±Renal failure (if rhabdomyolysis)	CK may ↑ WCC usually normal Dehydration

TIP: Explain that medications or drugs may be causing his symptoms. This may help Niruban to openly discuss drug use or non-adherence.

3. MSE, remembering …
- Affective/psychotic symptoms of primary psychiatric diagnosis
- Catatonic symptoms (Ch.68)
- Suicidal ideation (SS: is this a deliberate overdose?)
  NB: SS can resemble hypomania: restlessness, pressured speech.

4. Investigations
If Niruban is very unwell, site the largest cannulae possible and transfer straight to ED.
- CK (>200IU/L in NMS, and often in the thousands)
- Blood cultures, FBC, U&E, LFT, CRP, glucose
- ECG – especially if
  - (Es)citalopram/tricyclic antidepressant (TCA)
  - High dose antipsychotics
- UDS if possible.

Management

1. Milder symptoms/subacute presentations
Mild cases may be managed on your ward, if seniors ± medical registrar agree, e.g.
- NMS – e.g. alert but low-grade fever and slightly stiff
- SS – e.g. mild shakes and sweating.

Medications
- NMS – stop all antipsychotics and antidepressants
- SS – stop serotonergics
- Both: start regular benzodiazepines, e.g. lorazepam 0.5–1 mg bd.

Nursing advice
- 1:1 nursing
- Cooling, e.g. fans, cool cloths, ice packs
- Oral hydration
- At *least* hourly physical obs with scoring system, e.g. EWS
- Staff to contact you if concerned (give clear parameters)
- Avoid restraint if possible – it raises CK *and* carries an increased risk of death
  - Restrain for the least possible time, checking obs during and after
  - Supervised confinement may be safer than repeated restraints

Reviews
- In person 4-hourly, repeating bloods (check results/handover to the next doctor).
- If *very mild* SS – within the next 24 hours

Documentation
Document clearly and add an alert to the drug chart
- Transfer to the medics if:
  - No improvement
  - Deterioration (e.g. rising CK)
  - Suspect encephalitis/meningitis

2. Very unwell
Reasons for transfer include:
- Clear NMS/severe SS
- Deteriorating
- Very confused/drowsy
- High fever, e.g. >38.5°C
- Tachycardic, fluctuating BP
- Can't accept oral fluids

- Rising CK
- Suspected overdose (particularly TCA/(es)citalopram, where ECG monitoring is required)

Immediate action
- Stop all antipsychotics and antidepressants
- Ask the nurse in charge to organise:
  - Ambulance (blue-light to ED)
  - 1:1 nursing; RMN to stay with Niruban in the general hospital
  - Cooling
  - Photocopy of the drug chart.
- Insert the largest cannula you can and start IV fluids
- Write a brief cover letter and call the ED registrar to handover:
  - Suspected NMS/SS, not to receive antipsychotics/antidepressants
  - Use benzodiazepines for agitation
  - PMHx, PPHx
  - Your contact details
- Stay with Niruban until the ambulance arrives
- Handover to paramedics
- Document clearly. Add a medication alert to the notes.
- Handover to liaison psychiatry for urgent follow-up

In the general hospital (explain to relatives)
Severe presentations need supportive care ± ITU (cooling, fluid resuscitation ± ventilation and circulatory support). Both NMS and SS risk rhabdomyolysis.
- NMS – dantrolene, lorazepam, amantadine or bromocriptine may help
- SS – lorazepam; occasionally serotonin antagonists, e.g. cyproheptadine, chlorpromazine.

Prognosis
- NMS usually worsens for 24–72 hours, then improves within 2 weeks (longer if depot)
- SS usually resolves within 24–36 hours

3. Longer-term management

NMS: if antipsychotics are still needed:
- Niruban and his family will be anxious about the risks: discuss fully
- Wait at least 5 days *and* until NMS has fully resolved
- Use an SGA, e.g. quetiapine, aripiprazole, clozapine
  - Start low, go slow
  - Keep hydrated and monitor closely
  - Avoid polypharmacy (especially lithium/antidepressants)
  - Avoid depots.

SS: before reintroducing a serotonergic agent
- Consider other options, e.g. Cognitive Behaviour Therapy (CBT) instead of an antidepressant
- Avoid combining serotonergics, including OTC medications
- Allow at least a two week washout period (four to five weeks if fluoxetine)
- Cautiously reintroduce with close monitoring.

Take-Home Message

Stiff, feverish patients should worry you. Have a low threshold for transfer to the medics. Prevention is better than cure: if patients know to contact you with early signs, you can prevent full-blown disasters.

Further reading

Resuscitation Council (2011) *Immediate Life Support*, 3rd edn, Resuscitation Council UK, London.

Gurrera, R.J., Caroff, S.N., Cohen, A. *et al.* (2011) An international consensus study of neuroleptic malignant syndrome diagnostic criteria using the Delphi method. *Journal of Clinical Psychiatry* **72** (9), 1222–1228.

Taylor, D., Paton, C. & Kapur, S. (2015) *The Maudsley Prescribing Guidelines in Psychiatry*, 12th edn, Wiley-Blackwell, Chichester.

Ahuja, R. and Cole, A.J. (2009) Hyperthermia Syndromes in Psychiatry. *Advances in Psychiatric Treatment*, **15**, 181–191.

Sternbach, H. (2003) Serotonin syndrome: How to avoid, identify, and treat dangerous drug interactions. *Current Psychiatry* **2** (5), 15–24.

CHAPTER 68

Catatonia

Anna M Burnside

East London NHS Foundation Trust, London, England

> **RELATED CHAPTERS:** medical emergencies (65), stiff, feverish patients (67)

Lorena is 32 and has schizoaffective disorder. Relatives found her immobile in bed last week, and she was admitted under Section 3. She didn't eat or drink over the weekend, and your consultant has asked you to assess Lorena and present a management plan.

Catatonia is a syndrome of movement disorders, characterised by marked changes in muscle tone and activity. Sufferers may fluctuate between extremes, e.g. of excitement and stupor; automatic obedience and oppositional behaviour. Though originally described as a subtype of schizophrenia, catatonia actually occurs most commonly in mania. Differentials include:

- Catatonia caused by:
  - Mania, depression, psychosis
  - Organic illness, e.g. epilepsy, infections, metabolic disturbance
  - Drugs, e.g. cocaine, ecstasy
  - Medication, e.g. ciprofloxacin; sudden cessation of clozapine
- Hysteria (psychogenic catatonia)
- Malignant catatonia (extreme, life-threatening version of catatonia)
- Neuroleptic Malignant Syndrome (NMS; Ch.67)
- Serotonin Syndrome (SS; Ch.67)

It's been argued that malignant catatonia, NMS and SS are a spectrum of related disorders. They can certainly share core symptoms (hyperthermia, autonomic instability, rigidity and drowsiness). NMS and malignant catatonia both raise CK and worsen with antipsychotics. When in doubt, treat with benzodiazepines ± transfer to the medics.

Preparation

1. Gather information – notes, drug chart, obs chart, GP/Community Mental Health Team (CMHT), ward staff

- Previous catatonia and treatment, including electroconvulsive therapy (ECT)
- PMHx/recent symptoms (?organic cause)
- Recent medication changes/additions?
- Risks: dehydration, aggression

Psychiatry: Breaking the ICE – Introductions, Common Tasks and Emergencies for Trainees, First Edition.
Edited by Sarah Stringer, Juliet Hurn and Anna M Burnside.
© 2016 John Wiley & Sons, Ltd. Published 2016 by John Wiley & Sons, Ltd.
Companion Website: www.psychiatryice.com

2. Arrange to interview Lorena's family

Assessment

You must decide whether Lorena has catatonia (functional or organic), and whether a medical or psychiatric ward is most appropriate.

1. Approach
- If Lorena can't speak, don't assume she can't understand you
- Catatonic psychopathology is fascinating, but please remain respectful and gentle. Lorena isn't a science experiment, and may be terrified.

2. Collateral history, remembering …
- What preceded the catatonia?
  - Stressful life events
  - Manic, depressive or psychotic symptoms
  - Physical illness
  - Medication changes (especially antipsychotics)
- Duration of starvation, dehydration, immobility
- Previous episodes – what helped?
- Views on ECT (Lorena and carers)

3. MSE (especially if Lorena can't give a history), remembering …
Look for evidence of an underlying disorder (e.g. mania, psychosis), plus *catatonic symptoms*:
- Excitement – extreme, constant, purposeless hyperactivity
- Stupor – immobile, unresponsive to external stimuli
- Posturing – adopting and holding non-functional bodily positions
- Repetitive movements
  - Stereotypies – non-goal oriented, e.g. rocking, rubbing self
  - Mannerisms – goal-oriented, e.g. pointing
- Obstruction – stops inexplicably in the middle of a movement (motor version of thought block)
- Grimacing
- Staring
- Mute/inaudible whispering
- Echolalia – repeats your words
- Repetition of phrases/words
- Logorrhoea – endless, incoherent, speech
- Clouded consciousness (?malignant catatonia/NMS/SS)

4. Physical examination, remembering …
- Obs (and see Table 67.2, p410)
- Full neurological exam (increased resting tone)
- Catatonic signs (Table 68.1)

TIP: Catatonic patients may not only resist instructions, but do the opposite. This isn't 'bad behaviour' – they can't control it. Examples include clenching their mouth shut in response to food, soiling themselves *after* having sat on the toilet, sleeping *under* their bed …

Table 68.1 Catatonia physical examination.

Sign	Example test	Pathological response
Grasp reflex	Firmly place two fingers in her palm	Tightly grasps your fingers (±even if asked not to)
Opposition (gegenhalten)	Move her arm horizontally back and forth by the wrist, with varying degrees of strength	Automatically resists movement in each direction, matching your strength with each move
Negativism	Ask her to look at you	Turns away
Echopraxia	Scratch your head in an exaggerated way	Copies (±even if asked not to)
Waxy flexibility	Reposition her arm, into an unusual (but painless) position	Initial resistance, then allows herself to be repositioned and holds the pose, e.g. >1 minute
Mitgehen	Say, "*Don't* let me move your arm", then push her arm in different directions with just your finger	You can move her arm with the lightest touch ("like an anglepoise lamp")
Automatic obedience	Reach into your pocket and say: "Poke out your tongue, I need to stick a pin in it".	Sticks tongue out (Don't *actually* poke her with a pin!)
	Extend your hand, saying, "Please *don't* shake my hand"	Shakes your hand (± won't let go)
Ambitendence	Extend your hand, saying, "Please *don't* shake my hand"	Oscillates, e.g. reaching out then retracting her hand repeatedly
	Instruct: "Please walk to the end of the room and back"	Takes a step away, then back, then away again

5. Investigations
- FBC, U&E, LFT, TFT, glucose, CK
- UDS
- If diagnostic doubt, consider:
  - Blood and urine cultures
  - HIV and syphilis testing
  - Caeruloplasmin (Wilson's disease)
  - Heavy metal screen
  - Autoantibody screen
  - CT/MRI head
  - Lumbar puncture
  - EEG (TLE/non-convulsive status epilepticus)

6. Risk assessment, remembering...
- Self-harm/violence during excitement
- Dehydration/collapse
- Self-neglect
- Death from medical consequences of stupor, e.g. DVT/PE, renal failure

Management

1. Decide where to treat her
Transfer to the medics if:
- Suspected malignant catatonia, NMS or SS (Ch.67)
  - Hyperthermia, autonomic instability, rigidity, drowsiness ±↑CK
- Needs IV hydration/parenteral nutrition
- Otherwise severely ill

2. Supportive management
- Correct dehydration and malnutrition
- Start a food and fluid chart; monitor urine output
- Consider thromboembolism prophylaxis if immobile

3. Medication
Avoid/stop antipsychotics, at least initially.

Start lorazepam
- 1 mg PO/IM, and monitor response
- Repeat after 3 hours and up to 4 mg/day
- If no response after 1–2 days, your consultant may prescribe above-British National Formulary (BNF) doses, e.g. 8–24 mg/day, monitoring closely for respiratory depression

If catatonia has occurred after abruptly stopping clozapine, consider restarting clozapine (consultant decision; see Ch.37 for practicalities).

4. Treatment resistance
ECT (Ch.47) is the next step, if
- Higher dose lorazepam isn't effective within three to four days
- Life-threatening
- Malignant catatonia

5. Longer-term
Once better, ask Lorena how she'd like to be treated, should catatonia recur, e.g. early ECT. If the underlying cause was psychosis, you may need to cautiously treat with an SGA, but advise Lorena on the symptoms of NMS, and monitor closely for this.

Take-home message

Catatonia isn't as rare as once thought, and early detection and treatment improves outcomes.

Reference

Bush-Frances scale: http://abbottgrowth.ru/doctors/tables/files/f1261158827703.pdf

Further reading

Caroff, S.N., Mann, S.C., Francis, A., Fricchione, G.L., (2004) *Catatonia: From Psychopathology to Neurobiology.* American Psychiatric Press.

Rajagopal, S. (2007) Catatonia. *Advances in Psychiatric Treatment*, **13**, 51–59.

Taylor, D., Paton, C. & Kapur, S. (2015) *The Maudsley Prescribing Guidelines in Psychiatry*, 12th edn, Wiley-Blackwell, Chichester.

CHAPTER 69

Lithium toxicity

Noreen Jakeman[1] and Katherine Beck[2]

[1] Lewisham & Greenwich NHS Trust, London, England
[2] Yet to supply.

RELATED CHAPTERS: Bipolar affective disorder (BPAD) (25), medical emergencies (65)

You're on-call one weekend. The nursing staff ask you to review Lucy Taylor, 69. She relapsed with mania 6 weeks ago, after stopping her lithium suddenly. She's been in the wars: having suffered a sprained ankle a week ago, she's now 'gone down with a tummy bug' and has diarrhoea. She's weak, wobbly and shaky.

Always consider lithium toxicity before more benign causes of ill health in anyone using lithium. Lithium has a narrow therapeutic index: it doesn't take much to tip someone from therapeutic to toxic levels (Box 69.1).

Box 69.1 Lithium toxicity key facts.

Kidneys excrete lithium in exchange for sodium. Anything lowering sodium levels or renal function can raise lithium levels.
- *Therapeutic lithium levels: 0.4–1.0 mmol/l* (optimum 0.6–0.8; higher for mania)
- *Toxicity:* >1.5 mmol/l (severe >2.0 mmol/l)
  - Diarrhoea, nausea/vomiting, anorexia
  - Coarse tremor, ataxia, slurred speech, weakness, myoclonus
  - Lethargy, drowsiness
  - Higher levels:
    - Fits, confusion, coma
    - Renal failure/circulatory collapse
    - Death
- *Triggers include:* low-salt diets, dehydration, hot weather, fever, infection, medication changes, ageing (levels rise in the elderly)
- NB: some patients show signs of toxicity at <1.5 mmol/l

Preparation

1. On the telephone
- Ask the nurse to repeat physical obs and offer clear fluids

---

Psychiatry: Breaking the ICE – Introductions, Common Tasks and Emergencies for Trainees, First Edition.
Edited by Sarah Stringer, Juliet Hurn and Anna M Burnside.
© 2016 John Wiley & Sons, Ltd. Published 2016 by John Wiley & Sons, Ltd.
Companion Website: www.psychiatryice.com

2. On the ward – look specifically for causes of toxicity:

- *Obs chart* – signs of dehydration?
- *Drug chart:* especially
  - Lithium: dose increases; administration or prescribing errors (e.g. lithium carbonate and citrate aren't equivalent – have they been confused?)
  - ACE inhibitors, e.g. lisinopril, ramipril
  - Angiotensin II receptor antagonists, e.g. candesartan, irbesartan, losartan
  - Thiazide diuretics, e.g. bendroflumethiazide, indapamide
  - Non-steroidal anti-inflammatory drugs (NSAIDs)/COX-2 inhibitors,
    - *Was ibuprofen prescribed for Lucy's sprained ankle?*
  - Medications causing hyponatraemia, e.g. SSRIs, carbamazepine
  - Loop diuretics (e.g. furosemide, bumetanide) are safer, but patients are often advised to follow a *low-salt diet*
- *PMHx*: diarrhoea, vomiting, renal problems, Addison's disease
- *Recent bloods:* last lithium level, renal function, hyponatraemia

Assessment

1. Focused history, remembering ...
- Onset and type of symptoms
- Changes to diet, fluid intake, medications (including OTC)

2. MSE, remembering ...
- Slurring/dysarthria
- Mania, depression
- Suicidal? (Could this be a deliberate overdose?)
- Confusion

3. Physical examination, remembering ...
- Hydration status
- Neurological examination
  - Ataxia, coarse tremor, decreased power, hyper-reflexia
  - Fasciculations, myoclonic jerks, chorea
- Hypotension/arrhythmias (precede circulatory collapse)

4. Investigations
- U&E, eGFR
- Lithium level (immediately; repeat 12h post-dose for accurate level)
- ECG (QTc prolongation/arrhythmia)

Management

1. Decide where to treat
Discuss every case with Toxbase: telephone 0844 892 0111

Very mild symptoms
• May be monitored and treated on the unit
• *But* you must have a low threshold for transfer to ED
Always transfer (p403) if:
• Lithium levels >2.0
• Ongoing vomiting/diarrhoea (she'll continue to dehydrate)
• Hypotension/arrhythmia
• Severe neurological symptoms, including gross tremor, fits
• Confusion
• Renal failure

2. Stop responsible medications

Stop lithium and NSAIDs. Discuss stopping diuretics or presumed culprits with the medical registrar/Toxbase.

3. Rehydrate and flush out excess lithium

Push fluids. Severe toxicity needs IV hydration $\pm$ forced pressure alkaline diuresis or peritoneal/haemodialysis.

4. Ongoing management

If admitted to the general hospital, Lucy's medical team will need advice around future lithium prescribing. Remember that manic symptoms may recur when lithium is suddenly stopped.
• Lithium can *usually* be restarted once trough levels are below 1.0mmol/l, if Lucy's happy with this and there's no renal damage. Discuss first with a consultant psychiatrist and senior pharmacist, as a lower dose may be needed.
• Repeat trough levels 5 days after each increase
• Handover to liaison psychiatry for review if staying in hospital/ICU
• Decrease risks of future toxicity
  ◦ Replace her lithium booklet if she's lost it from her lithium pack (p421)
  ◦ Explain toxicity symptoms
  ◦ Advise her to contact her doctor early if worried
  ◦ Avoid low-salt diets
  ◦ Avoid dehydration, e.g. drink plenty, especially if hot weather /exercising; avoid saunas; care with alcohol
  ◦ Check all OTC medications (especially painkillers) with a pharmacist before use
  ◦ Three-monthly lithium levels are needed once stable
• For community patients – would a dosette box prevent dosing mistakes?
• Check for residual cognitive or cerebellar dysfunction (involve neurology, if so)
• Add an alert to her notes and explicitly state contraindicated medications on the allergies section of her drug chart.

What if ... ?

... It was a deliberate overdose?

This is more likely in the community, though inpatients can hoard lithium for an overdose. Remember there'll be a delay before full symptoms show. Management is the same, but extra care must be taken to contain the suicide risk, including 1:1 RMN care while in the general hospital, increased obs when back on the unit, and consideration of the longer-term safety of lithium. Remember that lithium lowers suicide rates in BPAD, so may be an important part of risk management. If stopping lithium, try to do so gradually, to prevent a manic relapse.

Take-home message

Always consider lithium toxicity in a physically unwell patient using lithium.

Further reading

Waring, W.S. (2006) Management of lithium toxicity. *Toxicology Review*, **25** (4), 221–230.
Finley, P.R., Warner, M.D. and Peabody, C.A. (1995) Clinical relevance of drug interactions with lithium. *Clinical Pharmacokinetics* **29** (3), 172–191.
Taylor, D., Paton, C. & Kapur, S. (2015) *The Maudsley Prescribing Guidelines in Psychiatry*, 12th edn, Wiley-Blackwell, Chichester.

Toxbase:

- www.toxbase.org
- UK: 0844 892 0111
- Ireland: (01) 809 2566

Patient resources:

Information leaflet on safe lithium usage http://www.patient.co.uk/medicine/lithium#
NSPA Lithium booklet for patients: http://www.nrls.npsa.nhs.uk/EasySiteWeb/getresource.axd?AssetID=65431

CHAPTER 70

Alleged sexual assault

Anna M Burnside[1], Sarah Stringer[2], and Penelope Brown[3]

[1] East London NHS Foundation Trust, London, England
[2] King's College London, London, England
[3] South London & Maudsley NHS Foundation Trust, London, England

RELATED CHAPTERS: adult safeguarding (63), child protection (64)

A nursing student, Emma, reports that her patient, Priya, has disclosed sexual assault by another patient, Alf.

Patients have a right to sexual expression, and often have relationships with each other. Problems arise when there's doubt about consent or where one person's mental state causes them to consent when they'd usually refuse. Your job isn't to decide whether a sexual assault has occurred – it's to keep both patients safe and involve the experts.

TIP: Never be judgemental. Hardly ever be prescriptive.

Alex Langford, CT3

Preparation

Involve the most senior nurse and follow your Trust's sexual assault policy.

1. Contain risk
- Separate Priya and Alf (consider 1:1 for both)
- If Priya's been injured, assess her need for transfer to ED

2. Preserve evidence until a decision is made about police involvement
- Secure the alleged site of assault as a crime scene
- Neither patient should wash, toilet, eat/drink, change clothes, brush teeth/hair
- If Priya's desperate to wash, keep samples where possible, e.g.
  - Gargle with water and spit into a specimen pot
  - Wipe affected areas with disposable cloths before showering – keep these and any clothing from the assault

Psychiatry: Breaking the ICE – Introductions, Common Tasks and Emergencies for Trainees, First Edition.
Edited by Sarah Stringer, Juliet Hurn and Anna M Burnside.
© 2016 John Wiley & Sons, Ltd. Published 2016 by John Wiley & Sons, Ltd.
Companion Website: www.psychiatryice.com

- ○ Collect first urine sample (especially if 'date rape' drugs suspected)
- ○ Sanitary towels, tampons ± faecal samples can all provide evidence
- If Priya lost a shoe/ear-ring at the crime scene, keep the remaining one of the pair

3. Gain further information
- Ask Emma exactly what Priya said and tell her to write a verbatim account
- Familiarise yourself with both patients' histories
- Find out if you have a local Sexual Assault Referral Centre (SARC – Box 70.1)
  - ○ www.thesurvivorstrust.org/sarc/
- Plan to interview Priya with a female colleague and Alf with a male colleague. Outline this plan to your consultant and check if anything else is needed.

Box 70.1 Sexual Assault Referral Centres (SARCs).

These specialist centres provide advice, assessment and support for victims of rape or sexual assault (male or female). They can coordinate:
- Full interview
- Physical examination ± evidence collection
- Police involvement (immediate / delayed / none)
- Post-coital contraception ('morning after pill')
- Prophylactic antibiotics/antiretrovirals
- Follow-up support, e.g. counselling referral.

Evidence of rape can be recovered for up to:
- 2 days – oral
- 3 days – anal
- 7 days – vaginal (3 days if pre-pubertal).

Where victims are ambivalent about involving the police, SARCs can collect and store evidence, keeping options open for later.

Assessment

1. Approach (Priya)
- Be gentle, calm and kind
- Give choices where possible, e.g. to speak to a senior/female doctor
- Reassure: she's safe; staff will support her and maintain her confidentiality
- Avoid touching her to comfort her
- Don't dismiss her story, even if she's psychotic or has a history of similar allegations

2. Physical assessment
Check for pain or injuries, but explain that you *won't* conduct an intimate examination. A trained expert can do this more gently than you, whilst following protocols to preserve and record evidence.

3. Sexual assault history
Ask her to *briefly* describe what happened, making verbatim notes.
- Perpetrator, part(s) of her body involved, place, time, witnesses
- Don't probe for details – you may jeopardise evidence
- If Priya *needs* to talk, listen without prompting.
If she's reported the assault to anyone else, they must write a statement.

4. Next steps

Check what *she* wants to do now:

- Contact the nearest SARC
- Involve police
- Nothing
- *Harm herself/Alf*

Briefly assess her capacity (p102) to make decisions about:

- Sexual contact
- Police/SARC follow-up

Note whether her mental state places her at risk of further assault, e.g. disinhibition.

5. Assess Alf

See Alf with a male colleague.

- Unless you think it'll place Priya at risk of harm, inform Alf that a *female patient* has made an allegation of sexual assault (don't name Priya)
- Stay calm, and remember that Alf may be innocent; it's not your job to judge or punish him
- Reassure him that the hospital has a duty of care to him, and will provide support if he must go through police proceedings
- Ask him for his version of events (make verbatim notes)
- Assess MSE, especially:
  - Disinhibition
  - Thoughts of harm to self/others (Priya?)

Management

1. Discuss with seniors

Your consultant or registrar should attend as soon as possible if:

- You've *any* concerns about Priya's capacity
  - They should formally assess this, as best interests decisions may need to be taken if she lacks capacity
- Priya wants to involve the police
  - They should assess Priya *and* Alf for Fitness for Interview (Box 70.2).

Try to observe these assessments. If either patient is unfit for interview, their particular interview should be postponed. Inpatients should have an Appropriate Adult who'll attend the interview to protect their rights and ensure it's conducted fairly when it happens.

Box 70.2 Fitness for police interview.

Check:
- Fully oriented
- Understands the consequences of their answers and actions
- A police interview wouldn't worsen existing physical/mental illness
- Their answers couldn't be misconstrued
- Their words or behaviours now couldn't be considered unreliable in a subsequent court hearing (e.g. due to suggestibility)
- *Perpetrator only:* understands the allegation/police caution.
Always consider whether an Appropriate Adult is needed.

(*Source:* Adapted from Rix, 2011.)

2. Priya's management

Ideally, locate your nearest SARC, and discuss Priya's case with them. They can advise on the best next steps, e.g. for Priya to attend immediately/next day; whether they'll attend the ward. If Priya wants to go to the SARC, offer to contact a friend, relative or female colleague to go with her. Alternatively, if Priya wants to involve the police immediately, they can attend, interview her ± refer her on to the local SARC.

Even if Priya refuses contact with the SARC or police, she may want to discuss the risks of pregnancy or STIs. Seek advice from the SARC, GUM clinic, or on-call pharmacist.

Consider 1:1 nursing or transferring Priya to a female ward if her mental state places her at high risk of further assault, e.g. sexual disinhibition.

3. Alf's management

Even if Priya chooses not to press charges, the incident should be discussed with the Trust legal team ± reported to the police.

Meanwhile, manage Alf's risk of sexual assault (or of being *accused* of sexual assault):
- Set clear boundaries on appropriate behaviour
- Consider increased obs (1:1/2:1) or transfer, e.g. to a male-only ward/PICU.

He may also need GUM follow-up, e.g. post-exposure prophylaxis, STI screening.

4. Documentation and follow-up

- Document the event in both patients' notes (referring to the *other* patient only by their initials)
- The nurse(s) who helped with interviews should complete an event and an incident form
- Update both patients' risk assessments
- Consider Priya's ongoing need for support
  - www.rapecrisis.org.uk/centres.php
  - Raise an adult safeguarding alert (Ch.63)
- The team should request a forensic opinion if:
  - Alf has a history of sexual assaults *or*
  - This was a very serious assault, e.g. rape.

What if ... ?

... A staff member is assaulted?

The principles of support, risk management and damage limitation are the same. Inform the senior nurse, involve the police and complete incident forms. Be kind and ensure your colleague has support at home, e.g. friend/relative.

... A staff member is accused of assault?

Inform the consultant, ward manager and unit manager. Don't interview the alleged perpetrator. Your colleague should be taken off duties while the allegation is investigated. Advise them to contact their indemnity provider/union for legal support.

... You're asked to assess a sex offender?

Sex-offending in mental health settings can be associated with mental disorder, including paraphilias, or may be completely unrelated. (Paraphilias are disorders of sexual preference, i.e. being sexually aroused by unusual stimuli. Most are legal and simply spice up consensual adult sex lives.) Problems arise when sexual behaviour causes:
- Distress, e.g. embarrassment, relationship problems
- Law-breaking/harm, i.e. sex offending
  - Paedophilia, exhibitionism, voyeurism, bestiality
  - Sadomasochism motivating rapes/assaults.

People rarely present primarily to discuss their sexual fantasies or behaviours. Instead, you'll assess people who:

- Have a history of sex offending – which may be closely related to mental illness, or have absolutely nothing to do with it
- Have become depressed/suicidal, e.g. due to discovery, prosecution, shame
- Currently pose sexual risks due to their mental state, particularly …
  - Mania, e.g. disinhibition, raised libido, impulsivity
  - Psychosis, e.g. responding to command hallucinations, erotomanic delusions
- Behave in a way which could be *misinterpreted*, e.g. approaching children in public, due to delusions that they need rescuing from abusive parents
- Wrongly believe they've committed a sexual offence, e.g. OCD (Ch.56), delusions of guilt in psychotic depression.

Assessment

Take a colleague. The patient may show anxiety, hostility or denial in order to cope with guilt or shame – it's OK to let them vent, if so. To assess thoroughly, you must gain rapport and hold an unshockable, non-blaming stance – even if their history upsets or disgusts you. Explain your duty to share information if you believe someone's at risk (±pass information to MAPPA if already known to them). Explore non-threatening areas of the history before focusing on sexual elements.

Know your limits: *don't* go into such detail that you're distressed or they're aroused; if you've been raped or sexually abused yourself, consider whether you can cope with the assessment.

- Sexual behaviour/fantasies
  - Onset, changes, escalation over time
  - Acts and plans
  - Sexual partner(s)/victims: *who, what, where, when?*
    - Profile, e.g. gender, age
    - Consent
    - Views of victim response? (Distorted?)
    - Domestic violence/sadomasochism.
  - *What do you think about when you're masturbating?*
    - Specifically check if fantasies are aggressive/involve children
  - Associated behaviours, e.g. seeking access, watching, grooming, stalking; internet habits, pornography; acts alone or with others?
- What do they feel/believe about the situation?
  - Motivations
  - Justifications
  - Guilt, fear? Empathy for victim?
  - Do they want help of any sort?
    - Motivation/barriers to seeking treatment (for mental illness *and/or* sex offending)
    - Any previous treatments?
- MSE + identify underlying/co-morbid illness
  - Organic – especially new behaviours in adults/elderly, e.g. dementia, delirium, dopaminergics in Parkinson's disease
  - Mania, depression, substance misuse, personality disorder, psychosis
  - LD/ASD – problems understanding appropriate sexual behaviour?
- Forensic history – convictions, charges (including dropped); unreported crimes
- Risk assessment
  - Sexual offending, particularly links between offending and mental state/substance misuse
  - Self-harm/suicide – especially if shame
  - Violence (to/from others).

> **TIP:** Think carefully about how you document and cascade information to other staff. Separate your emotional response from the facts, and be careful of stigmatising people. Off-hand comments and thoughts can easily be incorporated into the notes and amplified as a factual 'headline' when talking about sex offenders, or worse, *alleged* sex offenders. This can greatly affect people's experiences of psychiatric care – and subsequent engagement.
>
> Penny Collins, Forensic AMHP

Management

Discuss with seniors *before* sharing your plan with the patient. Consider:
- Admission – if mental disorder and high risks (psychosis or mania are particularly concerning)
- Disclosure to police, social services, MAPPA (p42)?
- Referral:
  - Specialist psychotherapy – if no immediate risk and help-seeking. Discuss with local forensic team.
  - Community LD service – if LD ±ASD
  - CMHT – if comorbid disorders, including ASD without LD
  - Forensic psychiatry – especially if serious/violent offending.

Afterwards, debrief *emotionally* as needed, with on-call seniors, or your consultant in supervision.

> **TIP:** Sex-offending patients are *still* people, who have problems, and have often been victims of sexual abuse themselves. They deserve the same respect and appropriate management as anyone else. Always assess how any mental illness affects sexual risk.
>
> Penny Brown, Consultant Forensic Psychiatrist

Reference

Rix, K.J.B. (2011) *Expert Psychiatric Evidence*. RCPsych publications, London.

Further reading

Houston, J.C. and Galloway, S. (2008) Sexual offending and mental health: multidisciplinary management in the community (Forensic Focus 28). Jessica Kingsley Publishers.

Lawn, T. and McDonald, E. (2009) Developing a policy to deal with sexual assault on psychiatric inpatient wards. *The Psychiatric Bulletin*, **33**, 108–111.

Yakeley, J. and Wood, H. (2014) Paraphilias and paraphilic disorders: diagnosis, assessment and management. *Advances in Psychiatric Treatment* **20**, 202–213.

CHAPTER 71

Self-harm on the ward

Jane Bunclark and Abigail Steenstra
South London & Maudsley NHS Foundation Trust, London, England

> **RELATED CHAPTERS:** self-harm (51), medical emergencies (65), hanging (72), death (73)

Catriona was admitted last week after deeply cutting both arms. She's 26, and well known to services, with depression and recurrent self-harm. She's cut herself on the ward.

Self-harm on psychiatric wards is fairly common, ranging from tiny scratches to life-threatening injuries. Address both medical and psychological management.

Preparation

1. On the telephone, ask staff to ...
- Describe urgency: site, severity, blood loss, obs
- If severe attend immediately, and advise staff to:
  - Call 999 + ERT
  - Stop bleeding ± start ILS
  - Fetch resus bag/trolley
- Locate and remove the cutting equipment (call police if risky)
- Basic first aid – stop the bleeding
- Repeat obs
- Fetch: sterile gloves, gauze, saline, dressings, steristrips.

2. On the ward
- *Briefly check Catriona for urgency – is she conscious and stable? Need for immediate medical attention?*
- *Nurses*
  - Catriona's recent presentation and stressors
  - Did she report the self-harm or await discovery?
- *Notes*
  - Symptoms ± working diagnosis
  - MHA status
  - Past self-harm: triggers, planned/impulsive, methods, severity; management.
  - Recognised *function(s)* of her self-harm, including suicide (Table 51.1, p321)
  - Existing self-harm management plans (follow as closely as possible).

Psychiatry: Breaking the ICE – Introductions, Common Tasks and Emergencies for Trainees, First Edition.
Edited by Sarah Stringer, Juliet Hurn and Anna M Burnside.
© 2016 John Wiley & Sons, Ltd. Published 2016 by John Wiley & Sons, Ltd.
Companion Website: www.psychiatryice.com

Assessment

1. Approach

Assess Catriona with a nurse. Aim for compassion and composure, rather than panic, drama or a sense of spectacle. Think about how your response might reinforce her behaviour (p77). Don't be punitive, e.g. being irritated, disgusted, dismissive or sighing heavily. Emphasise that you want to understand what happened and how the team can *support* her.

Try to actively involve Catriona in finding solutions and taking responsibility for self-harm.

PATIENT VIEW:

I was hacking into my arm. I didn't want to be doing it. I couldn't stop. This was in my room, so I went out into the ward, and asked the doctor to help me … I genuinely wanted to stop but he just thought I was doing it to get attention and I wasn't. I don't like blood.

'Claire'

---

2. Immediate self-harm assessment and treatment

- What did she cut with? (Clean/contaminated? Has it been removed?)
- Has she harmed herself in any other way? (Suspect overdose if drowsy)
- Tetanus vaccination history (full course = 5 injections before the age of 18)
- Examination:
  - Full obs
  - Assess the wound (Box 71.1)
  - Focused examination for signs of overdose or hypovolaemia
- Clean and dress the wound ± steri-strips

Box 71.1 Urgent transfer to ED if …

- You can't fully assess the wound
- Sutures are needed, but you lack resources/skills
- Possible vessel, nerve or tendon damage
- Bleeding won't stop
- Foreign body, e.g. broken glass, dirt
- Involves face/genitals
- Stabbing/deep laceration
- Objects inserted into the anus/vagina or under the skin
- Swallowed sharps, magnets or chemicals

3. Focused self-harm history (p320–322), remembering …

- *Triggers*: can Catriona say what happened beforehand?
  - Conflict, frustration?
  - Feeling ignored, rejected, criticised?
  - Pseudohallucinations, flashbacks, dissociation?
- How/where did she get the cutting equipment?
- Did she cut secretly or publicly?
- Function of self-harm (including suicide attempt)
- Is this her usual self-harm pattern?
- What support would she find helpful?

4. MSE, remembering ...

- Agitation/distress
- Ongoing self-harm/suicide plans
- Pseudohallucinations/hallucinations (especially commands)
- Dissociation
- Motivation to self-harm/abstain.

5. Risk assessment (p38)

Assess the risk of further self-harm, including factors that affect:
- Likelihood of repetition, *or*
- Severity of self-harm.

Catriona's risk will be affected by her ability to seek help (before or after self-harm).

Management

Don't make management decisions alone. A team response is essential, especially when working with people who have personality difficulties or who recurrently self-harm; consider a formal MDT meeting. Actively involve Catriona wherever possible, and explain the plan to her in the presence of her named nurse/ward manager to ensure everyone hears the same message.

1. Ongoing medical management

Involve Catriona, e.g. alerting staff to signs of infection, how to manage bathing.
Consider:
- Analgesia – don't leave her in pain
- Antibiotics or tetanus treatment (discuss with ED if unsure)
- Review and monitoring, e.g. dressing changes, when to remove sutures.

2. Identifying triggers and alternatives

Discuss how the team can best help her stay safe on the ward, e.g.
- Problem-solve
- Remove self-harming equipment
- Recognise that she may feel very stressed, especially if self-harm is a coping strategy. Explore her worries, and try to let her suggest what's helped previously.
- Encourage her to speak to nursing staff *before* self-harming, e.g. request 1:1 time
- Her named nurse could draw up a care plan, identifying antecedents and triggers – especially if Catriona has difficulties with impulsivity or mentalisation
- Consider harm-minimisation approaches *with* Catriona (p325)
- Ward psychologist may offer ongoing work.

The team should positively reinforce help-seeking, e.g. through praise, empathy, offering prompt attention/1:1 time.

TIP: There's no evidence base for giving benzodiazepines or clean blades as harm-minimization; both can cause more harm than good. Likewise, a 'behavioural contract' to *not* self-harm (e.g. in exchange for continued leave) *may* be perceived as punitive or unrealistic.

3. Observations and leave
You need to keep Catriona safe, but changes can feel punitive.
- Increased obs may be needed if Catriona's at risk of serious self-harm
  - However, close observation won't help her develop self-management skills, and *may* increase self-harming risks through positive reinforcement/raising stress and frustration levels
  - General obs may be the best way forward
- Review leave status
- If informal and asking to leave, discuss with the consultant. Section 5(2) *may* be counter-productive (p286).

4. Documentation and handover
- Update risk assessment
- Handover to the ward doctor, if not your patient.

> **TIP:** We enter psychiatry presuming that the line between staff and patients equals the line between health and illness. Then we make all sorts of interesting discoveries, and begin to suspect all sorts of dynamics we had no clue about. We're human, we get affected by what's happening around us. If we didn't, we wouldn't be able to do this job. In fact, we'd be dangerous. But those dynamics can affect us in ways that we don't always understand. That's why attending Case Based Discussion (Balint) groups early and consistently is essential to create and maintain the thinking space which differentiates the competent clinician from everyone else.
>
> Anastasia Apostolou, ST5 Psychodynamic Psychotherapy

What If ... ?

... She dies?
See Ch.73.

... It's an overdose?
Consider overdose in anyone with unexplained drowsiness, confusion or arrhythmia. Transfer to ED immediately if very drowsy, unconscious, or likely to have taken a serious overdose.
Clues to what's been taken include:
- Asking the patient (!)
- Full examinations, obs, ECG, UDS
- Drug chart – these medications are easily stockpiled (clozapine or lithium are particularly worrying)
- Empty medication packets in their bedroom
- Unescorted leave – may have taken *anything*.
Toxbase (0844 892 0111/www.toxbase.org) can advise on management/risk and may suggest likely drugs, based on the presentation.
- Don't induce vomiting
- If asymptomatic and a significant overdose is unlikely:
  - Monitor closely – obs, GCS, physical symptoms and signs of overdose
  - FBC, U&E, LFT, INR, bicarbonate
  - Salicylate levels
  - Paracetamol levels 4h post-ingestion
  - Other as suspected, e.g. lithium levels.

Take-home message

Take a team approach to managing risk *with* the patient, and don't be afraid to ask for help.

Further reading

NICE (2004) CG16 Self-harm: The short-term physical and psychological management and secondary prevention of self-harm in primary and secondary care. NICE, England.

James, K., Bowers, L. and Stewart, D. (2012) Self-harm and attempted suicide within inpatient psychiatric services: a literature review. *International Journal of Mental Health Nursing* **21** (4), 301–309.

Royal College of Psychiatrists (2006) *Better Services for People who Self harm: Quality Standards for Healthcare Professionals*. RCPsych, London.

CHAPTER 72

Hanging

Anna M Burnside

East London NHS Foundation Trust, London, England

> **RELATED CHAPTERS:** self-harm (51, 71), medical emergencies (65), death (73)

You're asked to clerk John Spencer. On entering his room, you find him hanging.

Cut down and oxygenate – most people die from cerebral hypoxia.

Immediate management

1. Shout for help – ERT, crash bag and 999

2. Cut John down
- Team: support his neck and weight (C-spine injury?)
- Cut noose with ligature cutters/wire cutters
- Lower to floor – don't drop.

3. Start ILS
- Stabilise C-spine
- Airway – *jaw-thrust* (*not* head tilt, chin-lift)
- *If breathing* – give 100% O_2 via oxygen mask
- *If not breathing*
  - Site I-gel (supraglottic) airway/guedel/nasopharyngeal airway
  - Bag-valve-mask + 100% O_2
- *No pulse: start CPR*
- Delegate colleagues to:
  - Keep a timed list of *all* actions taken
  - Guide the paramedics in
- Attempt IV access
- Handover to paramedics
  - If transferring to ED, send an RMN and photocopy of his drug chart
  - If John has died, go to Ch.73
- Lock John's room as a crime scene until discussed with the police.

Psychiatry: Breaking the ICE – Introductions, Common Tasks and Emergencies for Trainees, First Edition.
Edited by Sarah Stringer, Juliet Hurn and Anna M Burnside.
© 2016 John Wiley & Sons, Ltd. Published 2016 by John Wiley & Sons, Ltd.
Companion Website: www.psychiatryice.com

Afterwards

1. Staff debrief

Discuss what happened and how the team handled it. This is an important break from one of the most stressful things you'll deal with as psychiatrist, and an opportunity to share feelings, e.g. shock, sadness, anger. It also helps you plan next steps, e.g.
- Support for patients who witnessed the hanging
- Contacting senior staff, e.g. ward manager/out-of-hours hospital manager
- Locate and follow Trust policy.

2. Contact seniors

Contact the ward (or on-call) consultant.
- Talk them through your actions
- Ask what else you should do
- *They* should lead on liaison with relatives – don't do this alone
- *They* must ensure you feel safe and supported, whether by telephone or face-to-face support. If you're very distressed, discuss whether you should stay at work, or go home after completing your documentation.

If on-call, don't struggle on alone – ask your registrar to attend and help.

3. Documentation

Write a comprehensive account of the hanging and your management: expect a Serious Incident (SI) investigation, and scrutiny of your notes. Update John's risk assessment and help nursing staff complete incident report forms.

Ongoing management

1. If John survives

- He'll need brain and C-spine imaging, and observation/management of delayed airway and pulmonary complications
- Contact Liaison Psychiatry for review, especially if John's informal (may need MHA assessment)
- When he returns to your ward:
  - Start on 1:1 *arm's reach* obs
  - Explore the attempted hanging and assess suicide risk (Ch.51)
  - Review MSE, especially ongoing suicidal ideation, depression, psychosis
  - Consider MHA if he wants to leave or refuses treatment.

2. Longer-term

- A formal staff debrief will occur within 7–10 days to provide emotional support and learn from the event
- Expect an SI (p108), and don't worry when the investigating team contact you: they're seeking facts, not a scapegoat
- Talk through the hanging in supervision. Your consultant should provide reassurance, practical/emotional support, and a chance to reflect.
- Seek further emotional support if needed, via your GP or Occupational Health.

TIP: If and when you work with suicide, remember that you're not *expected* to be unaffected, and may need support dealing with the emotional impact. My first experience of suicide was a really likeable young woman, who I was working with closely. One morning, she threw herself under a train. It shattered me: the shock, grief, anger and guilt were awful. Meeting with her parents afterwards was probably the hardest thing I've ever done – they were heartbroken, and although they didn't blame me, *I* felt I'd let them down, and cried. Afterwards, I kept thinking I must have missed something, could have done something better, should have protected her. I lost my confidence and became anxious about sending anyone home if they sounded even slightly suicidal. It took me a long time – with my team's support – to *believe* it wasn't my fault. It took longer to feel I could trust myself or my patients again. I still think of her. I wish she'd come to see me that morning, but she'd made up her mind – her life was unbearable, and there was nothing I could do about that.

Sarah Stringer, S.12 Approved Doctor

What if ... ?

... The hanging wasn't 'serious'?
The only case where you wouldn't transfer to ED would be a 'near miss' where you are certain that *no* strangulation *or* a drop from height actually occurred.
- Remove ligature and give 100% oxygen
- Transfer to ED if *any* signs of damage
  - Neck: bruising, abrasions, swelling; petechiae above the ligature line
  - Cough, stridor or voice changes, e.g. muffled/hoarse
  - Pain on gentle palpation of the larynx (?laryngeal fracture)
  - Subconjunctival petechiae
  - Respiratory distress or hypoxia
  - GCS <15
  - Any neurological impairment
- At least hourly physical obs
- Have a low threshold for transfer to ED for 24h observation (delayed airway obstruction and pulmonary complications)
- Assess risk, including evidence of other self-harm
- Place on 1:1/2:1; suspend leave and consider assessment under s.5(2).

Take-home message

Attempted hangings are among the most stressful emergencies you'll encounter. Airway management is key, and transfer to ED is nearly always required.

Further reading

Resuscitation Council (2011) *Immediate Life Support* 3rd edn, Resuscitation Council UK.

CHAPTER 73

Death

Katherine Beck

South London & Maudsley NHS Foundation Trust, London, England

---

RELATED CHAPTERS: self-harm (71), hanging (72)

Robert Taylor, 28, has been found dead in his room.

Deaths on psychiatric wards are uncommon, and dealt with differently to deaths in general hospitals.

Preparation

1. On the telephone, ask staff to …
- Call an ambulance and the ERT
- Start/continue Immediate Life Support (ILS) (*unless* Do Not Attempt Resuscitation order).
- Delegate someone to keep a timed list of *all* actions taken.

2. State how long you'll be. *Run* to the ward.

Assessment

On the ward
Go straight to Robert and decide whether to:
- *Continue ILS*
  - Delegate staff to let paramedics in, gather the notes and drug chart
  - Transfer to ED
- *Stop ILS and verify the death (if you've any doubt at all, continue ILS)*
  - Sternal rub – no response to painful stimulus
  - Pupils – fixed, dilated
  - 1 minute
    - No carotid/brachial pulse
    - No heart and breath sounds
  - Record time and date.

Psychiatry: Breaking the ICE – Introductions, Common Tasks and Emergencies for Trainees, First Edition.
Edited by Sarah Stringer, Juliet Hurn and Anna M Burnside.
© 2016 John Wiley & Sons, Ltd. Published 2016 by John Wiley & Sons, Ltd.
Companion Website: www.psychiatryice.com

Management

1. Immediate
On psychiatric wards, most deaths are *unexpected* (e.g. suicide/heart attack). Follow Trust guidelines.
- *Lock the room/close off the area: this is now a crime scene*
  - Don't further disturb the body
  - Equipment (e.g. defibrillator pads) can only be removed with the Coroner's permission
- Check your team's OK and plan next steps
- Call the Coroner (in Scotland, the procurator fiscal and Mental Welfare Commission). They will:
  - Arrange for Robert's body to be removed for post-mortem
  - Advise on cultural issues, e.g. how the process affects Islamic or Jewish burial customs.
- Call the police, who act on the Coroner's behalf
  - They'll interview staff and search for evidence, e.g. suicide note
- Ask the RMO/on-call consultant to attend
  - If on-call, ask your registrar to cover your other work
- The lead nurse should contact the ward/hospital manager ± organise extra staff cover.

2. Working with the family
Someone senior or with previous family contact should inform the relatives. Arrange a meeting as soon as possible. The consultant or senior nurse will lead.
- Use Robert's name (not *the patient/the body*)
- Apologise and express sorrow
- Explain the *facts* of the event, clearly and compassionately. You have a Duty of Candour to provide all directly relevant information, giving as much detail as the relatives want *now*.
- Note any questions you can't confidently answer yet, and remember you still owe Robert a duty of confidentiality
- If circumstances suggest suicide, don't say he 'committed suicide'. Firstly, it sounds like a crime; secondly, it's a *suspected* suicide until the Coroner says otherwise.
- Allow space for venting: guilt, anger, despair, shock, blame …
- Avoid clichés, e.g. *Time's a healer; I know how you feel; there's lots to be grateful for …*
- Agree further action:
  - The Coroner will conduct a post-mortem and inquest. They give permission for viewing the body, organ donation, burial/cremation.
  - The Trust will conduct a Serious Incident (SI) investigation, to understand why and how this happened, and prevent recurrence where possible (p108)
  - Explain how the family will be kept involved.
Offer ongoing support:
- Give them contact details of:
  - Coroner's office
  - Senior staff
  - *Appropriate* services, e.g. hospital chaplains, SOBS (Survivors of Bereavement by Suicide)
- Offer bereavement leaflets (if available)
- Try to understand what support they'd appreciate, e.g. would a letter, card or attendance at the funeral be helpful or inflammatory?
If you *can't* contact the next of kin within six hours, ask the police to do this.

3. Documentation and dissemination
Record the time, date and circumstances of the death
- Clearly document *all the facts* of the event (use the timings recorded by the nurse). Your notes are essential to the SI and Coroner's Inquest.
- Help the nurses complete critical incident documentation.

A senior colleague should lead a formal staff debrief. This should:
• Be constructive and supportive
• Allow expression of emotions and worries
• Address team blame, guilt or splitting
• Identify distressed colleagues, e.g. junior staff who haven't dealt with death before; those close to Robert/who discovered him
• Agree the best way to inform, support and reassure other patients.

4. Longer-term
Depending on the nature of the death and your relationship with the patient, you may need support, e.g. for self-blame, anger, or loss of confidence in your clinical abilities. Discuss this in supervision with your consultant, and consider extra help via:
• Your GP
• Occupational health
• Trust staff support policy, e.g. post incident support groups
• Doctor-specific support services (p30).

You'll usually attend a fact-finding interview or submit a written statement for the internal SI investigation (p108). You may also need to prepare a report or attend Coroner's Court. Plan this with your consultant in supervision, and check your Trust's guidelines. Coroner's Court can be stressful, even though it's not apportioning blame, so ask your consultant or a Trust representative to attend and support you.

Ultimately, something should be learned from the death, and changes made, e.g. staff training, removal of ligature points. Try to be a part of this change if possible.

> **TIP:** Don't be put off by your first year in Psychiatry training – it can all feel a bit overwhelming at times – but does get better!
>
> Lucinda Richards, CT3

What If...?

...The death was expected?
• Document the date and time of death
• You may still need to report the death to the Coroner, e.g. deaths while under the MHA/DoLS are always investigated. If in doubt, call the Coroner's office immediately.
• Inform seniors
  ○ RMO and senior nurse on the unit
  ○ If on-call, your registrar, unit manager and on-call manager
• It may still need to be documented as a clinical incident
• Inform the GP. They or the RMO may issue the death certificate (local protocols vary).
• Inform the family and arrange to meet them. Once they receive the death certificate, they should register the death within five days at the Register Office in the borough where he died.

Take-home message

Deaths in psychiatric units are uncommon, usually unexpected, and usually formally investigated. Don't underestimate the emotional ramifications – particularly of suicide – on you, other staff, relatives and patients.

Further reading

Resuscitation Council (2011) *Immediate Life Support* 3rd edn, Resuscitation Council UK.

Hodelet, N. and Hughson, M (2001) What to do when a patient commits suicide. *Psychiatric Bulletin*, **25**, 43–45.

Høifødt, T.S. and Talseth, A. (2006) Dealing with suicidal patients – a challenging task: a qualitative study of young physicians' experiences. *BMC Medical Education*, **6**, 44.

CHAPTER 74

Aggression

Abigail G Crutchlow[1], Christina Barras[2], Noreen Jakeman[3], Sean Lubbe[4], Vivienne Mak[1], Rachel Thomasson[5], and Abigail Steenstra[1]

[1] *South London & Maudsley NHS Foundation Trust, London, England*
[2] *South West London & St George's Mental Health NHS Trust, London, England*
[3] *Lewisham & Greenwich NHS Trust, London, England*
[4] *UNSW Black Dog Institute, New South Wales, Australia*
[5] *Manchester Royal Infirmary, Manchester, Lancashire, England*

RELATED CHAPTERS: safety (8) aggressive children (75), violent threats (80)

You're called urgently to ED: 'Harry' is shouting, punching walls, threatening staff and destroying equipment.

Don't panic – you're not expected to physically tackle Harry. Contain the risks, then assess and manage the underlying cause:
- **Organic, e.g. head injury, delirium, alcohol withdrawal**
- **Functional illness, e.g. psychosis, mania**
- **Challenging behaviour, e.g. dementia, learning disability (LD)**
- **Antisocial behaviour, e.g. poor coping strategies, personality disorder, drunk.**

Preparation

1. On the telephone – tell caller to ...
- Contact hospital security ± police (ward: Emergency Response Team, ERT)
- Fetch notes, obs chart, drug chart
- Move other patients and potential weapons, e.g. chairs.
Always call the police if a weapon's involved (See What If ... ?)

2. On arrival – assess ...
- Who's leading?
  - If *someone*, support them
  - If *no-one* has expertise/knows Harry, you should lead
- Immediate risks – if too dangerous, withdraw and await police
- Verbal handover
  - Symptoms or diagnoses: psychiatric/medical/substance misuse
  - Legal status: informal/Mental Health Act (MHA)/Mental Capacity Act (MCA)
  - Why's he angry? What does he want?

Psychiatry: Breaking the ICE – Introductions, Common Tasks and Emergencies for Trainees, First Edition.
Edited by Sarah Stringer, Juliet Hurn and Anna M Burnside.
© 2016 John Wiley & Sons, Ltd. Published 2016 by John Wiley & Sons, Ltd.
Companion Website: www.psychiatryice.com

- Specific threats, actual assaults, access to weapons
- Known risks/forensic history
- Past aggression: known triggers, necessary interventions.

3. Ensure other staff *don't* leave; delegate roles

- Check security ± police are coming
- Identify staff trained in restraint, e.g. psychiatric liaison nurse (PLN), registered mental health nurse (RMN), security
- *Keep* other patients and weapons out of reach
- Read notes: missing details, existing aggression management plans
- Find your Trust's rapid tranquilisation (RT) protocol.

Assessment and verbal de-escalation

1. Approach
Use verbal de-escalation (p20)
- Observe for escalating aggression (p19)
- 1 person should speak to Harry
- Aims:
  - Keep everyone safe
  - Help Harry manage his emotions and regain control
  - Problem solve *with* Harry
  - Avoid restraint/RT
  - Gain history and MSE – underlying medical/psychiatric problem?
- Try to meet Harry's demands or find compromises without contradicting existing team plans
- If feeling unsafe, withdraw and discuss next steps as a team.
If Harry attacks:
- Trained staff – restrain
- Untrained staff – run out of reach.

2. Focused history, remembering ...
- Why's Harry upset? What does he need/want?
- Triggers, e.g.
  - Recent stressors
  - Frustration with staff/treatment
  - Psychiatric relapse
  - Physical problems, e.g. pain, head injury, hypoglycaemia, epilepsy
  - Substance misuse

3. MSE, remembering ...
- Aggression, agitation, impulsivity
- Intoxication/withdrawal
- Slurred speech/thought disorder
- Irritable, elated, afraid, suspicious; labile/unstable
- Thoughts of harm to others – direct threats, specific plans or victims?
- Delusions, especially persecutory, passivity, thought insertion, jealousy
- Hallucinations, especially commands
- Confusion, poor judgment
- Willing to work with the team/particular staff?
  - What usually helps when angry, e.g. medication, admission?
  - Blaming others/'not responsible' for his actions.

4. Risk assessment, remembering ...

- Violence, considering:
  - Targets, e.g. staff, patients; particular characteristics, e.g. race, gender
  - Anything you can change to lower risk, e.g. meet immediate needs, call family, medication
- Retributive violence
- Self-harm, suicide
- Absconding.

Management

1. Think: what's going on here?

Decide the cause of Harry's behaviour – if unsure, call your senior.

No acute medical/psychiatric problem

A member of the public is breaking the law. Drunkenness or personality disorder aren't excuses.

- Don't offer medication
- Remove Harry from ED (police/security)
- If ED want to press charges, police can arrest him, e.g. for assault, damage to property, threats to kill, drunk and disorderly behaviour (Box 74.1)
  - Psychiatric assessment can still be arranged from the police station later, e.g. once sober.

Physical illness

Address significant medical concerns, e.g. head injury, alcohol withdrawal. If Harry refuses urgent input, but lacks capacity, ED can investigate and treat in his best interests under the MCA, including sedation and proportionate restraint, if required (Ch.76).

Mental illness

If physically well, does Harry show signs of major mental illness? Manage the underlying problem as usual, and deal with ongoing agitation as needed (below).

2. Rapid tranquilisation (RT; 'rapid trank')

If ongoing aggression, continue verbal de-escalation, but consider *RT* (Figure 74.1, Table 74.1).
Use Trust protocols if available, otherwise, use the following advice, involving seniors urgently.

- RT is medication to prevent harm from acute agitation
- It's always a *team decision*, but as prescriber, *you* carry the medico-legal risk
  - If you feel it's inappropriate, don't prescribe – seek senior advice
- Always offer oral medication (PO) first
- Intramuscular medication (IM) is a last resort
  - Both IM and restraint are frightening and can kill
- Get senior advice before ...
  - Exceeding British National Formulary (BNF) maximum doses
  - Treating elderly/pregnant/under-18s or patients with LD/brain damage
  - Using IV medications.

Box 74.1 Pressing charges

> Police may be reticent to get involved when someone's mentally ill, but teams should decide if this would be helpful, especially if there's been an assault. Pressing charges reinforces the message that aggression is unacceptable, and may facilitate appropriate care, e.g. forensic team input. Always discuss with senior colleagues, and involve the local mental health police liaison officer, if available.

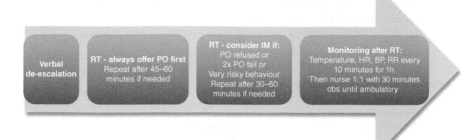

Figure 74.1 RT overview protocol.

Table 74.1 Factors affecting RT choice.

	Specifics

Legal	Local guidelines (NB: NICE only recommends lorazepam, promethazine and haloperidol, but other medications are not excluded)
	Proportionality (e.g. offer PO before IM)
	Legal status
	• Informed consent *always* try with every patient
	• If informal / s5(2)::
	  ∘ Use MCA if lacks capacity and RT's in *their* best interests
	  ∘ Common law if RT to prevent harm to *others*
	  ∘ *RT in informal patients should always trigger a MHA assessment*
	• Section 2 or 3 (see p101 if detained >3 months)

Historic	Allergies PMHx: cardiovascular, hepatic/renal impairment, respiratory, hypotension (see Appendix A7 for details) Medication exposure • Response • Side effects, especially extrapyramidal side effects (EPSE) / Neuroleptic malignant syndrome (NMS) • Antipsychotics (avoid if neuroleptic naive)
Current	Team plan/Advance Directive Medications: regular ± PRN = 24h total doses • Recent Acuphase? • Don't introduce a *second* antipsychotic Psychosis (antipsychotics more appropriate) Substance misuse • Causing agitation? • Alcohol/GBL withdrawal (Ch.77) – need detox • Amphetamines – increase risk arrhythmia • Benzodiazepines – less effective as RT if already tolerant Physical concerns (Appendix A7) Normal ECG (ideal before IM antipsychotics; *essential* before haloperidol PO/IM)

3. Co-ordinate a team

Clarify roles, e.g. negotiating, giving medication, holding particular body parts.
* Even if you're restraint-trained, don't restrain as the only on-call psychiatrist
* Prepare medication – oral and IM (Table 74.2)
* Gather crash bag/trolley, obs monitor, flumazenil, ECG machine ± procyclidine.

4. Offer oral medication (Table 74.2)

Give Harry choices, becoming firmer as needed, e.g.
* *What's helped when you've felt like this before?*
* *Medication might help you feel more relaxed. What do you think?*
* *I need to keep everyone safe, and think medication would help that*
* *You're very unsettled and I'm going to get some emergency medication*
* *I need to insist that you take medication now - will you take tablets?*
* *If you won't take a tablet, we will need to give you an injection.*

5. Restraint

Restraint reinforces the idea that action – not talking – solves problems. If used, it must be:
* Performed by trained staff
* Proportionate – using the least restrictive approach for the least time possible
* Explained – throughout the restraint, someone (often you) must talk to Harry; he'll be frightened/angry/confused.

Table 74.2 RT options in fit adults (see *What if ... ?* for elderly/LD/frail).

Medication	Stat dose	Maximum dose 24 h	Notes
Non-antipsychotics	**Use first-line if neuroleptic naive or regular antipsychotic already prescribed**		
Lorazepam	1–2 mg PO/IM	4 mg	*Must have flumazenil available*
Promethazine	25–50 mg PO/IM	100 mg	Sedating antihistamine – useful if benzodiazepine tolerant
			Wait longer to assess effect before repeating (IM = onset 1–2 h; PO longer)
Midazolam	2.5–7.5 mg IM	15 mg	Controlled Drug
			Must have flumazenil available
Antipsychotics	**Don't combine different antipsychotics (arrhythmia risk)**		
Olanzapine	5–10 mg PO/IM	20 mg	Give lower dose if neuroleptic naive/other risk factors
			IM: must leave at least 1–2 h between this and IM benzodiazepine
Risperidone	1–2 mg PO	16 mg (*rarely* >10 mg)	No IM option
Aripiprazole	5.25–15 mg IM (usually 9.75mg)	30 mg	Less sedating antipsychotic
			Better than olanzapine if hypotensive
			IM – wait 2 h before repeat; max 3 doses in 24 h
Haloperidol	5 mg PO/IM	20 mg PO 12 mg IM	Must have normal ECG first
			Avoid if another antipsychotic already in use
			High risk EPSE - must have procyclidine available (5–10 mg PO/IM)

Police and security are often trained in non-therapeutic (prone, i.e. face-down) restraint – *this can kill*. Monitor closely for positional asphyxia! Tell staff to move off if:
- Applying pressure to his torso
- Harry shows *any* signs of asphyxia:
  - *"I can't breathe!"*
  - Noisy breathing/gasping
  - Blue lips
  - Goes silent/still.

Move Harry from prone as soon as possible, e.g. turn over / restrain in arm holds while seated.

PATIENT VIEW:

I was held down, they had my arms held behind my back. I don't know what I'd done … He pulled my shoulder back so I felt my arm was coming out of my socket. Do you know how painful that is? You have no idea, because you haven't had it done to you.

'Sarah'

---

6. IM medication (Table 74.2)
- Aim to contain risky behaviour, not knock Harry out. Monitor closely.
- *Never use 'Acuphase' for RT (see What If..?)*
- In severe agitation, combinations are:
  - Benzodiazepine ± promethazine
  - Benzodiazepine ± antipsychotic (*not* olanzapine if using IM)
  - Promethazine ± antipsychotic (recommended if using haloperidol).
- If these options (and Figure 74.1) don't resolve the aggression, seek urgent senior help.

PATIENT VIEW:

They might have said to me, "you need medication." But no one said to me that if you don't have medication we will have to force you to have an injection. If someone had […] explained what my choices were … there would have been no need to hold me down and inject me, which I interpreted as a physical assault …

Clare Ockwell, *Experiences of Mental Health In-Patient Care*, p49

PATIENT VIEW:

I saw them doing control and restraint and it's barbaric…. There's like eight of them, and they've got their knee in his back and holding the man's hands behind … It's horrible and I thought, *If that's my brother I'd join in, punching them up!* It's soul destroying.

'Marco'

Afterwards

Breathe.

1. Team discussion and plan
Debrief, away from Harry
- Is everyone OK?
- What … went well/could have gone better/has been learned?

Immediate care plan
- Transfer to medical or psychiatric ward?
- Decide obs level, e.g. 1:1/2:1
- Physical monitoring ± ECG, outstanding bloods (Appendix A for details)
- Clarify ongoing legal framework
  - Assess for s5(2) if informal and *admitted* to hospital (not in ED)
  - Informal/s5(2): emergency treatment is under MCA or Common Law
  - Call seniors if MHA assessment is needed (±wait until Harry's alert)
- Advise behavioural management, e.g. boundaries, time-outs, praise if calm
- Drug chart
  - Prescribe safe RT options (Table 74.2): offer PO; IM if refused
  - Consider regular oral sedation if *recurrent* challenging behaviour, e.g.
    - Clonazepam 0.5–2 mg qds
    - Promethazine 25 mg qds
  - ±Omit regular medication if exceeding maximum doses
- Clarify time for next psychiatric review.

2. Debrief Harry
Once Harry's calmer, see him (± any carers) with a colleague:
- Let him explain how he was and is feeling
- Explain *your* actions
- Ask how he'd like to be managed if agitated again
- Teach ways to prevent agitation, e.g. asking staff for help, requesting a time out ± early use of sedative medication
- Feedback the plan. Be clear this is a team decision (use 'we' and 'the team' rather than 'I').
  - Set clear behavioural boundaries
  - Explain what the team will do if Harry's behaviour is unacceptable, to keep everyone safe (not punish him)
  - Fill assessment gaps.

3. Document clearly, including ...
- Staff involved
- RT: risks and reasons
  - Doses, times, response to treatment
  - Physical obs
  - Side effects and any management for these
  - Legal framework used
- In case the police request a statement, note whether you think Harry:
  - Was unwell
  - Understood his behaviour was wrong (Box 74.1)
- Ongoing plan ± handover to liaison if remaining in ED/general hospital
- Complete incident form
- Update risk assessment and add an aggression alert to notes
- Alert GP and other involved professionals to risks, if discharging.

PATIENT VIEW:

One time, The Controller told me, "Go and trash the computer in the office." So I went to the office and grabbed hold of the computer, but they grabbed me and they lay on me. I was terrified ... Worried for my life from The Controller and from the staff because they were laying on me. At the time I didn't [think the restraint was reasonable]. I only wanted to do what The Controller was telling me to do. Now, I do think it was reasonable, yeah, yeah, yeah, course! Well, I was going to trash it!

'Sarah'

What If ... ?

... He's armed?

Isolate Harry from all staff and patients and call the police. *Don't* try to remove the weapon, or ask him to hand it over – you'll get hurt. Encourage him to place the weapon somewhere neutral, then move both of you as far away as possible. Use verbal de-escalation from a safe distance, but abandon if risky.

Use common sense. The police won't be impressed if Harry's a frail, elderly man, wielding a slipper.

... Harry's elderly?

Use verbal de-escalation and environmental management before considering RT. Elderly patients need lower doses, and a lower threshold for considering organic causes, e.g. delirium. Check your Trust's RT protocol for elderly patients, but if there isn't one, see Table 74.3.
- Always offer PO first
- Consider IM if PO refused
- If repeated RT, he needs regular QTc checks and consideration of MHA
- *Consider ongoing care, e.g.*
  - Regular medication/night sedation to help manage delirium (p350)
  - 1:1 RMN
  - Handover to liaison for next-day follow-up. May need transfer to a psychiatric ward if persistent aggression can't be safely managed on a medical ward.

Table 74.3 RT in elderly/LD/frail patients.

Route	Indication	Medication	Dosestat (±maximum)	Notes
PO Repeat 1–2 hourly, if needed	If neuroleptic naive/already prescribed an antipsychotic	Lorazepam	0.5–1 mg (2 mg/24 h)	Can ↑confusion/falls Must have flumazenil available
		Promethazine	12.5–25 mg (100 mg/24 h)	Can ↑QTc Can ↑ confusion (anticholinergic)
	Oral antipsychotic possible if: • Normal ECG • ±No regular antipsychotic • ±No parkinsonism /DLB	Olanzapine	2.5 mg (7.5 mg/24 h)	
		Haloperidol	0.5–1 mg (5 mg/24 h)	ECG essential No concomitant antipsychotic; must have procyclidine available
IM Repeat 1–2 hourly if needed	If neuroleptic naive/already prescribed an antipsychotic ...	Lorazepam	0.5–1 mg (2 mg/24 h)	Can ↑confusion/falls risk. *Must* have flumazenil available
		Promethazine	12.5–25 mg (50 mg/24 h)	Useful if benzodiazepine tolerant
	Antipsychotic – only if meet criteria for oral antipsychotics (above)	Olanzapine	2.5 mg (7.5 mg/24 h)	*Never* with IM lorazepam (leave at least 1–2 h gap)
		Haloperidol	0.5–1 mg (3 mg/24 h)	ECG essential No concomitant antipsychotic Must have procyclidine available

Table 74.4 Managing aggression on psychiatric wards/CMHTs.

	Psychiatric ward	CMHT
Team leader	Nurse in charge ERT lead	Team manager/CC
Available	ERT staff trained in restraint RT medication BLS equipment	Staff may know patient well Some oral RT BLS equipment
Unavailable	Access to quick medical investigations	Restraint-trained staff Most RT medication Access to medical investigations
Your role	Medical expert: • Consider organic • ±Physical examination • Safe prescribing Support team	Medical expert: • Consider organic • ± Physical examination • Prescribe PO Support team
Risks	Stress/harm to staff Harm and distress to other patients	Stress/harm to staff Harm and distress to other patients Risk to general public if leaves

**Managing
   risks**
	ERT as needed
	Increase obs ± consider PICU
	Involve police if ERT can't cope, e.g.
	   patient is armed
		All staff attend if alarms sound
		Call 999 early

Take-home message	Always consider organic causes	Low threshold for 999

… Staff want to use 'Acuphase' (zuclopenthixol acetate)?

Never use Acuphase for RT because:
- Onset is too slow (two hours, but peaking *much* later)
- Duration up to three days: hard to assess while sedated, and interactions likely
  ○ E.g. respiratory arrest with benzodiazepines
- There are many contraindications, *including restraint* (risks intravasation and oil embolus).

Refer to seniors if pressured to prescribe. It's occasionally appropriate if an acutely psychotic patient has needed *repeated* IM medication.

… Aggression happens on a psychiatric ward or Community Mental Health Team (CMHT)?

See Table 74.4. Compared with aggression in the ED, management is:
- Easier on a psychiatric ward – you have the Emergency Response Team (ERT)
- Much harder in a CMHT.

In a CMHT …

- You can't restrain or give RT
- *Consider* oral medication if you have it on site, e.g.
  ○ Lorazepam 0.5–1 mg
  ○ Olanzapine 5 mg if psychotic symptoms
- The police can either arrest, or – if the CMHT is publically accessible – detain Harry under s136 and take him to a Place of Safety for assessment (p99; Ch.46)
- If he walks out, contact the police (p386) or consider organising a MHA assessment at home
- Ensure other patients are followed-up, e.g. if in the waiting room during aggression. They may have been in crisis themselves, but run away, unseen.

- Add aggression alert to his notes, and advise to see Harry in pairs
- Set boundaries with Harry on his return to the CMHT, e.g.
  - Written behavioural contract
  - Intention to press charges if violent
  - *If you discuss medication calmly we'll try to help you. If you threaten staff we'll end the meeting, ask you to leave, and involve police.*

... Harry was *brought* to ED by police ... ?

Ask the police to stay while you *swiftly* assess his needs, updating them on progress. Check:
- The legal framework they used, e.g. arrest, MCA, s136
- If ED can contain risks
- If Harry needs medical attention.

If Harry's detained under s136, and ...
- Doesn't need medical treatment, but is too risky to assess in ED, ask the police to transfer him to a s136 suite
- Needs medical treatment, negotiate with the police to stay. Liaise with seniors, e.g. s136 assessment may be possible *while* receiving treatment.

If not under s136:
- Discuss the best place to manage Harry
- The police must decide if they'll use s136 powers (implementation in ED is still a legal grey area).

... He's assaulted someone?

Assaults are usually low-level (e.g. slaps, pushes), but occasionally serious.
- Separate victim(s) from perpetrator(s)
- Medical staff should deal with victims
- You and the PLN ± security/police should handle perpetrators

In a CMHT/psychiatric ward, get a brief handover of victim(s) and any injuries: is anyone seriously ill, e.g. unconscious, bleeding heavily?
- Review victims with a colleague (preferably with first aid/general training)
- Make a quick, first pass review to prioritise patients
- Stabilise serious injuries while colleagues call 999
- Once stable, review and treat minor injuries
  - Bites need ED
- Review the perpetrator for injuries
- Document assaults in *both* patients' notes, referring to other patients by their initials. Help staff complete incident forms.
  - Victims need clear support plans, including separation from the perpetrator
- Inform the ward consultant/oncall senior of serious incidents.

... Staff are injured?

In ED, medics should treat staff. In CMHTs/psychiatric wards, provide emergency treatment yourself, but have a low threshold for ED referral. Then encourage staff to take a break/go home, rather than limping about.

If *you're* injured, inform your senior, get treatment and go home if you can't do your job properly. If just shaken up, take a break to settle your adrenaline levels. The Trust will have protocols around assaults on staff, and may press charges on your behalf.

... There are ongoing aggression issues?

Risk management should address:
- Relapse prevention
- ±Substance misuse work

- ABC (antecedent-behaviour-consequences) chart to inform behavioural management
- Need for forensic referral (Ch.28)
- Anger management:
  - Psychology input
  - Non-statutory e.g. Everyman Project (London).

TIP: Very few doctors handle aggression brilliantly *all* the time, especially initially. To improve:
- Review your management with the senior nurse present, or your consultant in supervision – include this as a reflective piece in your portfolio.
- Shadow senior ward nurses when they manage aggressive patients and hold team debriefs.
- When time allows, read the person's notes fully beforehand. Little annoys an aggressive patient more than a doctor who 'hasn't bothered' to understand their situation or treatment plan.

Take-home message

Management of agitation is a team effort, always involving verbal de-escalation before medication or restraint. Go with your gut: if feeling unsafe, get out.

Further reading

Nassisi D, Korc B, Hahn S, Bruns J, Jagoda A. (2006) The evaluation and management of the acutely agitated elderly patient. *Mt Sinai J Med* **73** (7), 976–984.

Richmond, J.S., Berlin, J.S, Fishkind, A.B. *et al* (2012) Verbal de-escalation of the agitated patient: consensus statement of the American Association for

Emergency Psychiatry Project BETA De-escalation Workgroup. *Western Journal of Emergency Medicine* **13** (1), 17–25.

Norfolk, Suffolk and Cambridgeshire Strategic Health Authority (2003) Independent Inquiry into the death of David Bennett. Available at: www.irr.org.uk/pdf/bennett_inquiry.pdf

Macpherson R, Dix R, Morgan S (2005) A growing evidence base for management guidelines: Revisiting… Guidelines for the Management of Acutely Disturbed Psychiatric Patients. *Advances in Psychiatric Treatment*, **11**, 404–415.

Taylor, D., Paton, C. & Kapur, S. (2015) *The Maudsley Prescribing Guidelines in Psychiatry*, 12th edn, Wiley-Blackwell, Chichester.

NICE (2015) NG10 Violence and aggression: short-term management in mental health, health and community settings. NICE, England.

Patient resources:

Help for men who are violent or abusive:
  - www.everymanproject.co.uk
  - www.everymanproject.co.uk/otheragencies.html

Mind patient information on anger, includes self-help advice and guidance for family and friends: http://www.mind.org.uk/information-support/types-of-mental-health-problems/anger/#.VChmfRY1DXM

CHAPTER 75

Challenging behaviour in children

Peter Hindley and Matthew Fernando
South London & Maudsley NHS Foundation Trust, London, England

---

RELATED CHAPTERS: child self-harm (52), child protection (64), aggression (74)

Joe is 10 and has diagnoses of ADHD and oppositional defiant disorder. His foster carer, Ali, has brought him to ED as his aggression at home and school has become unmanageable. ED staff are struggling to contain his behaviour.

Behavioural disturbance in children is challenging, especially if carers and staff feel helpless to intervene. Try to understand the causes and be a calming influence. When everyone's anxious, remember that the immediate priority of keeping Joe safe has already been partially achieved by bringing him to ED.

It's hard to know how long this will take – try to ensure other work is covered, so you can concentrate on Joe.

Preparation

1. Quick check
- If Joe's physically aggressive, consider the need for rapid tranquillisation (RT) (Box 75.1)
- Is Ali's presence a help or hindrance?

2. Gather information – notes, Ali, staff ± police/school
- Overview, including triggers and usual approaches to calm Joe
- Contact Joe's social worker urgently (duty social worker out-of-hours).

3. Involve experts
- Paediatricians – consider physical health ±RT options
- On-call Child and Adolescent Mental Health Service (CAMHS) senior – contact sooner, rather than later.

Assessment

1. Approach
Keep Joe at the centre of everything – his safety and wellbeing are your priority.
- Remember his aggression may communicate distress or fear

Psychiatry: Breaking the ICE – Introductions, Common Tasks and Emergencies for Trainees, First Edition.
Edited by Sarah Stringer, Juliet Hurn and Anna M Burnside.
© 2016 John Wiley & Sons, Ltd. Published 2016 by John Wiley & Sons, Ltd.
Companion Website: www.psychiatryice.com

- Stay calm and reassuring
- Use simplified verbal de-escalation (p20)
- Give Joe space to calm himself
- Clear other patients and potential weapons, e.g. chairs
- Set clear behavioural boundaries.

2. Full history, remembering…

Some history will be from Ali, but talk with Joe as much as possible.
- *HPC:* Onset and pattern of events leading to recent behaviour:
  - Sudden change or gradual deterioration with 'a final straw'
- *Recent stressors, including changes involving:*
  - Relationship with foster care family
  - Contact with biological family
  - School, e.g. bullying, getting into trouble, truancy, schoolwork
  - Friendships
- *PMHx* and physical symptoms
- *PPHx*, including recent management and medication changes
- *Substance misuse* (regardless of age)
- *Forensic history* and historic aggression.

3. MSE, remembering…

Observe Joe if too risky to approach.
- Relationship with Ali/other adults
- Response to social cues/norms
- Self-harm, neglect, impulsivity, over-activity
- Depression, elation, anxiety. Perplexed/suspicious?
- Thoughts of harm to self/others
- Psychotic symptoms
- Inattention, learning difficulties
- What help does he want?

4. Risk assessment

Which services are currently provided, and do they sufficiently manage risk?
- Aggression (including to carers)
- Self-harm
- Neglect/abuse (Ch.64)
- Retributive violence (from peers/carers).

Box 75.1 RT in children

In exceptional circumstances, if de-escalation fails, you'll need to consider RT.
- Follow local guidelines
- Work closely with CAMHS seniors/paediatricians
- *Always* offer PO before IM
- Monitor closely for adverse effects, including paradoxical agitation for benzodiazepines (especially if the child has autism or a learning disability)
- Benzodiazepines, e.g.
  - Lorazepam 0.5–1 mg PO/IM (<12y) *or* 0.5–2 mg PO/IM (>12y)
- Sedating antihistamines, e.g.
  - Promethazine 5–10 mg PO/IM (<12y) *or* 10–25 mg PO/IM (>12y)
- Antipsychotics: only with senior specialist advice.

Management

Your on-call CAMHS senior should probably attend and review Joe.
Wherever possible, management should include Joe's wishes and be acceptable to Ali. Care pathways vary, so refer to local guidelines and work closely with paediatrics.

1. Address triggers and increase support
- Investigate and treat physical health problems
- Problem-solve around social and emotional triggers
- Liaise with social services for additional support
  - A Common Assessment Framework (CAF) will help ensure Joe's needs are met. You wouldn't complete one in the acute ED setting, but should request that community staff undertake this as soon as possible.
- Enlist support, e.g. from extended family, friends, teachers.

> **TIP:** Parents and carers are experts on their children. Work closely with them, but *don't* overburden them with responsibility. When out of their depth, be clear that you wouldn't expect *anyone* to cope without extra support.

2. Child protection
Discuss any suspicions of abuse or neglect with the consultant paediatrician and social worker (Ch.64).

3. Address underlying mental health problems
Explain, but leave prescribing to CAMHS.
- *Challenging behaviour:*
  - Help carers manage behaviour, e.g. setting boundaries, rewarding good behaviour
  - Low dose risperidone is occasionally used for short-term aggression management in conduct disorder or autism
- *Depression/anxiety:*
  - Psychology, e.g. CBT
  - A trial of an SSRI might be considered
- *Psychosis:*
  - Antipsychotic trial – usually as an inpatient.

4. Admit or discharge?
Joe may be able to go home with CAMHS and social services follow up if he's calmer and triggers can be resolved. If discharge isn't safe and problems are ongoing, your options are:
- Paediatric ward admission – to treat medical problems or buy time to implement a package of care
- Alternative accommodation (respite or longer-term) – via social worker
- Inpatient psychiatric unit – sometimes necessary, if challenging behaviour *and* an underlying mental illness. This is the decision of the on-call CAMHS senior.
The law around treating young people is complex (p103), so involve your CAMHS senior and Duty AMHP as soon as possible.

5. Documentation
Clearly document in the medical and psychiatric notes. Decide with your seniors who will refer for CAMHS follow up, and remember to copy notes to GP, CAMHS and social services.

What If ... ?

... Ali refuses to take Joe home?

If Joe doesn't need admission but can't be taken home, social services will need to provide alternative accommodation.

... Joe also has autism or an LD?

These are common co-morbidities, and you'll need to modify your communication style (p276).
* Changes and unfamiliar environments may compound distress
* Beware diagnostic overshadowing (wrongly attributing *everything* to his LD or ASD).

... Joe is still in the care of his parents and doesn't have a social worker?

Refer to social services.

Take-home message

Seek senior CAMHS and paediatric support when working with disturbed children.

Further reading

Baren, J.M., Mace, S.E., Hendry, P.L. *et al.* (2008) Children's mental health emergencies – part 2: emergency department evaluation and treatment of children with mental health disorders. *Paediatric Emergency Care* **24** (7), 485–498.

Department of Health (2015) The Mental Health Act 1983: Code of Practice. The Stationery Office, Norwich (Chapter 19).

Taylor, D., Paton, C. & Kapur, S. (2015) *The Maudsley Prescribing Guidelines in Psychiatry*, 12th edn, Wiley-Blackwell, Chichester, Chapter 5.

CHAPTER 76

Refusal of urgent treatment

Vivienne Mak[1], Sean Cross[1], Sean Lubbe[2], and Rachel Thomasson[3]

[1] South London & Maudsley NHS Foundation Trust, London, England
[2] UNSW Black Dog Institute, New South Wales, Australia
[3] Manchester Royal Infirmary, Manchester, Lancashire, England

RELATED CHAPTERS: self-harm (51), delirium (55), learning disabilities (59), Video 1

You're urgently called to ED. Ben, 21, was admitted after his girlfriend dumped him: he cut both wrists and took 32 paracetamol. He initially accepted blood tests and N-acetylcysteine (NAC), but just pulled out his venflon and wants to leave.

All doctors can assess capacity, but you'll often be called in complex or mental health-related cases. Disagreements and confusion may arise, due to constantly evolving case law and grey areas (e.g. whether to use the MHA or MCA). Ultimately, medical treatment is the *medical* team's call. Your role is to assist their decision-making, not to take over. Get involved early, joint-work closely, and always involve seniors when unsure.

Preparation

1. On the telephone
- How soon will he leave?
- How urgent is the treatment?
- Say when you'll be there
- Ask for someone (e.g. PLN/security) to keep him talking and persuade him to wait (p340)
- If you *can't* attend before he leaves, an ED doctor should assess capacity.

Box 76.1 The law – leaving *before* capacity can be fully assessed.

"This is tricky – work with ED and the PLN to find a solution. Although you must *presume* capacity, allowing Ben to leave while there's reasonable belief he may lack capacity and might suffer serious harm *could* be judged a breach of his rights under the Human Rights Act (p104–5). Swiftly decide if his presentation suggests:
- He *may* have a disorder of the mind/brain, e.g. intoxication, confusion, history of mental illness, recent symptoms or behaviours
- Questionable capacity, e.g. sudden, inexplicable change of mind; evidence of poor understanding
- Serious risks without intervention.
If so, you have *some* evidence that capacity could be impaired. In this case, it's reasonable to try to hold him (using security /RMN/ other staff as available) until capacity can be fully assessed. You are unlikely to be criticized for trying to ensure a patient's safety – but call seniors as soon as possible."

Anna Burnside, Consultant Liaison Psychiatrist

Psychiatry: Breaking the ICE – Introductions, Common Tasks and Emergencies for Trainees, First Edition.
Edited by Sarah Stringer, Juliet Hurn and Anna M Burnside.
© 2016 John Wiley & Sons, Ltd. Published 2016 by John Wiley & Sons, Ltd.
Companion Website: www.psychiatryice.com

2. In ED
Consider greeting Ben and explaining how long you'll need to read his notes; this may reassure and settle him.
- *Don't* if likely to irritate him or start a lengthy discussion.

3. Gain further information
Ideally, read all notes as per Ch.55. If he's trying to leave, or this is a life-and-death matter, focus on key information/take a verbal handover from the treating doctor:
- Admission circumstances
- When and why did he change his mind about treatment?
- Current medical problems and intended treatment
  - ◦ The exact decision he must make
  - ◦ Urgency of decision (seconds/minutes/hours?)
  - ◦ Communication barriers, e.g. deaf, poor English
  - ◦ Medically: what are his best interests? Least restrictive option?
  - ◦ What's been explained so far? How (clear and simple)?
  - ◦ Risks and benefits of each option
  - ◦ Evidence of coercion, e.g. suicide pact with a partner?
- How has he been kept in ED so far?
- PPHx.

4. Take a colleague
- Joint capacity assessment with the treating ED doctor
- Security/ RMN/ other staff if potentially aggressive/absconding.

Assessment

1. Approach
- Explain you know he wants to leave, but you want to help and this will take time (e.g. 30 minutes)
- Empathise. If Ben's refusal is a protest against some part of his ED experience, showing concern and letting him vent may help him accept treatment.
- Clarify the consequences of treatment refusal: if he risks serious harm, say so!
  - ◦ *Your doctors say you could die if you leave now. Did they tell you that? What do you think about that?*
- Try to appeal to his intelligence/common sense/courtesy to stay a little longer.

2. Brief history
In an emergency, a lengthy history may aggravate Ben and introduce dangerous delays. Focus on:
- *Reasons for leaving* – if not forthcoming, check key areas ...
  - ◦ Wants to harm/kill himself
  - ◦ Practical problems, e.g. work, carer duties; needs to fetch keys ...
  - ◦ To resolve a conflict, e.g. by speaking to his ex-girlfriend
  - ◦ Alcohol/drug withdrawal
  - ◦ ED problems, e.g. noisy; feeling abandoned/disliked by staff
- *Self-harm*: reasons, planning, act, function
  - ◦ Future plans?
- *Mental illness:* screen for possible problems, e.g. delirium, depression, psychosis, adjustment disorder, emotionally unstable personality disorder (EUPD)/traits.

3. MSE, remembering ...

Look for an 'impairment of, or disturbance in, the functioning of brain or mind' – i.e. anything which *could* affect his decision-making, e.g.

- Intoxication/withdrawal
- Delirium/dementia
- Depression/mania/psychosis
- Strong emotional states, e.g. anxiety/anger/distress
- Severe pain
- Impulsivity (e.g. in EUPD).

Check for ongoing self-harm intent/plans.

4. Assess capacity to refuse current treatment

Ben lacks capacity if he has an impairment/disturbance of brain/mind *and* is unable to do *one or more* of:

- Understanding relevant information
- Retaining this information
- Weighing this information
- Communicating his decision

Enhance his capacity as needed, e.g. using an interpreter/signer, or written prompts.

Understanding

It's not unusual for someone to refuse treatment due to a clinician's bedside manner or poor explanation of the problem. By engaging and re-explaining well, you may solve the problem altogether.

- Start: *Tell me what you know about your physical health at the moment ... What do you know about the treatment?*
- Correct and add information as needed: risks and benefits of all options
- Chunk and check (give small bits of information, then check understanding)
- Don't rely on *"Do you understand?"* A "yes" answer means Ben can say "yes" – it doesn't prove understanding.
  - ○ Try: *Tell me in your own words what I've said about this treatment.*

Retention

He must hold this information *long enough* to properly weigh it and reach a decision. You don't need to demonstrate retention over a long period.

Weighing

Ben must show he can consider the risks and benefits of each option. This is all about his *process* of reasoning – regardless of whether you agree with his final decision.

- *Can you tell me the pros and cons of [each option in turn]?*
- *You've said you want to go home. Tell me why that seems a better idea than treatment.*
- *Is there anything that worries you about choosing X over Y?*

Suspect problems with weighing where Ben's answers either keep overlooking important issues, or he seems too impulsive in choosing an outcome. Mental illness may prevent him from giving adequate weight to important arguments, e.g.

- If depressed, severe worthlessness may prevent him from considering life-saving treatment
- If psychotic, delusions may compete unfairly with the truth, overwhelming his ability to weigh the information, e.g. believing NAC is poison.

TIP: Case-law will change, month-by-month. Stay up to date by attending training courses and keeping an eye on constantly updated resources, e.g. www.mentalhealthlaw.co.uk

Communication

Ben needs to communicate his decision. Refusal to engage with a capacity assessment is evidence of inability to communicate, so capacity can be deemed absent.

If uncertain whether Ben has capacity, seek senior advice. You only have to establish that it's *more likely than not* (i.e. balance of probability) that Ben lacks capacity to make this specific decision – in which case, he can be treated in his best interests under the MCA.

5. Risk assessment

Complete a risk assessment for immediate and longer-term risks to self and others.

Management

Take your time, seek advice and discuss plans with involved colleagues and on-call seniors.

1. Enhance capacity and problem-solve

Calm Ben's situation and help him focus on the key issue: treatment. Problem-solve immediate issues, as this may buy time or resolve his wish to leave, e.g.

- Child to pick up from school – contact the school or a responsible relative
- Pet needs feeding – can a friend pick up keys and pop in?
- Routine appointments – call and rearrange ± advocate, e.g. if he'll be in trouble with the Job Centre
- In pain – arrange analgesia
- Alcohol withdrawal (Ch.40) – benzodiazepine detox
- Friction with staff/patients – mediate or move him.

Don't underestimate the effect of negative emotions (distress, shame, regret, embarrassment) on Ben's capacity to make decisions. Think of this as a temporarily *locked* situation, which may be *unlocked* by decreasing distress and helping him to think clearly:

- Reassure/help him feel safe
- Involve allies, e.g. friends or family
- Instil hope.

Try to prevent the need for legislation by unlocking the situation, person-to-person.

2. Medical treatment

Clearly document your capacity discussion, including reasons *why* you assess Ben as having or lacking capacity. You *must* discuss any uncertainty with your on-call senior.

Has capacity and now agreeing to treatment

Great job! Tell the medics to go ahead.

Lacks capacity (whether accepting or refusing treatment)

If Ben's stopped trying to leave, the MCA is likely to be sufficient to provide treatment in his best interests. Capacity for each intervention should be assessed and documented. Where there are choices, use the least restrictive safe option.

- If refusing and actively trying to leave, consider the MHA. If *detained* under the MHA, this should be used to hold him, but medical treatment would still happen under the MCA.
- If refusing but likely to regain capacity soon (e.g. intoxication/acutely distressed), postpone interventions until capacity returns – *if safe to do so*
- Where you have time, advise a best interests meeting, involving family/close friends /Independent Mental Capacity Advocate (IMCA).

Refusing and has capacity

For minor matters, you can let Ben refuse and simply document clearly, e.g. if he's refusing sutures for a small wound, which will merely scar.

- If Ben's refusal may cause death or serious harm, you *must* discuss with on-call seniors, and request their review. *As a junior doctor, you should never leave someone to die because you deem them able to make this decision.*
- It's occasionally appropriate to use the MHA to treat the physical sequelae of self-harm, when secondary to a mental disorder. A senior psychiatrist – usually the Responsible Clinician (RC) – must make this decision, as it can be a controversial area of law.

3. Psychiatric treatment

Once medically stable, plan Ben's further psychiatric care, depending on the underlying diagnosis and level of risk (Ch.51):

- If medically admitted, refer to liaison psychiatry
- Low risk: discharge to GP/CMHT for follow-up within seven days. Some liaison psychiatry departments offer self-harm follow-up clinics (useful if available and not known to a CMHT)
- Medium risk: discharge to HTT/CMHT
- High risk: admit to psychiatric hospital, preferably informally. Arrange a MHA assessment if he refuses or lacks capacity to consent to admission.

What If ... ?

... He's already an inpatient?

Section 5(2) can be used once Ben's been admitted to hospital, but isn't legal in ED (minors/majors/ waiting room). Some hospitals admit patients to an assessment/ observation ward, which may count as an admission. See Table 50.2, p312 for details.

... He has an Advance Decision / Advance Directive?

Advance decisions are refusals of specific types of care, available to anyone over 18, under the MCA. They only apply once someone loses capacity to make the healthcare decision, and are controversial where suicidal behaviour is involved. If Ben has an advance decision, check it's valid:

- He had capacity when he made the statement
- It was witnessed *and* signed
- He hasn't withdrawn it while he had capacity to do so
- He hasn't made a Lasting Power of Attorney (LPA) for welfare (the LPA has the authority to make decisions)
- He hasn't done anything which clearly goes against the advance decision, suggesting a change of mind
- It applies to the situation at hand
- Where it involves a life-threatening situation, it must include a statement that the decision stands, *even if his life is at risk.*

Even if satisfied that the above criteria apply, you *must* take legal advice. Failure to follow an advance decision could lead to charges of battery or assault; failure to act when it's invalid could result in death or accusations of negligence. This isn't a lone trainee decision! Discuss with seniors, and remember you can involve Trust lawyers and/or your medical indemnity provider, if needed.

Take-home message

Involve seniors early on, especially where refusal of treatment may result in serious harm.

References

David, A.S., Hotopf, M., Moran, P. *et al.* (2010) Mentally disordered or lacking capacity? Lessons for management of serious deliberate self-harm. *British Medical Journal*, **341**, c4489.

Department for Constitutional Affairs (2007) Mental Capacity Act 2005 Code of Practice. The Stationery Office, Norwich.

Department of Health (2015) Mental Health Act 1983: Code of Practice. The Stationery Office, Norwich.

Jacob, R., Gunn, M. and Holland, A. (eds) (2013) Mental Capacity Legislation: Principles and Practice, RCPsych Publications, London.

Mental Health Law Online: a useful website explaining statute and particularly good for brief summaries of the cases which led to changes in the law:

o www.mentalhealthlaw.co.uk

CHAPTER 77

Delirium tremens

Rachel Thomasson[1], Isabel McMullen[2], and Lisa Conlan[2]

[1] Manchester Royal Infirmary, Manchester, Lancashire, England
[2] South London & Maudsley NHS Foundation Trust, London, England

> **RELATED CHAPTERS:** alcohol misuse (40), illicit drugs (41), delirium (55), treatment refusal (76)

Margaret was admitted three days ago for a femoro-popliteal bypass. She's diabetic and a known heavy drinker. Nursing staff report she's become increasingly confused and irritable, and is now shouting at a chair. They'd like you to 'section' Margaret and admit her to a psychiatric ward.

Some problems should *never* be managed in psychiatric units – and delirium tremens (DTs) is one of them (Box 77.1). Mortality rates are 5–35%, but higher without treatment or with comorbid physical illness. Consider DTs whenever assessing a recent-onset (<1 week) delirium, especially where alcohol intake may have been suddenly stopped or reduced, e.g. by hospital admission.

Box 77.1 Delirium Tremens

- *Prodrome:* restlessness, fear, insomnia
- *Onset:* 1–5 days after last drink; symptoms peak at 2–4 days
- *Duration:* ends by day 7–10
- *Presentation:*
  - Sweating, gross tremor, nausea, vomiting, dilated pupils
  - Fluctuating confusion
  - Hallucinations (auditory, visual, tactile)
  - Delusions
  - Affective changes, e.g. lability, terror, anger
  - Sympathetic overdrive ↑HR, BP, RR, temperature (later = cardiovascular collapse)
- *Differential: any* cause of delirium, hepatic encephalopathy, head injury, Wernicke's encephalopathy (WE)

Preparation

1. Gather information – notes, obs, drug chart, staff
- Clues to underlying cause of delirium, e.g. falls, intra-/post operative complications, infection
- Any evidence of confusion, agitation or psychosis before / at admission?
- Evidence of alcohol misuse:
  - Past contact with psychiatric/substance misuse services

Psychiatry: Breaking the ICE – Introductions, Common Tasks and Emergencies for Trainees, First Edition.
Edited by Sarah Stringer, Juliet Hurn and Anna M Burnside.
© 2016 John Wiley & Sons, Ltd. Published 2016 by John Wiley & Sons, Ltd.
Companion Website: www.psychiatryice.com

- ○ Documented alcohol history
- ○ Stigmata of chronic alcohol use
- ○ Fits since admission
- ○ Abnormal obs
- ○ ↑MCV, LFTs, GGT
- • Other substance misuse, particularly if cross-tolerant with alcohol, i.e.
  - ○ Benzodiazepines
  - ○ Gamma-butyrolactone (GBL) or gamma-hydroxybutyric acid (GHB) – see *What if...?*

2. Collateral (before or after assessment)

If possible, sensitively contact a friend or relative who knows Margaret well – especially if she's very confused or denies substance misuse. Check specifically:
- • PPHx, including cognitive impairment
- • Alcohol history
- • Other drug use

Assessment

1. Approach

Use general delirium approaches (p346) and remember that Maureen may be terrified. Spend time gaining rapport, addressing her concerns and giving reassurance before asking about alcohol.

TIP: If a full substance misuse history is impossible, try:
- • *Do you ever / usually drink alcohol?*
- • *When was your last drink?*
- • *Do you need a drink now?*

---

2. Focused history and MSE

- • *HPC:* reasons for agitation
- • *Current physical symptoms*
- • *Substance misuse* (p34–35)
- • *MSE:*
  - ○ Alcohol withdrawal symptoms
  - ○ Affective lability, hilarity, irritability, fear
  - ○ Psychotic symptoms: ask specifically about Lilliputian hallucinations (tiny people or animals)
  - ○ Clouded consciousness, disorientation
  - ○ Willing to stay in hospital and accept treatment? Assess capacity.

3. Risk assessment

- • Further deterioration of physical health
- • Wernicke's encephalopathy (WE; p253)
- • Wandering, falls, accidents
- • Self-neglect, malnourishment
- • Aggression
- • Retributive violence (if provocative)

Management

1. Delirium management

Benzodiazepines won't cure missed sepsis or an acute intracranial event. Ensure a full delirium screen is organized (Appendix A2), *specifically* including the tests in Table 77.1. Manage as any delirium: treating underlying causes, environmental management ± 1:1 nursing (p349).

Table 77.1 Extra delirium tests in suspected DTs.

Test	Reason
Amylase	Pancreatitis
Glucose	Hypoglycaemia
CXR	Pneumonia (commonly comorbid)
CT head	Bleeds/fractures (fits and falls more common)
Magnesium	Hypomagnesaemia common

2. Alcohol detoxification

If *any* evidence of alcohol withdrawal, she needs a detoxification. The ward team should manage this, but you may prevent delays by offering advice or (if allowed) prescribing directly. Follow Trust guidelines where available. Otherwise, see Ch.40, remembering:

- Prescribe flexibly over the first 24 hours according to withdrawal symptoms.
- Use short-acting benzodiazepines in liver disease, e.g. oxazepam
- DTs may require *very large* benzodiazepine doses
- Keep looking for other causes if Margaret doesn't settle.

TIP: If Margaret's already had chlordiazepoxide, this doesn't rule out DTs – the dose and duration may have been insufficient

3. Thiamine

WE can arise during or after DTs. Ensure:

- IV Pabrinex is started (Table 40.4, p256)
- That adrenaline 0.5 mg IM is available (*extremely rare* anaphylaxis risk).

4. Other treatments

- Diazepam 10 mg IV/PR PRN for withdrawal seizures
- Consider adding an antipsychotic (e.g. haloperidol/olanzapine) if distressing psychotic symptoms persist despite increasing benzodiazepines.

5. Further management

Ensure Margaret's referred to the alcohol liaison practitioner if there is one, or Liaison Psychiatry if not. They can explore alcohol use further, and offer support around her drinking once the delirium's resolved.

What If ... ?

... It's GBL/GHB withdrawal?

GBL (Gamma-butyrolactone) and GHB (gamma-hydroxybutyric acid) are increasingly common, and linked with the club and gay scenes and steroid use in gyms. Both drugs are swallowed as colourless liquids; GBL is quickly converted to GHB. They act on GABA pathways and *can be fatal in overdose and withdrawal*. Dependent users may dose as often as every 1–2h. Be aware that overdose can switch to withdrawal within a few hours (Table 77.2).

GBL withdrawal is terrifying, so be as calm and reassuring as possible. Take a full *substance misuse history (p34–35), particularly:*
- How do they behave when 'high'?
- What are they like if they don't use it for two to three hours?
  ◦ Is there a clear withdrawal state?
  ◦ Last GBL 'dose'
- Other drugs (commonly polyuse), especially:
  ◦ Solvent use, e.g. nail polish remover (contains GBL)
  ◦ Alcohol and benzodiazepines (GABA-ergic, so relieve withdrawal)
- Sleep pattern (severe withdrawal insomnia often triggers further use).

For diagnostic certainty, you ideally want a clear history of GBL dependence, with increasing tolerance and use of GBL/alcohol/benzodiazepines to relieve withdrawal.
- If the picture is mixed, consider other drugs (Appendix C6).

GBL withdrawal can kill, so a medical admission is required if dependent.
- Work closely with the medics to examine ± investigate for other causes of delirium
- Take senior advice and contact addiction services
- There are no standard protocols yet, but titrate diazepam against sweating, shaking and anxiety
  ◦ Much higher doses may be needed than in alcohol detox

Table 77.2 GBL/GHB.

Effect	Drowsiness, euphoria, disinhibition, ↑libido
Onset	Minutes
Duration	Intoxication 1–7 hours
Overdose	Easy, since narrow 'therapeutic index'
	Symptoms: sweating, dizziness, blurred vision, hot/cold flushes, memory lapses, agitation, ↓HR, ↓BP, coma
	Respiratory depression and death (especially combined with alcohol/ benzodiazepines)
Dependence	Can occur quickly, e.g. within weeks
	May use ≥2mls every couple of hours
Withdrawal	Starts within a few hours of the last dose and lasts for 4–10 days
	Sweating, tremor (fine then gross), ↑HR, insomnia
	Delirium
	Hallucinations (auditory, visual, tactile), paranoia
	Muscle rigidity (rhabdomyolysis, acute renal failure), seizures, death
Detection	Not on UDS
	Blood/urine within 12 hours (rarely performed, as needs a specialist laboratory)
Risks	Death (overdose *or* withdrawal)
	Black outs/collapses
	Aggression
	Sexual exploitation (sometimes used in drug-facilitated sexual assaults – 'date rape')
	Risky sexual encounters

- Add baclofen, e.g. 10 mg tds (more as needed; ±continue for 2–4 weeks)
- Have flumazenil available
- 1:1 RMN

Handover to liaison psychiatry:

- Psychoeducation around GBL/GHB risks
- Encourage addiction services ± GUM input
- Temporary, low dose antipsychotics may help if psychotic symptoms remain problematic (but also lower the seizure threshold)
- Acute psychiatric admission is occasionally needed if extreme agitation continues beyond the expected duration of withdrawal (seven to ten days)

> **TIP:** It's fairly common for GBL use to continue in hospital, complicating or prolonging withdrawal. Tell the ward to watch for the patient sipping little bottles of colourless liquid; they may need to search belongings and keep a close eye on any visitors.

... It's ketamine?

Acute intoxication produces a predominantly stimulant picture (Appendix A6). Whilst there's no clear withdrawal syndrome, patients may be anxious, agitated, and complain of pain (especially bladder-related). Unless acutely psychotic and in need of a psychiatric admission, these patients are best treated by addiction services.

... She suspects her drink was spiked?

Liaise with the police. They'll need blood and urine samples, and it may help to organize these while in ED. See Ch.70 if possible sexual assault.

Take-home message

DTs can kill and need urgent medical treatment.

Further reading

NICE (2011) CG115 Alcohol dependence and harmful alcohol use quality standard. NICE, England.

McKeon, A., Frye, M.A. and Delanty, N. (2008) The alcohol withdrawal syndrome. *Journal of Neurology and Neurosurgical Psychiatry* **79**, 854–862.

Winstock, A.R. and Mitcheson, L. (2012) New recreational drugs and the primary care approach to patients who use them. *British Medical Journal*, **344**, e288 pp. 35–40.

Patient resources:

NHS Choices information on alcohol misuse, including self-help and contacts:
  ◦ www.nhs.uk/Livewell/alcohol/Pages/Alcoholsupport.aspx

Information on drugs for patients and families, including advice on how to get support:
  ◦ www.talktofrank.com

CHAPTER 78

Puerperal psychosis

Anna M Burnside

East London NHS Foundation Trust, London, England

RELATED CHAPTERS: pregnancy (29 and 42), Bipolar affective disorder (25), mania (54)

Josie Soler, 27, presents to ED with her 5-day old son, Ezekiel. Staff describe her as disorganized and perplexed; their records show a puerperal psychosis after her first child's birth, two years ago.

Postpartum (puerperal) psychosis may resemble delirium, with rapid onset, fluctuating mental state, confusion, disorganization and hallucinations. It may be affective (manic/depressive) or resemble a paranoid psychosis (Table 78.1). Consider puerperal psychosis in any new mum who's:
- Confused
- 'Not herself'
- Got a history of psychosis, puerperal psychosis or bipolar affective disorder (BPAD).

Rapid deterioration is common, so treat urgently, and consider admission to the Mother and Baby Unit (MBU) to safely keep Josie and Ezekiel together.

Preparation

1. ED staff
- Josie's behaviour in ED
- Concerns about her/Ezekiel
- If Ezekiel hasn't been examined, request this, with Josie's consent.

2. Don't leave Josie alone
- Ask someone to sit with her: relative/PLN/ED staff *or*
- Assess immediately, asking the PLN to gather information for you

3. Gather information
- PPHx, PMHx, previous presentation
- Risk, including any child risk concerns

Psychiatry: Breaking the ICE – Introductions, Common Tasks and Emergencies for Trainees, First Edition.
Edited by Sarah Stringer, Juliet Hurn and Anna M Burnside.
© 2016 John Wiley & Sons, Ltd. Published 2016 by John Wiley & Sons, Ltd.
Companion Website: www.psychiatryice.com

Table 78.1 Post-partum differentials.

Diagnosis	Onset after birth	Duration	Symptoms	Treatment
Maternity blues/ 'baby blues'	3–10 days	1–2 days	Tearful, sad, anxious Labile Overwhelmed	• Reassurance: normal and self-limiting • Recruit family support • Ask GP to monitor for PND
Post natal depression (PND)	Within 1y, commonly first 6 weeks	>2 weeks	As for any depression Check for: • Not coping • Feeling like a 'bad mum' • 'Something wrong' with baby • Effect on caring for baby/self • Suicidal/infanticidal thoughts • Psychosis	As for any depression, *but*: • Involve perinatal psychiatry • Breast-feeding affects medication choice • May need HTT/MBU • Fast-track access to psychology
Post-partum (puerperal) psychosis	Usually ≤2 weeks		Subtypes: • Affective (depressive/manic) • Schizophreniform • Organic (delirium-like) Check suicidal/homicidal thoughts	Usually needs admission • Breast-feeding affects medication choice

Assessment

1. Approach
Normalise the stress of parenthood: *everyone finds it overwhelming at times, especially early on* (frequent feeds, sleep-deprivation, not knowing what's 'normal'). This may help Josie discuss difficulties without feeling judged or inadequate.

She may be very sensitive to any suggestion she's not coping, doing a 'bad job' or might harm Ezekiel. Be gentle, but *always* explore risk:
• *How do you feel when it's just you and Ezekiel together?*
• *Are there times when he won't stop crying? How do you cope with that?*
• *Are you worried about Ezekiel?*
  ○ *Do you think there's anything wrong with him?*
• *Do you ever feel Ezekiel would be better off without you?*
  ○ *Have you had any thoughts of killing or hurting yourself?*
• *Sometimes mums are so worried, they feel they must save their baby from something bad happening. Have you had any thoughts like that?*
• *This is a hard question, but do you ever wish you hadn't had Ezekiel?*
  ○ *Are you afraid/have you had any thoughts you might hurt him?*
Josie may be frightened of taking medication, being 'sectioned', or separated from Ezekiel. If able, reassure her, e.g. *Babies need to stay with their mums wherever possible – and I want to do everything I can to help you both.*

2. Full history, remembering ...
• *Triggers*: labour complications, social stressors, conflict with partner/relatives, disrupted sleep
• *Function:* how she's coping with childcare/self-care
• *PPHx:* mood, psychotic, perinatal illnesses
• DHx: current medications? What helped before?
  ○ Breastfeeding?

- *PMHx:* current physical health, obstetric complications
- *Substance misuse:* always ask!

3. MSE, remembering...

Although a baby may disrupt the assessment, keep Ezekiel present for at least part of the interview, unless at immediate risk of harm.

- Response to baby, e.g. excessive staring/ignoring his needs
- Abnormal behaviour, retardation/agitation
- Depression, elation; anxious, suspicious, perplexed
- Thoughts of harm to self/baby/others
- Delusions – including abnormal beliefs about Ezekiel, e.g. possessed/'special'/evil
  ○ Does she treat him differently because of this?
- Hallucinations, particularly commands
- Confusion
- Wants help?

TIP: Always put quotes in the notes. It's important to know what someone's delusions are, not just whether they are psychotic, depressed, etc.

Gemma Hopkins ST5

---

4. Risk assessment, including...
- Self-harm
- Suicide (leading cause of death in new mothers)
- Self-neglect
- Harm to baby/other children: violence, neglect.

5. Collateral

This is *essential*, especially for current concerns. If partner, friends or family haven't attended, tell Josie you'll call them. You don't need her consent (but should ask) to receive information. You *do* need consent to *share* information.

Management

1. Medical/obstetric review of any health problems

Don't miss a true delirium state, e.g. septicaemia following caesarean section. Treat under the MCA if refusing but lacks capacity (Ch.76).

2. Admit or discharge?

Puerperal psychosis can quickly deteriorate – what you see today may be *much* worse tomorrow. *Always* discuss with seniors and decide whether risks allow:

- Treatment at home (e.g. with HTT) *and*
- Contact with children.

If not, admit – preferably to an MBU, allowing Josie to stay with Ezekiel (the bed manager can guide you through this process). If unavailable, or child risks are unmanageable, admit to a general adult ward (the duty social worker will organise Ezekiel's care). Josie might await an MBU bed on a maternity ward – if the general hospital bed manager agrees risks can be managed with 1:1 RMN and daily liaison follow-up.

Contact seniors if Josie needs detention under the MHA.

3. Medication

The ward usually starts medication, but if there's an urgent need or delay in transfer, discuss with your senior/pharmacist. Breast-feeding should never prevent medication, but will guide drug choice.

- Consider restarting medications that previously worked
- Check BNF/Maudsley Prescribing Guidelines/Lactmed (see Resources)
- Use monotherapy where possible
- Try to include Josie's preferences, and don't be categorical about safety *or* harm – there simply isn't enough evidence.

4. Social services

Don't forget siblings: where is Josie's *other* child? Discuss input with the duty social worker and Josie's family.

5. Psychoeducation

Reassure Josie and her family of the good prognosis for BPAD/post-partum psychosis. With treatment, she's likely to recover quickly.

6. Handover

Document clearly, copy to the GP and handover to liaison psychiatry if remaining in the hospital.

> **TIP:** Everyone suffers and we're not trying to strive for an absence of suffering – just for it to be manageable.
>
> **Piers Newman, Family Therapist**

Take-home message

Always ask about thoughts of harm to self, the baby or other children.

Further reading

Centre for Maternal and Child Enquiries (CMACE) (2011) Saving mothers' lives: reviewing maternal deaths to make motherhood safer: 2006–08. The Eighth Report on Confidential Enquiries into Maternal Deaths in the United Kingdom. *British Journal of Obstetrics and Gynaecology*, **118** (Suppl. 1), 1–203.

Sit, D., Rothschild, A.J. and Wisner, K.L. (2006) A review of postpartum psychosis. *Journal of Womens Health*, **15** (4), 352–368.

Taylor, D., Paton, C. & Kapur, S. (2015) *The Maudsley Prescribing Guidelines in Psychiatry*, 12th edn, Wiley-Blackwell, Chichester.

Resources

The Lactmed database has up-to-date information on medications and breast-feeding:
  ◦ http://toxnet.nlm.nih.gov/newtoxnet/lactmed.htm

CHAPTER 79

Eating disorders

Christina Barras[1] and Sean Cross[2]

[1] *South West London & St George's Mental Health NHS Trust, London, England*
[2] *South London & Maudsley NHS Foundation Trust, London, England*

RELATED CHAPTERS: treatment refusal (76)

Emma Rigg, 19, has been dieting for 1 year. Her Body Mass Index (BMI) is now 13.5, but she's denied problems and refused CMHT contact. Emma's family have become so worried, they've brought her to ED.

People with eating disorders usually present to GPs/CMHTs, but you'll occasionally see them in ED due to physical complications or family crises. There's often professional anxiety that they'll 'end up in the wrong place' – on a medical ward which can't handle the psychological complexities and feeding, or a psychiatric ward ill-equipped to manage physical complications. Liaise closely with the medics to meet Emma's needs: first medical, then psychiatric.

Preparation

1. Gather information – notes, obs, investigations
- PMHx, including weight loss/vomiting complications
- PPHx, including CMHT/Eating Disorders team contact
- Ensure she receives a full physical, obs, ECG, bloods (Box 79.1 and Table 79.1)

2. Collateral
- Let relatives speak to you privately. Emma may not be entirely honest about her behaviour, but it may be difficult for carers to openly contradict her.
- See Table 79.2.

Box 79.1 Eating disorder examination

- Emaciation, breast atrophy/pre-pubertal physique
- Brittle hair/nails, dry skin
- Downy lanugo hair over body
- Peripheral cyanosis, delayed capillary refill

Psychiatry: Breaking the ICE – Introductions, Common Tasks and Emergencies for Trainees, First Edition.
Edited by Sarah Stringer, Juliet Hurn and Anna M Burnside.
© 2016 John Wiley & Sons, Ltd. Published 2016 by John Wiley & Sons, Ltd.
Companion Website: www.psychiatryice.com

- Anaemia/hypercarotenaemia
- Vomiting clues
  - Parotid/submandibular gland swelling; dental erosions
  - Russell's sign (calluses over interphalangeal joints)
  - Conjunctival haemorrhages
- Cardiac failure
- Distended, tender abdomen (constipation/poor gastrointestinal motility)
- Gastric dilatation (life-threatening)
  - Acutely painful, distended abdomen; loss of gastric bowel sounds; ↑HR, ↓BP
  - Caused by binge eating/refeeding
- Peripheral neuropathy

Assessment

1. Approach

Start by exploring/acknowledging any ambivalence, e.g. *How do you feel about being asked to talk to me?* This may help Emma express the (often complicated) feelings she may have about having a psychiatry assessment. Empathise with any frustration or distress.

Emma may be very sensitive to suggestions that her eating habits are abnormal.

- Try to avoid labelling her eating disorder
- Start with open questions and use her language (e.g. 'diet')
- Remember that eating disorders are *not* simply issues of eating too little (or too much) – they're more emotionally complex than that
- Be honest about her physical risks, but don't try to scare her with them: you'll only increase her resistance to change.

> **PATIENT VIEW:**
>
> I think a lot of it is really about compassion and about treating somebody as if they are a human being. People do have ideas about what has gone wrong for them, and it's about finding out what those ideas are.
>
> 'Ellie'

2. Full history, remembering Table 79.2 ...

3. MSE, remembering ...

- Overt signs of weight loss/vomiting
- Psychomotor agitation/retardation
- Self-harm scars
- Depression/irritability
- Thoughts of self-harm/suicide
- Low self-esteem; guilt, shame
- Overvalued ideas e.g. *I'm overweight and must lose more*
- Delusions (could this be psychotically-driven, e.g. is food *poisoned?*)
- Poor concentration, memory
- Insight may be superficially present, e.g. acknowledging low weight and risk
  - *But* may lack insight into the nature of the problem (i.e. mental *illness*, not lifestyle choice).

Table 79.1 Eating disorder medical risk assessment (adapted from Treasure (2009) *A Guide to the Medical Risk Assessment for Eating Disorders*).

Test	Concern	Alert	Notes
BMI (kg/m²)	<14	<13	Easily falsified Less reliable if rapid weight loss/extremes of height Not used for children
Weight loss/week	>0.5 kg	>1.0 kg	
Skin breakdown	<0.1 cm	>0.2 cm	
Purpuric rash		Present	
Temperature	<35	<34.5	
Systolic BP	<90	<80	
Diastolic BP	<70	<60	
Postural drop	>10	>20	
HR	<50	<40	NB: *Tachycardia* + other signs of severe risk may precede cardiovascular collapse
Squat test (stand from squatting)	Needs arms for balance	Needs arms for leverage	Proximal myopathy
Sit-up test (sit from lying flat)	Needs arms for leverage	Unable	
ECG		QTc >450 msec	Other abnormalities: bradycardia/heart block, ST segment changes, right axis deviation
		Arrhythmia	
WCC	<4.0	<2.0	Blood changes: • ↓Hb, WCC common in starvation • ↓Platelets = rare and worrying • Low Hb but ↑MCV and MCH suggests no acute drop
Neutrophils	<1.5	<1.0	
Hb	<11	<9.0	
Acute Hb drop		Present	
Platelets	<130	<110	
Potassium	<3.5	<3.0	↓ = vomiting/diuretics/refeeding syndrome
Sodium	<135	<130	↓ = water loading/laxatives/SIADH from neurogenic diabetes insipidus/ hyperaldosteronism
Magnesium	0.5–0.7	<0.5	Refeeding syndrome
Phosphate	0.5–0.8	<0.5	Refeeding syndrome
Urea	>7	>10	Urea and creatinine ↑ in dehydration, ↓ in starvation
Bilirubin	>20	>40	LFTs – commonly mildly ↑ in starvation; marked ↑ in critical starvation
ALP	>110	>200	
AST	>40	>80	
ALT	>45	>90	
GGT	>45	>90	
Albumin	<35	<32	Rarely drops. When low, associated with high mortality. NB: ↓albumin + ↓glucose + hypothermia in starvation may indicate infection despite normal/low WCC
Creatinine kinase	>170	>250	Excessive exercise
Glucose	<3.5	<2.5	
ESR			↑ = consider physical causes of weight loss
TFTs			Exclude hyperthyroidism May show euthyroid sick syndrome (↓T3/T4 and ↑rT3). This reverses with weight gain.

Source: Adapted from Treasure, 2009.

NB: Baselines may differ between laboratories, but *any* abnormal result should provoke monitoring and discussion with eating disorders specialists.

Table 79.2 Eating disorder history.

Ask about …	Particularly …
Triggers	• Bullying • Family/partner tensions • School/college problems, including peer pressure around appearance / weight • ± Abuse

Abnormal eating behaviour	• Detailed daily food and fluid intake
	• Dietary restriction
	  ○ *Rules* of diet, e.g. maximum calories per day; 'good' or 'bad' foods
	• Other weight control methods
	  ○ Vomiting
	  ○ Laxatives
	  ○ Exercise
	  ○ Slimming pills, stimulants
	  ○ Medication misuse e.g. diuretics, thyroxine; insulin omission in diabetes
	• Does she ever feel she's lost control of her eating?
	• Has she ever eaten an unusually large amount of food? (Explore – subjective 'binge' may amount to normal eating)

Body image distortion	• Extreme fear of weight gain/'fatness' ○ NB: may be absent, particularly in men/ethnic minority groups • Disturbed perception of own weight and shape • Extremely low target weight • Time looking in the mirror/measuring parts of her body?
Weight history	• Premorbid weight, current weight • Rate of weight loss • Target (ideal) weight
Hypothalamic–pituitary-gonadal axis dysfunction	• Delayed puberty • Loss of periods/morning erections • Low libido
Associated psychosocial issues	• Preoccupation with food, e.g. cooking/eating rituals; cooking for others; eating alone • Anxiety • Low mood • Obsessionality • Poor concentration • Insomnia • Impact on work/studies, relationships (especially family) • Substance misuse
Physical side effects	• Fatigue • Constipation • Dizziness/fainting on standing • Feeling cold (especially extremities) • Palpitations • Headaches

4. Risk assessment
- Self-harm and suicide
- Medical complications (Table 79.1).

5. Capacity

Assess capacity regarding investigations and treatment. Emma may be very articulate and readily understand and retain information at an intellectual level. However, her ability to *weigh* information may be impaired by poor insight or overwhelming illness beliefs, e.g. fear of weight gain; *vitamins will make me fat; I don't deserve care.* Risk minimization is characteristic, and again affects *weighing* of information.

Management

1. Admit or discharge?

Discuss Emma's case with the medics and your senior on-call: medical/psychiatric admission or discharge depends on risks and the support available at home (Table 79.3).

The Management of Really Sick Patients with Anorexia Nervosa (MARSIPAN, 2014) report advises that extremely unwell patients should be managed on a Specialist Eating Disorder Unit (SEDU) unless they need interventions only available in a medical hospital, e.g. IV fluids, cardiac monitoring.

Table 79.3 Choice of admission site/discharge.

Site	Criteria

SEDU
If unavailable,
    consider
    psychiatric/medical
    admission
	• High medical risk – evidence of one highly abnormal parameter, several significant abnormalities, or escalating risk (Table 79.1).
	• Needs nasogastric (NG) feeding
	• High psychiatric risk
	• Intolerable social circumstances prevent safe community management
	• Failed outpatient treatment for severe eating disorder

Medical admission	• Phosphate <0.7 • QTc >450 • Creatinine >150 • BP<80/50, HR<40 • Needs IVI/cardiac monitoring • Acute abdomen (gastric dilatation needs emergency decompression) • Acute comorbid physical health problem requiring treatment
General psychiatric admission	• Only if low medical risk (and no need for NG feeding) • Psychiatric comorbidity • High suicide risk • Intolerable social circumstances prevent safe community management • NB: occasionally appropriate to admit for safety whilst awaiting specialist assessment
Discharge home	• No acute risks • Good family support/willing to work with HTT • Prevents disruption of usual eating habits (dangerous in itself)

2. Medical treatment
- Treat urgent physical complications
- Use the MCA if she lacks capacity (Ch.76)
- The MHA *may* be used to treat medical complications *arising* from an eating disorder, but should be agreed first with a consultant psychiatrist.

3. Vitamins
If admitting, give Pabrinex to prevent Wernicke's encephalopathy (WE), especially if Emma vomits/misuses alcohol (see p255–6).
Start multivitamins (whether admitting or discharging), e.g.
- Sanatogen Gold *or* Forceval: 2 tablets od for 1 month, then 1 tablet od
- +Thiamine 50 mg qds *or* 100mg tds (see local protocol)
- +Vitamin B compound strong 1 tablet tds

4. Start feeding
If admission's required, feeding *must* be established safely and immediately to prevent death from malnutrition. *However*, feeding too rapidly causes refeeding syndrome, which can kill.
- Follow MARSIPAN guidance and involve a specialist dietician urgently
- Out-of-hours, most hospitals have an emergency feeding protocol (follow it)
- Consider 1:1 nursing to support feeding
- NG feeding should be provided under the MHA, if refused.
If admitting to a psychiatric unit out-of-hours, support Emma to continue her own eating plan, plus two pints of milk per day (high in phosphate).
- Daily weight, FBC, U & E, LFT, glucose, calcium, phosphate

5. Handover
Whether admitting or discharging, Emma's case must be referred and urgently discussed with eating disorder specialists. Include test results in any referral.
- Ask liaison psychiatry to review if admitting to a medical ward
- If discharging:
  - Consider HTT input
  - Liaise with GP for close physical health monitoring.
  - Urgently refer to a specialist eating disorder service (or CMHT if no direct care pathway).

What if ... ?

... It's bulimia nervosa?
More commonly treated in outpatients, but electrolyte abnormalities can be life-threatening, e.g. hypokalaemia/hyponatraemia. Explore the pattern of binges and vomiting/purging. An SSRI may be useful, but ask the CMHT/Eating Disorder team to start and monitor. If severe, follow guidance above.

Take-home message

Prioritise physical management and feeding, seeking early advice from eating disorder specialists.

References

The MARSIPAN group (2014) College Report CR189. *MARSIPAN:* Management of Really Sick Patients with Anorexia Nervosa (2nd edition). Royal College of Psychiatrists, London.
   ○ www.rcplondon.ac.uk/sites/default/files/cr189.pdf.
Palmer, R.L. (1996) The management of Anorexia Nervosa. *Advances in Psychiatric Treatment*, **2**, 61–68.
Treasure, J. (2009) A *Guide to The Medical Risk Assessment for Eating Disorders.* Section of Eating Disorders, Institute of Psychiatry and Eating Disorders Unit, South London and Maudsley NHS Foundation Trust.
   ○ www.kcl.ac.uk/ioppn/depts/pm/research/eatingdisorders/resources/guidetomedicalriskassessment.pdf.

CHAPTER 80

Threats of violence

Penelope Brown[1] and Rachel Thomasson[2]

[1] *South London & Maudsley NHS Foundation Trust, London, England*
[2] *Manchester Royal Infirmary, Manchester, Lancashire, England*

RELATED CHAPTERS: forensics (28 and 43), aggression (74)

Bradley is 26. He was treated in ED for a hand injury, then demanded to see a psychiatrist. The ED doctor didn't feel he was mentally ill, but when she tried to discharge him, Bradley calmly threatened to 'seriously hurt someone' unless admitted to hospital.

Violent statements may indicate frustration and poor coping skills and/or an underlying disorder, e.g. psychosis, OCD (Ch.56), antisocial personality disorder (ASPD), learning disability (LD). Focus on de-escalation (p20–21), boundary-setting, and understanding Bradley's motivation for making threats. You'll then be able to logically assess and manage the risks (Table 80.1).

Preparation

1. Safety
- If aggressive, see Ch.74
- Request security support
  - They should search Bradley if he's suspected of carrying weapons (e.g. bags/bulky clothing). Involve police if needed.
- Assess with a colleague, e.g. PLN.

2. Gather information – notes, staff
- Current:
  - Presenting problems, e.g. hand injury – accident, assault, self-inflicted?
  - Other physical health concerns
  - Substance misuse
  - Recent triggers, e.g. relationship/accommodation breakdown
- Previous presentations/recent increase in attendances
  - Triggers? Management?
- PPHx, known diagnoses
  - Existing care plan around aggression?
- Risks.

Psychiatry: Breaking the ICE – Introductions, Common Tasks and Emergencies for Trainees, First Edition.
Edited by Sarah Stringer, Juliet Hurn and Anna M Burnside.
© 2016 John Wiley & Sons, Ltd. Published 2016 by John Wiley & Sons, Ltd.
Companion Website: www.psychiatryice.com

Table 80.1 Risk factors for violence.

	Exacerbating factors	Protective factors
Demographic	• Male • Young • Socially isolated • Unemployed	• Good social support
Historic	• Past history of violence • Young age at first violent incident • Substance misuse • Childhood abuse/neglect; bullied or a bully • Unstable/no close relationships • Unstable/chequered employment • Personality disorder, especially EUPD, ASPD, psychopathy • Violence when unwell • Use of weapons	• Self-control/ability to walk away from conflict • Coping strategies • Stable, supportive relationships • Stable employment

Current clinical presentation	• Psychotic symptoms:
	  ◦ Feeling that others wish them harm
	  ◦ Command hallucinations
	  ◦ Passivity
	  ◦ Thought insertion
	  ◦ Suspiciousness
	  ◦ Grandiosity
	  ◦ Excitement
	  ◦ Delusional jealousy
	
	• Hostility
	• Impulsivity
	• Poor insight into illness/past violence
	• Violent fantasies (including sexual)
	• Current plans for violence
	• Named victim(s)
	• Access to weapons
	• Non-concordance/treatment resistance
	• Current stressors
		• Negative psychotic symptoms
		• Treatment concordance
		• Engaging with other services, e.g. probation officer

Assessment

1. Approach (also p19)

Be polite, formal and unthreatening – don't stride into the room as if ready for a fight. Model non-confrontational behaviour; Bradley may start to mirror you, e.g. uncrossed arms and legs, soft speech, attentive (not constant) eye contact.

Set boundaries early, e.g.

- *I want to help you, but I need to feel safe to do that, so we need some basic rules. Both of us need to stay respectful: no shouting, swearing or threatening behaviour. If either of us feels unsafe, we'll say so and end the interview.*
- *Our conversation is confidential, unless you tell me something suggesting you or someone else may get hurt. If that's OK, let's start.*

Give Bradley time to express himself. Empathise and agree wherever possible, whilst monitoring closely for escalating aggression.

- Positively reinforce calm behaviour, e.g. *I know it's been stressful, but you've done an excellent job of staying calm with me – so thank you.*
- Leave if worried he'll lash out, using excuses if needed, e.g. *I need to work out a plan with my team …*

Bradley may *enjoy* keeping you worried, e.g. telling you he'll hurt his partner, but refusing to say where she lives. There are numerous ways to gain potential victims' contact details:

- Use the administrative approach early on (*I have to get this from everyone …*), collecting details of all relevant professionals *and* personal contacts
- Explore plans, rather than directly requesting contact details, e.g.
  - *Do you know where she lives/works?*
  - *When is she there?*
  - *How would you get there? How would you get in?*
- Gain rapport: Bradley may directly offer contact details, especially if seeking psychiatric support
- Look for carers/next-of-kin details in old notes and ED contact sheet
- Contact the police

2. Full history, remembering …

- *HPC:* what does Bradley want from you/admission?
  - Does admission avoid something, e.g. prosecution, homelessness?
- *Violent threats*
  - Is a specific person at risk? Why?
  - Formed plans
  - Access to victim ± weapons
  - How likely does Bradley think he is to carry out plans?
  - Is anything stopping him from acting on his plans / thoughts?
- *Function of violence/threats*
  - Motives, e.g. revenge, emotional expression; gaining drugs/money
- *Screen for:* psychosis, substance misuse, LD
  - ASPD traits: callous, impulsive, low frustration tolerance, remorseless, tendency to blame others
  - EUPD traits may be relevant as seeking admission, e.g. mood instability, fears of abandonment, self-harm
- *Forensic history*
  - Convictions, charges
  - Current probation
  - Violence that hasn't been reported to the police
- *SHx* – stressors, social support.

3. MSE, remembering …

- Level of agitation
- Intoxication/withdrawal
- Irritability, depression; lability
- Psychotic symptoms
- Insight – can Bradley acknowledge if there's no clinical reason for admission?

4. Risks, including …

- Aggression/sexual assault
- Accidental, planned or impulsive self-harm
- Retributive violence.

Management

1. Address urgent psychiatric problems
If Bradley's psychotic, it would be unusual and extremely unwise to discharge him. Discuss admission (± MHA assessment) with your registrar. Inform ward staff of the risks *before* transfer.

2. High risk but no clear mental illness
Psychiatric admission rarely helps, and *may* place other patients and staff at risk of violence. However, consider asking your registrar to assess Bradley before deciding whether to admit or discharge, especially if there's a history of violence.
- Making threats to kill is a criminal offence. Have a low threshold for involving police.

3. Problem-solving
Try to problem solve *with* Bradley, finding ways to minimize frustration around current stressors, e.g.
- Alert involved parties to his presentation e.g. GP, CMHT, probation services
- Signpost to practical advice, e.g. Citizen's Advice Bureau.

Don't make promises you can't keep or paint an overly rosy view of services you recommend, e.g. *definite* accommodation help; swift access to anger management therapy. The reality may cause disappointment, frustration, and further threats or violence.

4. Discuss psychological options
If Bradley is amenable to psychological input, like anger management or stress management, consider:
- Asking his GP to refer to Improving Access to Psychological Therapies (IAPT) service or other local services, e.g.
  - www.everymanproject.co.uk (London)
  - www.everymanproject.co.uk/otheragencies.html
- CMHT referral – if comorbid mental health problems or high complexity
- Addiction service self-referral – if appropriate.

Your referral must state that he shouldn't be assessed alone. Clarify boundaries with Bradley, e.g. *When you see X, it's important that you stay calm and polite with them, like you have with me. Otherwise, they won't be able to help you, and may need to involve the police.*

5. Handover
Carefully document your assessment, and communicate your diagnosis and risk assessment to all involved agencies. Add an aggression alert to his notes.

> **TIP:** Imagine ahead to the worst-case scenario of serious harm to a victim. Would your plan be defensible? Probably, if discussed with seniors and relevant parties ...

What if ... ?

... He has ASPD?
This *is* a mental disorder and shouldn't be used to exclude Bradley from services. People with ASPD present high risks to themselves and others, including suicide. Risk management is needed. If Bradley

has a history of high-risk offending (e.g. serious assaults, sexual offending, attempted murder, arson, stalking) he may be appropriate for forensic service assessment. Discuss with your registrar.

... He makes more threats to harm someone?

If you've established that these threats are not driven by an acute mental health problem that could be treated in hospital, explain why admission isn't useful at this point and reiterate options that you think could be helpful. Explain that making threats to harm people (especially killing) is an offence, and that you'll need to inform the police.

... He storms out, shouting he'll now 'have' to do something bad?

Contact the police, giving as much information as possible: appearance, demographics, verbatim threats. You may need to break confidentiality and make reasonable efforts to warn a specific person if you believe Bradley will harm them. You're *not* expected to warn the general public of non-specific threats (e.g. if Bradley hates vegans), though should still contact the police if violence seems likely.

Tell ED staff – including receptionists – about Bradley's threats. They should call the police if he returns.

Take-home message

Significant violence is unusual but possible after such presentations. Don't shoulder the risk yourself – seek advice and share information with seniors and relevant agencies.

Further reading

NICE (2015) NG10. Violence and aggression: short-term management in mental health, health and community settings. NICE, England. – www.nice.org.uk/guidance/ng10

NICE (2009) CG77 Antisocial Personality Disorder: Treatment, Management and Prevention. NICE, England. http://guidance.nice.org.uk/CG77

Yakeley, J. and Williams, A. (2014) Antisocial Personality Disorder: new directions. *Advances in Psychiatric Treatment*, **20**, 132–143.

Appendices

Appendices

APPENDIX A

Investigations/Monitoring

Juliet Hurn[1], Noreen Jakeman[2], Anna M Burnside[3], and Abigail Steenstra[1]

[1] *South London & Maudsley NHS Foundation Trust, London, England*
[2] *Lewisham & Greenwich NHS Trust, London, England*
[3] *East London NHS Foundation Trust, London, England*

Table A.1 Overview of physical health monitoring in Severe Mental Illness (SMI).

Risk factor to be monitored at least *annually*	Part of GP Annual Health Check?	Needs intervention?
History/lifestyle		
Family history: vascular disease, diabetes, hypertension, hyperlipidaemia	✓	–
Smoker	✓	Brief intervention Nicotine Replacement Therapy (NRT) Refer to Smoking Cessation Clinic
Alcohol/drug misuse	✓	See Audit Questionnaire, Appendix C
Activity level		Brief Intervention - exercise
Diet		Dietary advice
Measurements/investigations		
Central obesity	✓ (BMI)	Initially diet/exercise advice
• Body Mass Index (BMI) (kg/m^2)		See NICE CG43
○ ≥25 – overweight		
○ ≥30 – obesity		
• Waist circumference		
○ Men ≥94 – high; ≥102 – very high		
○ Women ≥80 – high; ≥88 – very high		
Blood Pressure (2 separate measurements, at an interval)	✓	Lifestyle advice Discuss antihypertensive with GP
• ≥140/90 mmHg		See NICE CG127
Blood glucose (mmol/L)	✓	Lifestyle advice
• Fasting ≥5.5		Discuss oral hypoglycaemics/insulin with GP
• Random ≥11.1		See NICE CG87
HbA1c		
• ≥6%		
Total cholesterol: HDL ratio	✓	Dietary advice
• High (>10%) according to cardiovascular disease prediction charts (see BNF)		Discuss statin with GP NICE CG181

Source: Adapted from Lester UK adaptation 2014.

Psychiatry: Breaking the ICE – Introductions, Common Tasks and Emergencies for Trainees, First Edition.
Edited by Sarah Stringer, Juliet Hurn and Anna M Burnside.
© 2016 John Wiley & Sons, Ltd. Published 2016 by John Wiley & Sons, Ltd.
Companion Website: www.psychiatryice.com

Table A.2 Delirium investigations.

Investigation	Essential/ PRN	Notes/indications
Physical observations	E	HR, BP, RR, temperature, SaO$_2$
Physical examination	E	Include: • Neurological exam • PR (exclude constipation) • Pressure areas (sores/infection) • Evidence of pain • Visual acuity • Hearing • Swallow • Missed fractures (e.g. bruising, limited mobility)
ECG	E	Especially: • MI, arrhythmia • QTc – check normal before using antipsychotics, especially if on other QTc-prolonging drugs
Routine bloods	E	Minimum: • FBC, U&E, LFT, glucose • CRP • Calcium/phosphate
Septic screen	PRN	Remember that older adults don't always raise inflammatory markers or temperature, so have a low threshold for: • Urine dipstick ($\pm$MC&S) • Blood cultures • CXR
UDS	PRN	All younger patients; older adults if suspect drug misuse
CT head	PRN	*Urgent* if localising neurological signs *or* anything else indicating cerebral pathology It's otherwise reasonable to leave it until tomorrow.
Other bloods	PRN	• TFTs • Iron studies – especially if malnutrition/frail elderly • B12, folate – especially in drinkers, eating disorders, frail elderly • HIV, syphilis – remember HIV is increasingly common in older adults • ESR
MRI head	PRN	If suspect neuropathology, but CT NAD
LP	PRN	If suspect neuropathology/CNS infection
EEG	PRN	If diagnostic confusion/suspect non-convulsive status

Table A.3 First episode psychosis investigations.

Investigation	Essential/PRN	Notes/indications
Physical observations	E	HR, BP, RR, temperature, SaO$_2$
Physical examination	E	Include: • Neurological exam • Stigmata of alcohol/drug use • Missed concurrent illness
ECG	E	QTc - check normal before using antipsychotics, especially before rapid tranquilisation and always before using haloperidol
Routine bloods	E	More important to establish physical health status and any missed needs; occasionally pick up organic cause for psychosis (see Appendix A.2) • FBC, U&E, LFT, glucose • CRP
UDS	E	Carry a kit with you; ED often don't stock them
CT head	PRN	*Urgent* if: • Localising neurological signs *or* anything else indicating cerebral pathology It is not essential to scan everyone with FEP. Threshold for scanning decreases with age, e.g. consider scanning over-40s; definitely scan over-65s with FEP. Check local protocols. May need sedation to allow urgent scan – judge carefully, as you still need to assess MSE!
Other bloods	PRN	• TFTs – Results can take time; especially useful if affective component • Lipids – needed as baseline before starting antipsychotics; may not be practicable acutely, but do as soon as possible • HIV – almost routine now, depending on risk/sexual history and demographic • Syphilis – increasingly prevalent • Calcium / phosphate (especially if elderly) • ANA/Anti-dsDNA – consider lupus • ESR – if systemic illness suspected
Weight, BMI	PRN	Needed for antipsychotic monitoring – do as soon as possible
MRI head	PRN	May not be practicable acutely, but more sensitive than CT head. Use only when clear suspicion of neuropathology.
Lumbar puncture	PRN	If suspicion of neuropathology/CNS infection
EEG	PRN	If diagnostic confusion/suspect non-convulsive status
Pregnancy test	PRN	If possibly pregnant, especially before starting medication

Antibody-mediated encephalitis ("autoimmune psychosis") is increasingly being recognised. Discuss with liaison and neurology if a young person suffers an acute onset of a paranoid psychosis, with any of the following markers: a prodromal physical illness (malaise, headache, fever); spontaneous movement disorder (e.g. catatonia, orofacial dyskinesia); cognitive impairment. Antipsychotics may have little effect, or cause adverse reactions (e.g. collapse) in these patients. Tests would include serum antibodies (NMDAR & VGKC), EEG and MRI. Treatment may include immunotherapy.

Table A.4 Baseline checks before starting psychotropics.

Group	Antipsychotics				Mood stabilisers				Antidepressants						
Test	Psychosis patients	Clozapine	Haloperidol	Quetiapine	BPAD patients	Lithium	Valproate	Carbamazepine	Depressed patients	SSRIs	SNRIs	TCAs	Mirtazapine	MAOIs	Agomelatine
FBC	R	E			R		E	E	R				R		
U&E	R				R	E			R	E†					
LFT	R				R		E	E	R					E	E
TFT				R	R	E			R						
PRL	R														
CK	R														
Lipids**	R				R							R	R		
Glucose**	R				R				R						
Troponin		R													
BMI	R				R				R				R		
BP	R				R				R		R			E	
Pulse	R														
Temperature		R													
ECG	R		E		R	E*			R			E		R	

Key: E = Essential; R = Recommended; * = If clinically indicated/cardiovascular risk factors; ** = Fasting if possible;
† in elderly patients

Sources of information: Maudsley Prescribing Guidelines, British National Formulary, Zaponex Treatment Systems & Lester UK Adaptation 2014

Table A.5 Ongoing monitoring - antipsychotics.

Test	All patients using antipsychotics	Clozapine	Olanzapine	Quetiapine	Phenothiazines, e.g. chlorpromazine, trifluoperazine
FBC	R: yearly	E: weekly for 18 weeks; then fortnightly until 1y; then monthly			
U&E	R: yearly				
LFT	R: yearly (not sulpiride/amisulpride)	R: at 6 weeks, 12 weeks			
TFT				R: yearly	
PRL	R: at 6 months then yearly (not clozapine, olanzapine or aripiprazole)				
CK	E: If suspect NMS (p408)				
Lipids	R: at 3 months then yearly	R: at 6 weeks, then 3-monthly for 1st year	R: 3-monthly for 1st year	R: 3-monthly for 1st year	R: 3-monthly for 1st year
G	R: at 4–6 months, then yearly	R: at 6 weeks, then 3-monthly for 1st year	R: at 1 month		
Troponin		R: Weekly for 1 month			
CRP		R: Weekly for 1 month			
BMI	R: frequently for 3 months, then yearly	R: at 6 weeks, then 3-monthly for 1st year	R: 3-monthly for 1st year		
BP	R: frequently in titration (not amisulpride, sulpiride, trifluoperazine, aripiprazole)	E: at least daily during titration, then at 6 weeks, 12 weeks, yearly			
Pulse		E: At least daily during titration			
Temperature		E: At least daily during titration			
ECG	R: yearly and after dose increases	E: If tachycardic			
EEG		R: If seizures			
Drug levels		During titration At steady state and yearly If poor response/suspected toxicity/changed smoking status			

Key: R = Recommended; E = Essential
Reference: Taylor, D., Paton, C. & Kapur, S. (2015) The Maudsley Prescribing Guidelines in Psychiatry (12th edition). Wiley Blackwell.

Table A.6 Ongoing monitoring - mood stabilisers.

Test	All BPAD patients	Lithium	Valproate	Carbamazepine
FBC	R: yearly		R: 6-monthly	R: 6-monthly
U&E	R: yearly	E: 6-monthly (more if interacting drugs)		R: 6-monthly
LFT	R: yearly		R: 6-monthly	R: 6-monthly
Albumin & clotting			R: if LFTs abnormal	
TFT	R: 6-monthly	E: 6-monthly		
PRL	R: if suspect ↑PRL			
Lipids	R: yearly if >40y			
G	R: yearly			
Calcium		R: if long-term treatment		
BMI	R: yearly	6-monthly	R: 6-monthly	R: 6-monthly
BP	R: yearly			
ECG	R: if CV risk factors or history	R: if CV risk factors or history		
Drug levels (trough)		E: 5–7 days after each dose change until stable levels; then 3-monthly Aim 0.4–1.0 mmol/L	R: Check toxicity/ adherence/ effect of other drugs on valproate levels Aim >50 mg/L	R: 2–4 weeks after start & any dose changes; then 6-monthly Aim: 7–12 mg/L

Reference: Taylor, D., Paton, C. & Kapur, S. (2015) The Maudsley Prescribing Guidelines in Psychiatry (12th edition). Wiley Blackwell.

Table A.7 Rapid tranquilisation (RT) cautions and contraindications.

Condition	Potential problem	Medication caution
Cardiovascular (CV): • Prolonged QTc • Cardiac history • Metabolic syndrome • Significant CV risk factors	Sudden CV collapse/death	Caution with antipsychotics, especially haloperidol
Hepatic/renal impairment	Reduced rate drug metabolism/excretion	Dose adjustment may be needed, especially if long half-life See BNF
Respiratory disease	Respiratory depression/arrest	Avoid benzodiazepines
Hypotension	Worsens hypotension Risk of falls	Olanzapine can cause vasovagal bradycardia/ syncope. Extra care if using regular medications which lower BP
History of: • NMS • Acute dystonia • Severe EPSE	High risk recurrence	All antipsychotics Avoid FGAs, especially haloperidol

Reference: Taylor, D., Paton, C. & Kapur, S. (2015) The Maudsley Prescribing Guidelines in Psychiatry (12th edition). Wiley Blackwell.

Table A.8 Monitoring after RT.

Monitoring	Concern	Action
Temperature	Pyrexia - NMS? (Ch.67)	Stop antipsychotics Benzodiazepine if RT needed Urgently check CK and WCC
Pulse	Arrythmia *or* bradycardia (<50 bpm)	Urgent transfer to ED Do ECG while waiting
BP	Diastolic <50 mmHg *or* systolic drop >30 mmHg on standing	Lie flat, legs raised Monitor closely ± discuss with medics

RR/SaO$_2$	Respiratory depression
	RR < 10
	SaO$_2$ < 90%
		Manage airway + give O$_2$
		If benzodiazepines involved, give flumazenil:
		
		• 200 mcg IV over 15 seconds
		• After 60s, if continued respiratory depression
		  ○ 100 mcg over 10 seconds
		  ○ Repeat (max 1 mg in 24 h)
		• Continuously monitor RR until returns to baseline (flumazenil half-life < most benzodiazepines)
		
		If not benzodiazepine-induced/RR doesn't return to normal with flumazenil
		• Urgent transfer to ED

GCS	Over-sedation	Continuous 1:1 nursing; maintain airway Monitor RR and SaO$_2$ Consider dehydration risk
General	Ongoing agitation	Discuss with seniors: benzodiazepine paradoxical agitation *or* missed organic cause *or* need for further RT?
	Acute dystonia	Procyclidine 5-10 mg IM
	Akathisia	Increases risk of violence/self-harm; consider benzodiazepine
	Dehydration	Offer fluids

Reference: Taylor, D., Paton, C. & Kapur, S. (2015) The Maudsley Prescribing Guidelines in Psychiatry (12th edition). Wiley Blackwell.

APPENDIX B

Medications

Noreen Jakeman[1] and Sarah Stringer[2]

[1] Lewisham & Greenwich NHS Trust, London, England
[2] King's College London, London, England

B.1 Common antipsychotics – approximate relative side effect profiles

Table B.1.1 Oral antipsychotics – approximate relative side effects.

Drug	↑QT	Sedation	↑Weight	Diabetes	↑Lipids	Dystonia / parkinsonism	Akathisia	Tardive dyskinesia	Anticholinergic	↓BP	↑Prolactin
FGAs											
Chlorpromazine											
Haloperidol											
Sulpiride		*			?				*	*	
Trifluoperazine	?										
Zuclopenthixol	?		?		?						
SGAs											
Amisulpride		*							*	*	
Aripiprazole	*	*	*	*	*				*	*	*
Clozapine						*	*	*			*
Lurasidone	*		*	*	*			?	*	*	
Olanzapine											
Quetiapine						*					*
Risperidone								?			

Key (? = lack of data, so best guess)

	Low (* good choice if problems)
	Moderate
	Severe

NB: Hyperprolactinaemia is often (but not always) a proxy marker of sexual dysfunction.

Sources:

- Joint Formulary Committee (2014) British National Formulary (BNF) 68. Pharmaceutical Press.
- Taylor D, Paton C, Kapur S (2015). The Maudsley Prescribing Guidelines. 12th ed. Wiley-Blackwell, London.
- Bazire, S (2014) Psychotropic Drug Directory 2014: The professionals' pocket handbook and aide memoire. Lloyd-Reinhold Communications LLP.
- Clinician experience.

Psychiatry: Breaking the ICE – Introductions, Common Tasks and Emergencies for Trainees, First Edition.
Edited by Sarah Stringer, Juliet Hurn and Anna M Burnside.
© 2016 John Wiley & Sons, Ltd. Published 2016 by John Wiley & Sons, Ltd.
Companion Website: www.psychiatryice.com

Table B.1.2 Depot antipsychotics – approximate relative side effects.

Drug	↑QT	Sedation	↑Weight	Diabetes	↑Lipids	Dystonia / parkinsonism	Akathisia	Tardive dyskinesia	Anticholinergic	↓BP	↑Prolactin
FGAs											
Flupentixol					?						
Fluphenazine					?						
Haloperidol											
Zuclopenthixol	?				?						
SGAs											
Aripiprazole	*	*	*	*	*				*	*	*
Olanzapine											
Paliperidone	*							?			
Risperidone								?			

Key (? = lack of data, so best guess)

	Low (* good choice if problems)
	Moderate
	Severe

NB: Hyperprolactinaemia is often (but not always) a proxy marker of sexual dysfunction.

Sources:

- Joint Formulary Committee (2014) British National Formulary (BNF) 68. Pharmaceutical Press.
- Taylor D, Paton C, Kapur S (2015). *The Maudsley Prescribing Guidelines*. 12th ed. Wiley-Blackwell, London
- Bazire, S (2014) Psychotropic Drug Directory 2014: The professionals' pocket handbook and aide memoire. Lloyd-Reinhold Communications LLP.
- Clinician experience

Table B.2 Common oral antipsychotics – key information.

Name	Preparations	Dose (PO)			Notes *Emphasise to patient*
		Usual start	**Increase**	**Max daily**	
FGAs					
Chlorpromazine	Tablets Liquid IM	25 mg tds PO	25 mg increments as tolerated	1000 mg	Rarely used *Sedative* *Photosensitive rash – use sunblock*
Haloperidol	Tablets Liquid IM (p444) Depot (Table B3)	1.5–3 mg bd PO	As needed	20 mg	Mandatory ECG baseline High incidence EPSE *Report stiffness to doctor* *If eye fixation/lockjaw, attend ED*
Sulpiride	Tablets Liquids	200–400 mg bd	Positive symptoms: increase as needed, up to 1200 mg bd Negative symptoms: 200–400 mg bd for alerting effect Mixed picture 400–600 mg bd	2400 mg	Renally excreted, so useful in liver impairment ↑Prolactin problematic *Tell doctor if irregular periods, breast tenderness, sexual dysfunction*
Trifluoperazine	Tablets Liquid	5 mg bd	Increase to 15 mg daily after a week if needed, then 5 mg increases at ≥3 day intervals. Doses should be divided bd.	30 mg	High incidence EPSE
Zuclopenthixol	Tablets Depot (Table B3)	20–30 mg daily	Can continue at 20 mg or increase in 10–20 mg increments. Usual treatment dose is 20–50 mg.	150 mg	Don't confuse with zuclopenthixol acetate (*Acuphase*, p447)
SGAs					
Amisulpride	Tablets Liquid (£)	200 mg bd Negative symptoms, use lower range, e.g. 50 mg od	No specific titration. Adjust to clinical response. >300 mg, use bd dosing. Positive symptoms: aim for 400–800 mg/day Negative symptoms: aim for 50–300 mg	1200 mg	Renally excreted, so useful in liver impairment ↑Prolactin problematic (see sulpiride)

(*continued overleaf*)

Table B.2 (*continued*)

Name	Preparations	Dose (PO)			Notes
					Emphasise to patient
		Usual start	**Increase**	**Max daily**	
Aripiprazole	Tablets ODT Liquid (£) IM (p444) Depot (£; Table B3)	10–15 mg PO (try 5 mg if elderly or concerned re: side effects)	5–10 mg PO	30 mg (but little evidence >15 mg)	Often used if other antipsychotics cause metabolic, weight or cardiac side effects. Little/no effect on QTc Can cause insomnia + severe akathisia Drug interactions common - check BNF Lower doses used in adjunctive therapy *May feel restless – tell doctor* *Weight gain and sexual dysfunction unlikely*
Clozapine	Tablets Unlicensed liquid (£)	12.5 mg	Dosing schedule needed – ask pharmacist	900 mg	See Ch.37
Olanzapine	Tablets ODT IM (p444) Depot (£; Table 3)	Usually 5–10 mg od; may be 15 mg for mania	Rate of increase tempered by sedation, often 5 mg increments	20 mg	Monitor closely for hyperglycaemia. *Drowsiness, weight gain and raised blood sugar levels. Diet and exercise important.*
Quetiapine	Tablets (Immediate Release = IR) XL tablets Liquid (£)	IR Day 1: psychosis 50 mg; mania 100 mg XL tablets: start 300 mg od (psychosis /mania)	IR: Day 2 – 50 mg bd Day 3: 100 mg bd Day 4: 150 mg bd Then titrate up daily as needed XL: day 2: 600 mg For depression, see BNF	Psychosis 750 mg; mania 800 mg	Check TFTs Postural drop with initial doses (especially IR) *May feel dizzy initially - get up slowly*
Risperidone	Tablets ODT Liquid Depot (£; Table 3)	1 mg bd or 2 mg nocte	Increase from next day to 3 or 4 mg, if needed	16 mg, but no efficacy >10mg (usual dose 2–6 mg)	EPSE + ↑PRL – advice as for haloperidol & sulpiride *May feel dizzy initially - get up slowly.*

- Doses for psychosis, unless otherwise stated
- Rule of thumb for costs: liquids >orodispersible tablets (ODT) >modified release (MR/"XL") >regular tablets
- £ = Products costing >£200/month for maximum dose, at time of going to press

Table B.3 Common depot antipsychotics – key information.

Name (Trade name)	Dosing				Notes, including time to reach steady state (SS)
	Efficacy/ tolerability test	Next dose	Frequency	Max	
FGAs					
Flupentixol decanoate (Depixol)	Test dose 20 mg	≥7 days later, give 20–50 mg. Increase in 20–50 mg increments.	2–4 weeks	400 mg/week	Buttock/lateral thigh SS ~9 weeks Mild alerting effect
Fluphenazine decanoate (Modecate)	Test dose 12.5 mg	4–7 days later, give 12.5–100 mg	2–5 weeks	50 mg/week (single injection ≤100 mg)	Gluteal SS ~8 weeks
Haloperidol decanoate (Haldol)	Test dose 25 mg	≥7 days later. Increase in 50 mg increments	2–4 weekly	300 mg/month	Gluteal SS ~14 weeks High rate EPSEs ECG essential
Zuclopenthixol decanoate (Clopixol)	Test dose 100 mg	≥7 days later give 200–500 mg.	1–4 weeks	600 mg/week	Buttock/lateral thigh SS ~12 weeks More sedating Don't confuse with zuclopenthixol acetate (Acuphase; p447)
SGAs					
Aripiprazole (£) (Abilify Maintena)	Tablets, e.g. 10–20 mg for a fortnight	400 mg	4-weekly	400 mg /month	Continue oral aripiprazole for 2 weeks after depot started Gluteal SS 10–12 weeks Lower depot doses may be needed if 400 mg not tolerated

Olanzapine pamoate (£) (*ZypAdhera*)	Tablet, i.e. optimise olanzapine oral dose	Dose depends on effective PO dose (see BNF)	2–4 weeks	300 mg/ fortnight	Gluteal SS ~12 weeks Use limited, as must observe for 3 h after each injection
Paliperidone (£) (*Xeplion*)	Check past response to paliperidone or risperidone Then: loading dose 150 mg deltoid	100 mg on day 8	4-weekly	150 mg/month (doses: 50, 75, 100 or 150 mg)	If switching from another depot, loading dose unnecessary. Gluteal or *deltoid* (less embarrassing) SS ~20 weeks Complicated to restart if doses missed
Risperidone Long Acting Injection (LAI) (£) (*Risperdal consta*)	Check past response to risperidone No test dose needed	Usual starting dose 25 mg (higher if >2 mg PO daily)	2-weekly	50 mg/fortnight	Continue risperidone PO for at least 3 weeks after initial dose Gluteal or *deltoid* SS ~8 weeks

- Use smaller test doses in elderly or physically frail.
- All depots are expensive; £ = products costing > £200/month, at time of going to press
- The bigger the volume, the more it hurts; 3 ml volume usually maximum in a single injection
- Common trade names included, as often used by patients
- Test dose not required if previously treated with the depot, without problem

Table B.4 Selective Serotonin Reuptake Inhibitors (SSRIs) – key information.

Drug Preparations	Dose (mg)			Licensed uses							Notes
	Start (minimum effective)	Increases as needed (3–4 weeks)	Maximum	Depression	OCD	PTSD	Agoraphobia/panic	GAD	Social phobia	Bulimia nervosa	
Citalopram Tablets Liquid	20	10	40	✓			✓				QTc prolongation - consider ECG monitoring, especially at higher doses; avoid combining with other QTc prolonging drugs Liquid dose is different – see BNF!
Escitalopram Tablets Liquid	10	10	20	✓	✓		✓	✓	✓		See citalopram (except liquid dose *is* equivalent to tablet dose!)
Fluoxetine Capsules Liquid	20	20	60	✓	✓					✓	Long half-life – *can* often stop without discontinuation symptoms (reduce higher doses to 20 mg over 2 weeks, then stop)
Fluvoxamine Tablets	50	50–100	300	✓	✓						BD dosing over 150 mg Nausea more common Most likely to interact with other drugs
Paroxetine Tablets Liquid	20	20	50	✓	✓	✓	✓	✓	✓		Short half life – *can't* miss/delay dose More anticholinergic and sexual side effects Max dose in OCD = 60 mg
Sertraline Tablets	50	50	200	✓	✓	✓	✓			✓	Fewer significant drug-drug interactions than other SSRIs

- See p60 for side effects
- Prescribe mane unless the patient experiences drowsiness as a side effect
- If sensitive to side effects, start at half the usual dose and increase more slowly
- See BNF for elderly doses (often lower) *or* non-depression usage (often higher)
- Liquid preparations are more expensive than tablets
- For advice on changing between antidepressants, see Maudsley Prescribing Guidelines – Swapping and Stopping table.

Table B.5 Non-SSRI antidepressants – key information.

Group	Dosing			Other information
Examples	Start	Increases	Max	What patients must know
Tricyclic antidepressants (TCAs) Clomipramine Doxepin Imipramine Lofepramine Nortriptyline Trimipramine (Amitriptyline, Dosulepin)	Nocte See BNF	See BNF	See BNF	For: depression clomipramine used in OCD Liquids and tablets available Very toxic in overdose (amitriptyline and dosulepin no longer recommended for depress on due to OD risk) Caution in CVD and many physical conditions Tolerance to side effects may develop Anticholinergic side effects: • Dry mouth • Constipation • Urine retention • Blurred vision • Tremor • Postural hypotension • Tachycardia/arrhythmia • Confusion Sedation Weight gain Sexual dysfunction Overdose can kill!
Noradrenergic and specific serotonergic antidepressants (NASSAs) Mirtazapine	15–30 mg nocte	2–4 weeks, 15 mg increments	45 mg	For: depression Tablets, ODT, liquid (special order) Relatively safe where physical comorbidity (some caution in liver/renal disease) Don't combine with other weight-gaining medications, e.g. olanzapine Few sexual side effects/nausea Sedation (often wears off at higher doses) Increased appetite

(continued overleaf)

Table B.5 (*continued*)

| Group / Examples | Dosing | | | Other information |
	Start	Increases	Max	*What patients must know*
Serotonin and Noradrenaline Reuptake Inhibitors (SNRIs)				*Side effects similar to SSRIs, especially GI (constipation, dry mouth, nausea), sedation/insomnia.* *Added risk of hypertension*
Venlafaxine	37.5 mg bd or 75 mg MR	≥2 weeks, 75 mg increments	375 mg	For: depression GAD, social anxiety disorder Caution in CVD Monitor BP if CVD or higher doses GAD/social phobia, start at 75mg, max 225mg *Don't delay doses if non-MR (discontinuation symptoms)*
Duloxetine	60 mg	–	60 mg	For: depression, GAD; neuropathic pain and incontinence (see BNF) Mane if insomnia, nocte if sedation side effects GAD - start at 30mg; max 120mg
Serotonin Antagonist and Reuptake Inhibitors (SARIs) Trazodone	150 mg nocte (or divided doses) after food	≥2 weeks	300 mg daily (600 mg if inpatient)	For: depression, anxiety Tablets, capsules, liquid *Side effects:* • *Sedation* • *Dizziness/postural hypotension* • *Nausea/vomiting* • *Tachycardia* • *Headache* • *Tremor* • *Priapism - attend ED!* Anxiety dose is 75mg, max 300mg
Melatonergic Agomelatine	25 mg nocte	≥2 weeks	50 mg	For: depression Tablets Check LFTs baseline, then at 3, 6, 12 and 24 weeks Stop agomelatine if AST or ALT >3x normal range No tapering needed on stopping *Common side effects:* • *Drowsiness* • *Nausea* • *Dizziness* • *Headaches* *Rarely: liver problems*

| Monoamine Oxidase Inhibitors (MAOIs)
Phenelzine
Isocarboxazid
Tranylcypramine
Moclobemide | See BNF | See BNF | See BNF | See BNF | For: depression
Pressor effect can cause hypertensive crisis if MAOIs combined with certain foods and other medications
Moclobemide is a reversible MAOI, less likely to cause pressor effect (tyramine advice still applies); also licenced for social phobia.
Dangerous hypertension if eat high tyramine foods.
• *Need list of foods to avoid (including alcohol, processed foods, yeast extracts and gravies)*
• *Don't take OTC medicines without checking OK with pharmacist (e.g. decongestants)*
• *Report severe, throbbing headache immediately* |

- Advise all patients not to stop medication suddenly, as risk of discontinuation syndrome (p60)
- If sensitive to side effects, start at half the usual dose and increase more slowly
- See BNF for elderly doses (often lower) or non-depression usage (often higher)
- Rule of thumb for costs: liquids >orodispersible tablets (ODT) >modified release (MR/'XL') >regular tablets
- For advice on changing between antidepressants, see Maudsley Prescribing Guidelines – Stopping and Swapping Table

Table B.6 Mood Stabilisers – key information.

Drug	Preparations and dosing	Other information *What patients must know*
Lithium	Two formulations • Carbonate = tablets/MR • Citrate = liquid	*Patient information – p61, p418.* *Offer a lithium treatment pack - contains an information leaflet, lithium alert card to carry constantly, and record book.* • Available through pharmacy • Explains side effects, how to avoid/spot toxicity (Ch.69)
	Be careful! These are not equivalent and bioavailability varies widely between different brands. See BNF for dosing, and always prescribe formulation *and* brand. Start at 400 mg daily *carbonate equivalent*, increase by 200–400 mg, according to levels.	Check trough levels (12h post dose) 5–7 days after starting, and 5–7 days after each dose increase until steady state: • Usual aim 0.4–1.0 mmol/L • 0.4 mmol/L may work in unipolar depression • 0.6–1.0 mmol/L for BPAD • >1.5 mmol/L = toxicity (Ch.69) • >2.0 mmol/L = emergency When monitoring levels on wards, ensure the patient has their blood test *before* their morning dose (mark on drug chart and tell nurses). Monitoring: • Pregnancy test before starting in women • Baseline then 6-monthly: eGFR, U&E, TFTs, BMI • ECG (if CV risk factors/PMHx) • Lithium levels 3-monthly • Check calcium in long-term treatment Discontinue slowly to avoid relapse • Decrease over 1–3 months • Try to lower lithium levels less than 0.2 mmol/L at a time
Valproate	Suggested starting doses: • Semi-sodium valproate 750 mg daily in 2–3 divided doses • Sodium valproate MR, 500–600 mg od • Sodium valproate GR 300 mg bd Increase every 3 days (faster if tolerated), in 200–250 mg increments. NB: Can initiate all preparations at 20 mg/kg for rapid effect.	*Patient information – p61* Monitoring: • Pregnancy test before starting in women • Baseline and 6-monthly FBC, LFT, BMI • If LFTs abnormal, do albumin and clotting • Valproate levels if suspect non-concordance/toxicity/other drugs lowering valproate levels (>50 mg/L is effective) Avoid in women of child-bearing age; if unavoidable, use reliable contraception and take prophylactic folate Valproate can give a false positive for ketones on urine dip
Carbamazepine	Tablets (plain, chewable or MR) Liquid • Start 100–200 mg bd • Increase in 100–200 mg increments fortnightly • Dose guided by response + levels • Usually 400–600 mg daily • Max 1.6 g • Always bd dosing	*Patients should know:* • Immediately report rash, fever, mouth ulcers, bleeding or easy bruising • Common side effects: minor rash, nausea, dizziness, sedation, double vision, ataxia, dry mouth, swollen ankles, low sodium • Rare side effects: very low WCC, liver disease or dangerous allergic rash.

(continued overleaf)

Table B.6 (*continued*)

Drug	Preparations and dosing	Other information *What patients must know*
		CBZ induces liver enzymes and interacts with many medications (check BNF before prescribing).

Uses:
- Sometimes used if no response to lithium in mania
- Less effective than lithium for BPAD prophylaxis
- Some use in depression

Monitoring
- Pregnancy test before starting in women
- Baseline and 6-monthly FBC, U&E, LFT, weight
- CBZ levels
  - Aim for 7–12 mg/L and symptoms controlled
  - Take trough levels (before morning dose)
  - Check two weeks after increase (induces own metabolism, so levels can drop)
  - 6-monthly once stable

Other:
- LFTs (+GGT) commonly rise (don't worry if less than 3x normal)
- Chronic low WCC common
- Watch for agranulocytosis/aplastic anaemia (1 in 20,000)
- Rarely: multiorgan hypersensitivity reaction ($\downarrow$WCC, $\uparrow$LFTs, skin reactions). Stop CBZ immediately and never rechallenge *or* use TCAs
- $\uparrow$Risk Stevens-Johnson syndrome in people of Han-Chinese/Thai descent (*must* ensure HLA-B*1502 allele negative if prescribing)

Drug	Preparations and dosing	Other information
Lamotrigine	Tablets ODT • Start 25 mg od for 2 weeks (or alternate days if on valproate) • Increase by 25 mg, fortnightly (slower if on valproate) • Max 200 mg bd (if on valproate, max 100 mg bd)	*Patients must know:* • Report rash, fever or easy bruising immediately Some use in bipolar depression prophylaxis Risk of hypersensitivity reaction increased by fast titration, especially if using valproate Stop immediately if rash occurs, unless clearly unrelated Monitoring: • Pregnancy test before starting in women • Nil else

Table B.7 Sedatives – key information.

Drug	Preparations	Dosing (mg)		Notes
		Start	**Max daily**	
Clonazepam	Tablets / liquid	0.5–2	8	Used off-label for sedation in some units
Diazepam	Tablets / IV / PR	2.5–5	30	Sedation
				Alcohol detoxification/seizures (>BNF doses may be needed)
				IV rarely used in psychiatric units, for RT
Lorazepam	Tablets / IM	0.5–1	4	IM commonly used in RT (p442)
				Higher doses used in catatonia (Ch.68)
Oxazepam	Tablets	15–30	120	Useful if hepatic impairment
Promethazine	Tablets / liquid / IM	25–50	100	Used off label for sedation/insomnia
				RT in some units (p444)
Zopiclone	Tablets	3.75	7.5	Give sleep hygiene advice
				Other 'Z-hypnotics' are zolpidem and zaleplon (see BNF)

• NB: all should be short-term (2–4 weeks) as risk dependency

Alcohol and drugs

Table C.1 Quick guide to alcohol units (*Cheryl Kipping*).

Drink	% ABV	Amount	Units
Beers (lager, bitter)			
Regular lager	4%	440 ml can	1.8
E.g. Carlsberg, Carling, Foster's		1 pint	2.3
Premium lager	5%	275 ml bottle	1.4
E.g. Budweiser, Kronenbourg, Stella, Grolsch, Peroni, Becks		330 ml bottle	1.7
		440 ml can	2.2
		1 pint	2.9
Super Strength Lager	9%	500 ml can	4.5
E.g. Skol Super, Tennent's Super, Special Brew, Kestrel			
Bitter	3.8%	440 ml can	1.7
E.g. Tetley, John Smith's		1 pint	2.2
Guinness	4.2%	440 ml can	1.8
		1 pint	2.4
Ciders			
Regular	4.5%	440 ml can	2
E.g. Magner's, Bulmer's		1 pint/568 ml bottle	2.6
Strongbow	5.3%	440 ml can	2.3
		2 litre bottle	10.6
Scrumpy Jack	6%	500 ml	3
Strong	7.5%	275 ml bottle	2
E.g. Diamond White, White Star		500 ml can	3.8
Wine commonly 12–13.5%			
Small glass	12%	175 ml	2.1
Large glass		250 ml	3
Bottle		750 ml	9
Spirits usually 37.5–40% ABV			
Gin, vodka, whisky, brandy	37.5%	25 ml (single) measure	1
		75 cl bottle	28–30
Other			
Alcopops	4%	275 ml bottle	1.1
E.g. Bacardi Breezer, WKD, Smirnoff Ice			

The % ABV for other drinks is: Martini 15%, Baileys 17%, Sherry 17.5%, Tia Maria 20%, Port 20%

- This is a rough, practical guide to the number of units of alcohol in common drinks (units rounded to the nearest 0.1u)
- Strength varies between brands - always check % (Alcohol By Volume; ABV)
- To more accurately calculate units $= \dfrac{\text{volume (litres)} \times \text{ABV (\%)}}{1000}$

Psychiatry: Breaking the ICE – Introductions, Common Tasks and Emergencies for Trainees, First Edition.
Edited by Sarah Stringer, Juliet Hurn and Anna M Burnside.
© 2016 John Wiley & Sons, Ltd. Published 2016 by John Wiley & Sons, Ltd.
Companion Website: www.psychiatryice.com

Table C.2 Alcohol Use Disorders Identification Test (AUDIT) questionnaire.

1. How often do you have a drink containing alcohol? (0) Never [Skip to Qs 9–10] ☐ (1) Monthly or less ☐ (2) 2 to 4 times a month ☐ (3) 2 to 3 times a week ☐ (4) 4 or more times a week ☐	**6. How often during the last year have you needed a first drink in the morning to get yourself going after a heavy drinking session?** (0) Never ☐ (1) Less than monthly ☐ (2) Monthly ☐ (3) Weekly ☐ (4) Daily or almost daily ☐
2. How many drinks containing alcohol do you have on a typical day when you are drinking? (0) 1 or 2 ☐ (1) 3 or 4 ☐ (2) 5 or 6 ☐ (3) 7, 8, or 9 ☐ (4) 10 or more ☐	**7. How often during the last year have you had a feeling of guilt or remorse after drinking?** (0) Never ☐ (1) Less than monthly ☐ (2) Monthly ☐ (3) Weekly ☐ (4) Daily or almost daily ☐
3. How often do you have six or more drinks on one occasion? (0) Never ☐ (1) Less than monthly ☐ (2) Monthly ☐ (3) Weekly ☐ (4) Daily or almost daily ☐ *Skip to Questions 9 and 10 if Total Score for Questions 2 and 3 = 0*	**8. How often during the last year have you been unable to remember what happened the night before because you had been drinking?** (0) Never ☐ (1) Less than monthly ☐ (2) Monthly ☐ (3) Weekly ☐ (4) Daily or almost daily ☐
4. How often during the last year have you found that you were not able to stop drinking once you had started? (0) Never ☐ (1) Less than monthly ☐ (2) Monthly ☐ (3) Weekly ☐ (4) Daily or almost daily ☐	**9. Have you or someone else been injured as a result of your drinking?** (0) No ☐ (2) Yes, but not in the last year ☐ (4) Yes, during the last year ☐
5. How often during the last year have you failed to do what was normally expected from you because of drinking? (0) Never ☐ (1) Less than monthly ☐ (2) Monthly ☐ (3) Weekly ☐ (4) Daily or almost daily ☐	**10. Has a relative or friend or a doctor or another health worker been concerned about your drinking or suggested you cut down?** (0) No ☐ (2) Yes, but not in the last year ☐ (4) Yes, during the last year ☐
Total score:	

Table C.2 Alcohol Use Disorders Identification Test (AUDIT) questionnaire. (*continued*)

Audit Score Guidance		
AUDIT score	**Drinking category***	**Intervention**
0–7	Lower risk	No specific intervention.
		Consider offering information and promote continued drinking within 'safe' levels.
		If working towards abstinence, encourage continued reduction.
8–15	Increasing risk (hazardous use)	Above recommended levels
		Simple brief advice: provide information.
		Encourage to reduce
16–19	Higher risk (harmful use) e.g. women 35+u or men 50+u/week	Extended brief intervention.
		Offer sessions to help reduce drinking and risk-taking behaviour.
		Focus on enhancing motivation to change.
20–40	Possible dependence (very likely with higher scores)	Community - complete SADQ (Severity of Alcohol Dependence Questionnaire, p508)
		Inpatient – monitor using CIWA-Ar (withdrawal assessment scale, p509).
		Consider specialist advice and referral to alcohol service if person wants to stop drinking.

*Thresholds are lower for some groups (e.g. elderly, some BME, SMI) - consider the *next* level up if concerned.

- *Read questions as written. Record answers carefully. Begin the AUDIT by saying, "Now I am going to ask you some questions about your use of alcoholic beverages during this past year."*
- *Explain what is meant by 'alcoholic beverages' by using local examples of beer, wine, vodka, etc. Code answers in terms of 'standard drinks'. Place the correct answer in the box at the right.*

Source: Babor, T.F., Higgins-Biddle, J.C., Saunders, J.B. and Moterio, M.G. (2001). The Alcohol Use Disorders Identification Test: Guidelines for use in primary care (2nd edition). World Health Organisation. Reproduced with permission of the World Health Organisation.

Table C.3 Severity of Alcohol Dependence Questionnaire (SADQ).

SADQ
Please recall a recent month when you were drinking in a way that was typical of a heavy drinking period for you. Please fill in the month and year:

Month....   **Year.....**

We want to know more about your drinking during this time and how often you experienced certain feelings. Please put a tick to show how frequently each of the following statements applied to you during this typical period of drinking.

Question	Score			
	Almost never 0	Sometimes 1	Often 2	Nearly always 3
The day after drinking alcohol ...				
1. I woke up feeling sweaty				
2. My hands shook first thing in the morning				
3. My whole body shook violently first thing in the morning				
4. I woke up absolutely drenched in sweat				
5. I dreaded waking up in the morning				
6. I was frightened of meeting people first thing in the morning				
7. I felt on the edge of despair when I woke up				
8. I felt very frightened when I woke up				
9. I liked to have an alcoholic drink in the morning				
10. I always gulped down my first few morning drink(s) as quickly as possible				
11. I drank in the morning to get rid of shakes				
12. I had a very strong craving for a drink when I awoke				
13. I drank more than 1/4 bottle of spirits or 4 pints of beer or 1 bottle of wine a day				
14. I drank more than 1/2 bottle of spirits or 8 pints of beer or 2 bottles of wine a day				
15. I drank more than 1 bottle of spirits or 15 pints of beer or 4 bottles of wine a day				
16. I drank more than 2 bottles of spirits or 15 pints of beer or 8 bottles of wine a day				
Imagine the following situation: you have been completely off drink for a few weeks and then you drink heavily for two days. *How would you feel the morning after those drinking days?* *(If person has not been abstinent for a period of 2 weeks, score 3 for remaining items).*				
17. I would start to sweat				
18. My hands would shake				
19. My body would shake				
20. I would be craving a drink				

Total score	
≤15	**Mild dependence**
16–30	**Moderate dependence**
31+	**Severe dependence**

Source: Adapted from Stockwell, T., Murphy, D. & Hodgson, R. (1983). The severity of alcohol dependence questionnaire: Its use, reliability and validity. *British Journal of Addiction, 78(2)*, 45–156. Free to reproduce.

Table C.4 Clinical Institute Withdrawal Assessment of Alcohol Scale, Revised (CIWA-Ar).

Patient	
Date	**Time**
Heart rate	**BP**
Nausea & vomiting	**Tactile disturbances**

Nausea & vomiting
Do you feel sick to your stomach?
Have you vomited?
Observation
 	
0   No nausea or vomiting
1   Mild nausea, no vomiting
2
3
4   Intermittent nausea + dry heaves
5
6
7   Constant nausea, frequent dry heaves + vomiting
	Tactile disturbances
	Have you any itching, pins and needles sensations, any
	burning, any numbness, or do you feel bugs crawling on or
	under your skin?
	Observation
	
	0 None
	1 Very mild itching, pins and needles, burning or
	     numbness
	2 Mild itching, pins and needles, burning or numbness
	3 Moderate itching, pins and needles, burning or
	     numbness
	4 Moderately severe hallucinations
	5 Severe hallucinations
	6 Extremely severe hallucinations
	7 Continuous hallucinations

Tremor Arms extended and fingers spread apart. Observation 0 No tremor 1 Not visible, but can be felt fingertip to fingertip 2 3 4 Moderate, with patient's arms extended 5 6 7 Severe, even with arms not extended	**Auditory disturbances** *Are you more aware of sounds around you? Are they* *harsh? Do they frighten you? Are you hearing anything that* *is disturbing to you? Are you hearing frightening things you* *know are not there?* Observation 0 Not present 1 Very mild harshness or ability to frighten 2 Mild harshness or ability to frighten 3 Moderate harshness or ability to frighten 4 Moderately severe hallucinations 5 Severe hallucinations 6 Extremely severe hallucinations 7 Continuous hallucinations
Paroxysmal sweats Observation 0 No sweat visible 1 Barely perceptible sweating, palms moist 2 3 4 Beads of sweat obvious on forehead 5 6 7 Drenching sweats	**Visual disturbances** *Does the light appear to be too bright? Is its colour* *different? Does it hurt your eyes? Are you seeing anything* *that is disturbing to you? Are you seeing things you know* *are not there?* Observation 0 Not present 1 Very mild sensitivity 2 Mild sensitivity 3 Moderate sensitivity 4 Moderately severe hallucinations 5 Severe hallucinations 6 Extremely severe hallucinations 7 Continuous hallucinations

Table C.4 Clinical Institute Withdrawal Assessment of Alcohol Scale, Revised (CIWA-Ar). (*continued*)

Anxiety	Headache, fullness in head
Do you feel nervous? Observation 0 No anxiety, at ease 1 Mildly anxious 2 3 4 Moderately anxious, or guarded, so anxiety is inferred 5 6 7 Acute panic	Ask, *Does your head feel different? Does it feel like there is a band around your head?* Do not rate for dizziness or light-headedness. Otherwise, rate severity. 0 Not present 1 Very mild 2 Mild 3 Moderate 4 Moderately severe 5 Severe 6 Very severe 7 Extremely severe
Agitation	**Orientation and clouding of sensorium**
Observation 0 Normal activity 1 Somewhat more than normal activity 2 3 4 Moderately fidgety and restless 5 6 7 Paces back and forth during most of the interview, or constantly thrashes about	*What day is this? Where are you? Who am I?* 0 Oriented and can do serial additions 1 Cannot do serial additions or is uncertain about date 2 Disoriented for date by no more than 2 calendar days 3 Disoriented for date by more than 2 calendar days 4 Disoriented for place/or person
Total CIWA-Ar score: Maximum possible score 67	**Rater's initials:**
Scores: ≤ 10 – mild withdrawal (does not need additional medication) ≤ 15 – moderate withdrawal > 15 – severe withdrawal	

Source: Sullivan, J.T., Sykora, K., Schneiderman, J., Naranjo, C.A., & Sellers, E.M. (1989) Assessment of alcohol withdrawal: The revised Clinical Institute Withdrawal Assessment of Alcohol scale (CIWA-Ar). *British Journal of Addiction*, 84: 1353–1357. Free to reproduce.

Table C.5 Clinical Opiate Withdrawal Scale (COWS).

Patient name:	Time of observation/Score			
Resting pulse rate: *record beats per minute after patient is sitting or lying for 1 minute* 0 = ≤80 1 = 81–100 2 = 101–120 4 = >120				
Sweating: *over past 1/2 hour, not accounted for by room temperature/patient activity* 0 = no report of chills or flushing 1 = subjective report of chills or flushing 2 = flushed or observable moistness on face 3 = beads of sweat on brow or face 4 = sweat streaming off face				
Restlessness: *observation during assessment* 0 = able to sit still 1 = reports difficulty sitting still, but is able to do so 3 = frequent shifting or extraneous movement of legs/arms 4 = unable to sit still for more than a few seconds				
Pupil size 0 = pupils pinned or normal size for room light 1 = pupils possibly larger than normal for room light 2 = pupils moderately dilated 5 = pupils so dilated that only the rim of the iris is visible				
Bone or joint aches: *If patient was having pain previously, only the additional component attributed to opiate withdrawal is scored.* 0 = not present 1 = mild diffuse discomfort 2 = patient reports severe diffuse aching of joints/muscles 4 = patient is rubbing joints or muscles and is unable to sit still because of discomfort				
Runny nose or tearing: *Not accounted for by cold symptoms or allergies* 0 = not present 1 = nasal stuffiness or unusually moist eyes 2 = nose running or tearing 4 = nose constantly running or tears streaming down cheeks				
GI upset: *over last 1/2 hour* 0 = no GI symptoms 1 = stomach cramps 2 = nausea or loose stool 3 = vomiting or diarrhoea 5 = multiple episodes of diarrhoea or vomiting				

(continued overleaf)

Table C.5 (*continued*)

Patient name:	Time of observation/Score			
Tremor: *observation of outstretched hands* 0 = no tremor 1 = tremor can be felt, but not observed 2 = slight tremor observable 4 = gross tremor or muscle twitching				
Yawning: *observation during assessment* 0 = no yawning 1 = yawning once or twice during assessment 2 = yawning three or more times during assessment 4 = yawning several times/minute				
Anxiety or Irritability 0 = none 1 = patient reports increasing irritability or anxiousness 2 = patient obviously irritable/anxious 4 = patient so irritable or anxious that participation in the assessment is difficult				
Gooseflesh skin 0 = skin is smooth 3 = piloerection of skin can be felt or hairs standing up on arms 5 = prominent piloerection				
TOTAL SCORE				
Observer's initials				

Total score	Withdrawal level
5–12	Mild
13–24	Moderate
25–36	Moderately severe
> 36	Severe

- *For each item, write in the number that best describes the patient's signs or symptom*
- *Rate on just the apparent relationship to opiate withdrawal. For example, if heart rate is increased because the patient was jogging just prior to assessment, the increase pulse rate would not add to the score.*

Source: Wesson, D.R. & Ling, W (2003). The clinical opiate withdrawal scale (COWS) Journal of Psychoactive Drugs, 35, 253–259. Free to reproduce.

Table C.6 Common illicit drugs summary.

Drug Examples	Intoxication	Withdrawal	Notes
Cannabis *(weed, skunk, hash, ganja)*	Relaxation, sedation Euphoria, giggling Anxiety, paranoia Perceptual/time distortion Nausea/vomiting Hunger ("the munchies") Dry mouth, bloodshot eyes ↓ Attention, short-term memory ↓ Reactions, coordination ↓ BP ↑ HR	Irritability, anxiety Restlessness Insomnia/vivid dreams (can last three weeks) Shaky, sweaty; cold chills ↓ Appetite Stomach pains	Can trigger psychosis. Usually smoked, sometimes eaten/drunk. Skunk is a particularly potent form.
Stimulants Amphetamines *(speed)* Cocaine *(coke)* Crack cocaine Khat	Energy, euphoria, alertness Overactive, agitation Insomnia ↓ Appetite ↑Confidence ↑Impulsivity ↑HR, BP Arrhythmia	'Crash': dysphoria, fatigue	Can trigger psychosis. Khat – leaves, commonly chewed in Somali/Yemeni communities. Poor dentition common.
Benzodiazepines *(downers, jellies)*	Relaxation/sedation Ataxia, slurred speech ↓ RR, HR, BP Respiratory arrest/coma	Anxiety, panic Insomnia Agitation Tremor Headache Nausea/vomiting ↑HR Fits	Deaths from respiratory depression, especially in combination with alcohol/opiates. Often used to cope with withdrawal from other drugs. See p254–255
Ketamine *(K, special K, super K)*	Euphoria, stimulation, anxiety Synaesthesia, dissociation Floating/"spiritual" experiences Psychosis ↑HR, BP, ↓ RR, GCS Dilated pupils Ataxia Nausea/vomiting Dizziness, diplopia Insomnia Confusion Inability to speak/move	Agitation, anxiety Abdominal/bladder pain (lose analgesia)	Chronic use: bladder problems Urinary frequency, haematuria Accidental injury during intoxication (anaesthetic and psychotic effects)
Ecstasy *(MDMA, E)*	Stimulant effects Empathy, talkativeness Overactivity Teeth-grinding Nausea/vomiting Sweating ↑Temperature Dehydration	*No clear withdrawal syndrome*	Deaths related to dehydration, hyperthermia *and/or* excessive fluid intake

Table C.6 (*continued*)

Drug Examples	Intoxication	Withdrawal	Notes
Hallucinogens E.g. lysergic acid diethylamide (LSD; *acid*), magic mushrooms	Synaesthesia Depersonalisation/derealisation Illusions, hallucinations Anxiety	*No clear withdrawal syndrome*	
Solvents E.g. aerosols *(glue, gas)*	Euphoria Ataxia, dizziness Disinhibition Confusion Hallucinations Nausea/vomiting Coma	Headaches Fits	Often inhaled by teenagers, e.g. from a plastic bag/clothing Deaths usually from asphyxiation of vomit

- For opiates, see Ch.41
- For GBL/GHB, see p464

APPENDIX D

Cognitive testing

Appendix D.1 The Montreal Cognitive Assessment (MOCA)

MONTREAL COGNITIVE ASSESSMENT (MOCA)
Version 7.1 Original Version

NAME:
Education: Date of birth:
Sex: DATE:

VISUOSPATIAL / EXECUTIVE			POINTS
Trail making test	Copy cube [ ]	Draw CLOCK (Ten past eleven) (3 points) [ ] Contour [ ] Numbers [ ] Hands	__/5

NAMING

[ ] [ ] [ ] __/3

MEMORY Read list of words, subject must repeat them. Do 2 trials, even if 1st trial is successful. Do a recall after 5 minutes.		FACE	VELVET	CHURCH	DAISY	RED	
	1st trial						No points
	2nd trial						

ATTENTION Read list of digits (1 digit/ sec.).	Subject has to repeat them in the forward order [ ] 2 1 8 5 4	__/2
	Subject has to repeat them in the backward order [ ] 7 4 2	

Read list of letters. The subject must tap with his hand at each letter A. No points if ≥ 2 errors
[ ] FBACMNAAJKLBAFAKDEAAAJAMOFAAB __/1

Serial 7 subtraction starting at 100 [ ] 93 [ ] 86 [ ] 79 [ ] 72 [ ] 65 __/3
4 or 5 correct subtractions: **3 pts**, 2 or 3 correct: **2 pts**, 1 correct: **1 pt**, 0 correct: **0 pt**

LANGUAGE	Repeat : I only know that John is the one to help today. [ ] The cat always hid under the couch when dogs were in the room. [ ]	__/2
	Fluency / Name maximum number of words in one minute that begin with the letter F [ ] _____ (N ≥ 11 words)	__/1

ABSTRACTION Similarity between e.g. banana - orange = fruit [ ] train – bicycle [ ] watch - ruler __/2

DELAYED RECALL	Has to recall words	FACE	VELVET	CHURCH	DAISY	RED	Points for UNCUED recall only	__/5
	WITH NO CUE	[ ]	[ ]	[ ]	[ ]	[ ]		
Optional	Category cue							
	Multiple choice cue							

ORIENTATION [ ] Date [ ] Month [ ] Year [ ] Day [ ] Place [ ] City __/6

© Z.Nasreddine MD **www.mocatest.org** Normal ≥ 26 / 30 | TOTAL __/30 |
Administered by: _____ | Add 1 point if ≤ 12 yr edu |

Copyright Z. Nasreddine MD. Reproduced with permission. Copies are available at www.mocatest.org

Psychiatry: Breaking the ICE – Introductions, Common Tasks and Emergencies for Trainees, First Edition.
Edited by Sarah Stringer, Juliet Hurn and Anna M Burnside.
© 2016 John Wiley & Sons, Ltd. Published 2016 by John Wiley & Sons, Ltd.
Companion Website: www.psychiatryice.com

Appendix D.2 The Addenbrooke's Cognitive Examination-III (ACE-III)

UK ACE-III Administration and Scoring Guide – 2012

The Addenbrooke's Cognitive Examination-III (ACE-III) is a brief cognitive test that assesses five cognitive domains: attention, memory, verbal fluency, language and visuospatial abilities. The ACE-III replaces the previous Addenbrooke's Cognitive Examination-Revised and was developed at Neuroscience Research Australia (NeuRA; www.neura.edu.au). The total score is 100 with higher scores indicating better cognitive functioning. Administration of the ACE-III takes, on average, 15 minutes and scoring takes about 5 minutes.

These instructions have been designed in order to make the questions and their scoring clear for the tester. Please read them carefully before giving the test. If possible, leave the scoring until the end of the session, since the participant will not be able to check whether the tester is ticking for correct answers or crossing for wrong ones. This might avoid anxiety, which can disturb the participant's performance on the test.

To download the ACE-III, as well as updates on publications and language translations, please go to the following website: http://www.neura.edu.au/frontier/research

ATTENTION – Orientation – score 0 to 10

Administration: Ask the participant for the day, date, month, year, season as well as the name of the hospital (or building, or number if an address), floor (or room, or street if an address), town, county and country.
Scoring: Score 1 point for each correct answer. A mistake of ± 2 days is allowed for the date (e.g., 5th when the actual date is the 7th). If the participant says "23rd of the 3rd", then prompt for the name of the month. If the participant is at home, ask for the name of the place such as the apartment complex/retirement village and, for the floor, you might ask for the name of the room (e.g., kitchen, living room, etc). If at a single storey health setting, you could ask about a local landmark. When the season is changing (e.g., at the end of August) and the participant says, "Autumn" then ask, "could it be another season?" If the answer is "Summer", give 1 point since the two seasons are in transition. Do not give 1 point if the answer is "Winter" or "Spring". If participants come from another county, orientation for suburb can be scored somewhat more liberally.

Seasons: Spring – March, April, May; Summer – June, July, August; Autumn – September, October, November; Winter – December, January, February.

For aphasic patients: Allow patients to write down their answer, if unable to give verbal responses.

ATTENTION – Registration of 3 Items – score 0 to 3

Administration: Ask the participant to repeat and remember the three words. Speak slowly. Repeat the words if necessary but up to a maximum of 3 times only. Tell the participant that you will ask for this information later.
Scoring: Score the first attempt only. Record the number of trials it takes to learn all 3 words.

ATTENTION – Serial 7 Subtraction – score 0 to 5

Administration: Ask the participant to subtract 7 from 100, record the answer, and then ask the participant to keep subtracting 7 from each new number until you ask them to stop. Stop the participant after 5 subtractions.
Scoring: Record responses and do not stop the participant if they make a mistake. Allow them to carry on and check subsequent answers for scoring (e.g., 92, **85**, 79, **72**, **65** – score = 3).

MEMORY – Recall of 3 Items – score 0 to 3

Administration: Ask the participant to recall the words that you asked them to repeat and remember earlier.
Scoring: Record responses and score 1 point for each correct item. Do not prompt the participant for the items.

Appendix D.2 The Addenbrooke's Cognitive Examination-III (ACE-III) (*continued*)

VERBAL FLUENCY – Letter and Category – score 0 to 14

Letters – score 0 to 7

Administration: Tell the participant: *"I'm going to give you a letter of the alphabet and I'd like you to generate as many words as you can beginning with that letter, but not names of people or places. For example, if I give you the letter "C", you could give me words like "cat, cry, clock" and so on. But, you can't give me words like Catherine or Canada. Do you understand? Are you ready? You have one minute. The letter I want you to use is the letter "P".*
Scoring: First, record the total number of words that the participant generates. Then, count the total number of correct words, which do not include: (1) repetitions, (2) perseverations (e.g., pay, paid, pays – score = 1), (3) intrusions (i.e., words beginning with other letters), (4) proper names (i.e., names of people or places) and (5) plurals (e.g., pot, pots – total = 2, correct = 1). Use the table provided on the ACE-III sheet to obtain the final score for this test.

Animals – score 0 to 7

Administration: Tell the participant: *"Now can you name as many animals as possible. It can begin with any letter."*
Scoring: Again, record the total number of animals that the participant generates. Then, count the total number of correct words, which do not include higher order categories when specific exemplars are given (e.g., "fish" followed by "salmon" and "trout" – total = 3; correct = 2). All types of animals are accepted, including insects, humans, prehistoric, extinct as well as mythical creatures (e.g., unicorn). If the participant misunderstands the instructions and perseverates by naming animals beginning with "p" (e.g., panda, possum, platypus etc), then reiterate to the participant that they should name animals beginning with any letter.

MEMORY – Anterograde Memory – Name and Address – score 0 to 7

Administration: Instruct the participant: *"I'm going to give you a name and address and I'd like you to repeat the name and address after me. So you have a chance to learn, we'll be doing that 3 times. I'll ask you the name and address later."* If the participant starts repeating along with you, ask them to wait until you give it in full.
Scoring: Record responses for each trial but only responses in the third trial contributes to the ACE-III score (0-7 points).

MEMORY – Retrograde Memory – Famous People – score 0 to 4

Administration: Ask the participant for the name of the current Prime Minister, the woman who was Prime Minister, the president of the USA and the president of the USA who was assassinated in the 1960s.
Scoring: Score 1 point each. Allow surnames (e.g., "Obama") and ask for a surname if only the first name is given (e.g., "Maggie"). If the full name given is incorrect (e.g., "June Thatcher"), then the score would be 0. If there has been a recent change in leaders, probe for the name of the outgoing politician.

LANGUAGE – Comprehension – score 0 to 3

Administration: Place a pencil and a piece of paper in front of the participant. As a practice trial, ask the participant to *"pick up the pencil and then the paper"*. If this is incorrectly performed, score 0 and do not continue any further. Otherwise, continue onwards with the three other commands listed on the protocol. Before beginning each trial, always place the pencil and piece of paper in front of the participant.
Scoring: A score of 1 is given for each command performed correctly.

Appendix D.2 The Addenbrooke's Cognitive Examination-III (ACE-III) (*continued*)

LANGUAGE – Sentence Writing – score 0 to 2

Administration: Ask the participant to write two sentences and suggest a few topics (e.g., recent holiday, hobbies, family or childhood) if they are unable to come up with anything to write. Importantly, if the participant writes only one sentence, prompt for a second.
Scoring: Sentences must have a subject and a verb. We are looking for spelling and grammar errors. Sentences do not need to be about the same topic; they can be unrelated. If a patient can only write one sentence, despite prompting, then this will be penalized.

Points	Description of Sentence
2	Two sentences with no errors in grammar or spelling. Note that sentences do not need to be centred on the one topic. E.g., "I like to go to the beach. I have three grandchildren."
1	Two sentences with either incorrect grammar or spelling. One sentence with correct grammar and spelling. E.g., "I like to go to the beech. I also like dancing." "I like go beach. I like dance." I like swimming." (The patient does not write another sentence despite prompting)
0	One sentence with incorrect grammar and/or spelling. A few words that is a phrase (e.g., "like dancing"), place (e.g., "Royal Hospital" or a person's name. Unable to write a sentence

LANGUAGE – Single Word Repetition – score 0 to 2

Administration: Ask the participant to repeat each word after you, saying only one word at a time.
Scoring: If the repetition does not sound normal (e.g., halting, laboured, slurred) then it is incorrect. Only the first attempt is scored. Score 2 if all words are correct; 1 if only 3 are correct; 0 if 2 or less are correct.

LANGUAGE – Proverb Repetition – score 0 to 2

Administration: Ask the participant to repeat each proverb.
Scoring: Do not accept partially correct repetitions (e.g., "all that glistens is not gold"). Score 1 point for each proverb.

Note: Following the repetition of each proverb, the examiner may wish to ask the participant "What does this proverb mean?" or "How would you explain this proverb to someone who has not heard it before?" This additional measure can aid the clinician in the qualitative assessment of verbal abstract thinking.

Appendix D.2 The Addenbrooke's Cognitive Examination-III (ACE-III) (*continued*)

LANGUAGE – Object Naming – score 0 to 12

Administration: Ask the participant to name each picture.
Scoring: Correct answers are: spoon; book; penguin; anchor; camel or dromedary; barrel, keg, or tub; crown; crocodile or alligator; harp; rhinoceros or rhino; kangaroo or wallaby; piano accordion, accordion or squeeze box. Score 1 point for each item.

LANGUAGE – Comprehension – score 0 to 4

Administration: Ask the participant to point to the pictures according to the statement read. Do not provide any feedback regarding the word meaning.
Scoring: Score 1 point for each item. Self-corrections are allowed.

LANGUAGE – Reading – score 0 or 1

Administration: Ask the participant to read the words aloud.
Scoring: Score 1 point if all five words are read correctly. Record the mistakes using the phonetic alphabet, if possible.

VISUOSPATIAL ABILITIES – Intersecting Infinity Loops – score 0 or 1

Administration: Ask the participant to copy the intersecting infinity loops.
Scoring: A score of 1 is given if two infinity loops are drawn and overlap. Both infinity loops must come to a point/cross and do not look like circles.

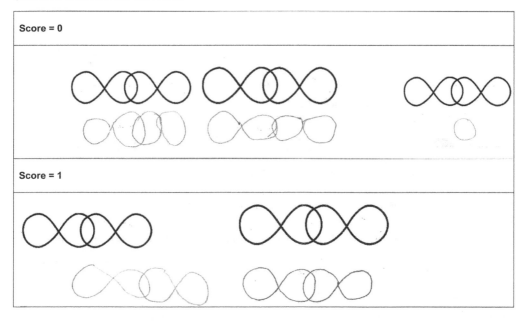

Appendix D.2 The Addenbrooke's Cognitive Examination-III (ACE-III) *(continued)*

VISUOSPATIAL ABILITIES – 3D Wire Cube – score 0 to 2

Administration: Ask the participant to copy the 3-D wire cube.
Scoring: The cube should have 12 lines to score 2 points, even if the proportions are not perfect. A score of 1 is given if the cube has fewer than 12 lines but a general cube shape is maintained.

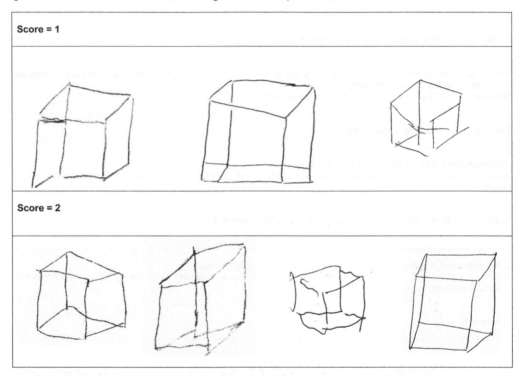

Score = 1

Score = 2

VISUOSPATIAL ABILITIES – Clock – score 0 to 5

Administration: Ask the participant to draw a clock face with numbers on it. When he/she has finished, ask them to put the hands at "ten past five". If the participant does not like their first drawing and would like to do it again, you can allow for that and score the second clock. Participants may correct their mistakes by erasing it while drawing.
Scoring: The following scoring criteria are used below to give a total of 5 points.

Circle	1 point maximum if it is a reasonable circle
Numbers	2 points if all numbers are included within the circle and numbers are evenly distributed. A slight rotation to the overall clock face is acceptable. 1 point if all numbers are included but the numbers are either outside of the circle or the numbers are unevenly spaced 0 points if not all numbers are included
Hands	2 points if both hands are drawn, lengths are correct and placed on correct numbers (you might ask which one is the small and big one) 1 point if both hands are drawn and placed on the correct numbers but lengths are incorrect

Appendix D.2 The Addenbrooke's Cognitive Examination-III (ACE-III) (*continued*)

1 point if both hands are drawn but only one hand is placed on the correct number and drawn with correct length
0 points if two hands are drawn but both lengths incorrect and one number is correct
0 point if two hands are drawn but both lengths and numbers are incorrect
0 point if one hand is drawn

Score 1	Score 2	Score 2
Circle (1); not clear that all numbers are present (0); not clear where the hands are positioned	Circle (1); one hand placed on the correct number and has the correct length (1)	Circle (1); all the numbers but not placed inside the circle (1)

Score 2	Score 3	Score 3
Circle (1); all the numbers but not placed inside the circle (1); two hands with one number correct but lengths are even (0)	Circle (1); all the numbers present and proportionally distributed (a slight rotation of the whole clock face is OK) (2); one hand only (0)	Circle (1); numbers are not inside the circle and there are 2 number 10s (0); hands placed correctly and correct lengths (2)

Score 3	Score 4	Score 4
Circle (1); numbers are unevenly spaced (1); one hand placed correctly and has the correct length (1)	Circle (1); all the numbers but not proportionally distributed (1); both hands placed correctly and has the correct length (2)	Circle (1); numbers are proportionally distributed (2); one hand placed correctly and has the correct length (1)

Appendix D.2 The Addenbrooke's Cognitive Examination-III (ACE-III) (*continued*)

Score 5
Circle (1); numbers proportionally distributed on both halves of the clock face (2); hands placed correctly (2) 

PERCEPTUAL ABILITIES – Counting Dots – score 0 to 4

Administration: Ask the participant for the number of dots in each square. The participant is not allowed to point.
Scoring: Score 1 point for each correct answer. Correct answers: 8, 10, 9 and 7.

PERCEPTUAL ABILITIES – Identifying Letters – score 0 to 4

Administration: Ask the participant to identify the letter in each square. The participant is allowed to point.
Scoring: Score 1 point for each correct answer. Correct answers: K, M, T and A.

For aphasic patients: If the participant is unable to say the number of dots or letter name, allow them to write their answer. For the letter, allow them to say the correct letter sounds (e.g., "mmm").

MEMORY – Recall of Name and Address – score 0 to 7

Administration: Say to the participant: *"Now tell me what you remember of that name and address we were repeating at the beginning"*.
Scoring: Score 1 point for each item recalled, using the score guide provided in the test.

Harry Barnes
73 Orchard Close
Kingsbridge
Devon

Example: 1a

Harry Bond	1 + 0	
78 Orchard Close	0 + 1 + 1	
Kingsbury	0	
....	0	**Score 3/7**

Example: 2a

Harry Barnes	1 + 1	
73 Kingsbridge Close	1 + 0 + 1	
....	0	
Devon	1	**Score 5/7**

Example: 3a

Harry Bond	1 + 0	
33 Kingsbury Way	0 + 0 + 0	
Kingsbridge Close	0 + 0	
Cambridge	0	
Devon	1	**Score 2/7**

Appendix D.2 The Addenbrooke's Cognitive Examination-III (ACE-III) (*continued*)

MEMORY – Recognition of Name and Address – score 0 to 5

Administration: This condition is given to participants if they fail to recall one or more items in the Recall condition. This task is given to allow the participant a chance to recognise items that he/she could not recall. If all of the items in the name and address are correctly recalled, this condition is not needed and the participant automatically scores 5 points. However, many participants will recall only parts of the name and address. First, tick the correctly remembered items on the shaded column (right hand side) and then tell the participant, "*Let me give you some hints. Was it x, y or z?*" and so on.
Scoring: Every item recognised correctly scores 1 point. Add the correctly recalled and recognised item to give a total of 5 points for this condition.

Example 1b (based on example 1a)

Tester ticks "Orchard Close" on the right hand side shadowed column because participant had recalled that item. The tester should then ask: - Was it Jerry Barnes, Harry Barnes or Harry Bradford? - Was it 37, 73 or 76? - Was it Oakhampton, Kingsbridge or Dartington? - Was it Devon, Dorset or Somerset?	Participant's answers: Harry Barnes 76 Kingsbridge Dorset	 1 0 1 0 + 1 (Orchard Close) **Score 3/5**

Example 2b (based on example 2a)

Tester ticks "Harry Barnes", "73" and "Devon" on the right hand side shadowed column because participant had recalled those items. The tester should then ask: - Was it on Orchard Place, Oak Close or Orchard Close? - Was it Oakhampton, Kingsbridge or Dartington?	Participant's answers: Orchard Close Kingsbridge	 1 1 + 3 (Harry Barnes, 73, Devon) **Score 5/5**

Example 3b (based on example 3a)

Tester ticks "Devon", on the right hand side shadowed column because participant had recalled that item. The tester should then ask: - Was it Jerry Barnes, Harry Barnes or Harry Bradford? - Was it 37, 73 or 76? - Was it Orchard Place, Oak Close or Orchard Close? - Was it Oakhampton, Kingsbridge or Dartington?	Participant's answers: Jerry Barnes 37 Orchard Place Oakhampton	 0 0 0 0 +1 (Devon) **Score 1/5**

S C O R E S – Domain and Total Score of the ACE-III

Scoring: Sum the items for each of the five domains (attention, memory, fluency, language and visuospatial) to give the Domain Scores for the ACE-III. The Total ACE-III score (/100) consists of the sum of the five domain scores. Sum together the shaded boxes for the Mini-ACE score (/30). Note: The Orientation score for the Mini-ACE is scored out of a maximum of 4 only; the Season item is not included.

ACE-III: Scoring <82 suggests dementia if other causes have been excluded. A global reduction across domains is usually seen in dementia; if scores are very skewed, more specialist assessment may be warranted (discuss with Old Age or Neuropsychiatry).

ACE-III: Scoring <82 suggests dementia if other causes have been excluded. A global reduction across domains is usually seen in dementia; if scores are very skewed, more specialist assessment may be warranted (discuss with Old Age or Neuropsychiatry).

See p530–531 for M-ACE and scoring.

Appendix D.2 The Addenbrooke's Cognitive Examination-III (ACE-III) (*continued*)

ADDENBROOKE'S COGNITIVE EXAMINATION – ACE-III
UK Version A (2012)

| Name:
Date of Birth:
Hospital No. or Address: | Date of testing: ___/___/___
Tester's name:_____
Age at leaving full-time education:_____
Occupation: _____
Handedness: _____ |

ATTENTION

(Sum together only the items in BOLD for the M-ACE score)

	Day	Date	Month	Year	Season	**Attention** [Score 0-5] *☐ ☐
➤ Ask: What is the						
➤ Ask: Which	No./Floor	Street/Hospital	Town	County	Country	**Attention** [Score 0-5] ☐

ATTENTION

➤ Tell: "I'm going to give you three words and I'd like you to repeat them after me: lemon, key and ball." After subject repeats, say "Try to remember them because I'm going to ask you later".
➤ Score *only* the first trial (repeat 3 times if necessary).
➤ Register number of trials: _____

Attention
[Score 0-3]
☐

ATTENTION

➤ Ask the subject: "Could you take 7 away from 100? I'd like you to keep taking 7 away from each new number until I tell you to stop."
➤ If subject makes a mistake, do not stop them. Let the subject carry on and check subsequent answers (e.g., 93, 84, 77, 70, 63 – score 4).
➤ Stop after five subtractions (93, 86, 79, 72, 65): ___ ___ ___ ___ ___

Attention
[Score 0-5]
☐

MEMORY

➤ Ask: 'Which 3 words did I ask you to repeat and remember?' _____ _____ _____

Memory
[Score 0-3]
☐

FLUENCY

➤ **Letters**
Say: "I'm going to give you a letter of the alphabet and I'd like you to generate as many words as you can beginning with that letter, but not names of people or places. For example, if I give you the letter "C", you could give me words like "cat, cry, clock" and so on. But, you can't give me words like Catherine or Canada. Do you understand? Are you ready? You have one minute. The letter I want you to use is the letter "P".

Fluency
[Score 0 – 7]
☐

≥ 18	7
14-17	6
11-13	5
8-10	4
6-7	3
4-5	2
2-3	1
0-1	0
total	correct

➤ **Animals**
Say: "Now can you name as many animals as possible. It can begin with any letter."

Fluency
[Score 0 – 7]
☐

≥ 22	7
17-21	6
14-16	5
11-13	4
9-10	3
7-8	2
5-6	1
<5	0
total	correct

Appendix D.2 The Addenbrooke's Cognitive Examination-III (ACE-III) (*continued*)

MEMORY

➤ Tell: "I'm going to give you a name and address and I'd like you to repeat the name and address after me. So you have a chance to learn, we'll be doing that 3 times. I'll ask you the name and address later."

Score only the third trial.

Memory
[Score 0 – 7]

	1*st* Trial	2*nd* Trial	3*rd* Trial
Harry Barnes 73 Orchard Close Kingsbridge Devon	___ ___ __ ___ ___ _____ _____	___ ___ __ ___ ___ _____ _____	___ ___ __ ___ ___ _____ _____

MEMORY

➤ Name of the current Prime Minister..
➤ Name of the woman who was Prime Minister ....
➤ Name of the USA president...
➤ Name of the USA president who was assassinated in the 1960s......................................

Memory
[Score 0 – 4]

LANGUAGE

➤ Place a pencil and a piece of paper in front of the subject. As a practice trial, ask the subject to "**Pick up the pencil and then the paper.**" If incorrect, score 0 and do not continue further.

➤ If the subject is correct on the practice trial, continue with the following three commands below.
  • Ask the subject to "**Place the paper on top of the pencil**"
  • Ask the subject to "**Pick up the pencil but not the paper**"
  • Ask the subject to "**Pass me the pencil after touching the paper**"
  Note: Place the pencil and paper in front of the subject before each command.

Language
[Score 0-3]

LANGUAGE

➤ Say: "I want you to write two sentences. It can be about anything that you like. I want you to write in full sentences and avoid abbreviations." If the subject does not know what to write about, you could suggest a few topics. "For instance, you could write about a recent holiday, your hobbies, your family or childhood." If the subject writes only one sentence, then prompt for a second one.

Sentences must contain a subject and a verb. Spelling and grammar are penalized. Sentences do not need to be about the same topic. See scoring guidelines for more information.

Language
[Score 0-2]

LANGUAGE

➤ Ask the subject to repeat: '**caterpillar**'; '**eccentricity**; '**unintelligible**'; '**statistician**'
Score 2 if all are correct; score 1 if 3 are correct; and score 0 if 2 or less are correct.

Language
[Score 0-2]

Appendix D.2 The Addenbrooke's Cognitive Examination-III (ACE-III) (*continued*)

LANGUAGE	
➤ Ask the subject to repeat: **'All that glitters is not gold'**	**Language** [Score 0-1]
➤ Ask the subject to repeat: **'A stitch in time saves nine'**	**Language** [Score 0-1]

LANGUAGE	
➤ Ask the subject to name the following pictures:	**Language** [Score 0-12]

LANGUAGE	
➤ Using the pictures above, ask the subject to:	**Language** [Score 0-4]

- Point to the one which is associated with the monarchy   ....
- Point to the one which is a marsupial   ....
- Point to the one which is found in the Antarctic   ....
- Point to the one which has a nautical connection   ....

Appendix D.2 The Addenbrooke's Cognitive Examination-III (ACE-III) (*continued*)

LANGUAGE	
➢ Ask the subject to read the following words: (Score 1 only if all correct) ### sew ### pint ### soot ### dough ### height	**Language** [Score 0-1]

VISUOSPATIAL ABILITIES	
➢ Infinity Diagram: Ask the subject to copy this diagram.	**Visuospatial** [Score 0-1]

➢ Wire cube: Ask the subject to copy this drawing (for scoring, see instructions guide).	**Visuospatial** [Score 0-2]

➢ Clock: Ask the subject to draw a clock face with numbers. Then, ask the subject to put the hands at ten past five. (For scoring see instruction guide: circle = 1, numbers = 2, hands = 2 if all correct).	**Visuospatial** [Score 0-5]

Appendix D.2 The Addenbrooke's Cognitive Examination-III (ACE-III) (*continued*)

VISUOSPATIAL ABILITIES

> Ask the subject to count the dots without pointing to them

Visuospatial
[Score 0-4]

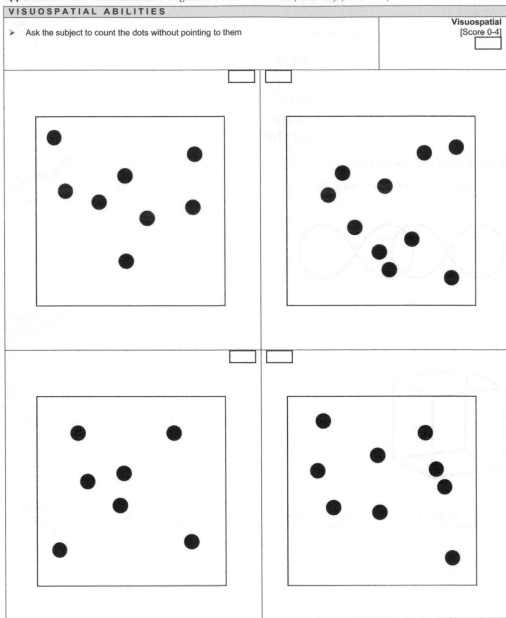

Appendix D.2 The Addenbrooke's Cognitive Examination-III (ACE-III) (*continued*)

VISUOSPATIAL ABILITIES

> Ask the subject to identify the letters

Visuospatial
[Score 0-4]

MEMORY

> Ask "Now tell me what you remember about that name and address we were repeating at the beginning"

Harry Barnes	....	**Memory** [Score 0-7]
73 Orchard Close	....	
Kingsbridge	....	
Devon	....	

MEMORY

> This test should be done if the subject failed to recall one or more items above. If all items were recalled, skip the test and score 5. If only part was recalled start by ticking items recalled in the shadowed column on the right hand side; and then test not recalled items by telling the subject "ok, I'll give you some hints: was the name X, Y or Z?" and so on. Each recognised item scores one point, which is added to the point gained by recalling.

Memory [Score 0-5]

Jerry Barnes	Harry Barnes	Harry Bradford		recalled	
37	73	76		recalled	
Orchard Place	Oak Close	Orchard Close		recalled	
Oakhampton	Kingsbridge	Dartington		recalled	
Devon	Dorset	Somerset		recalled	

SCORES

TOTAL ACE-III SCORE	/100
TOTAL M-ACE SCORE	/30
Attention	/18
Memory	/26
Fluency	/14
Language	/26
Visuospatial	/16

Appendix D.3 The Mini-Addenbrooke's Cognitive Examination (M-ACE)

MINI – ADDENBROOKE'S COGNITIVE EXAMINATION UK Version A (2014)

Name: Date of Birth: Hospital No. or Address:	Date of testing: ____/___/___ Tester's name:_____ Age at leaving full-time education:_____ Occupation: _____ Handedness: _____

ATTENTION

➢ Ask: What is the	Day	Date	Month	Year	**Attention** [Score 0-4]
	_____	_____	_____	_____	☐

MEMORY

➢ Tell: "I'm going to give you a name and address and I'd like you to repeat the name and address after me. So you have a chance to learn, we'll be doing that 3 times. I'll ask you the name and address later."

Score only the third trial.

Memory
[Score 0 – 7]
☐

	1ˢᵗ Trial	*2ⁿᵈ Trial*	*3ʳᵈ Trial*
Harry Barnes	_____ _____	_____ _____	_____ _____
73 Orchard Close	____ _____ _____	____ _____ _____	____ _____ _____
Kingsbridge	_____	_____	_____
Devon	_____	_____	_____

FLUENCY – ANIMALS

➢ **Animals**
Say: "Now can you name as many animals as possible. It can begin with any letter. You have one minute. Go ahead."

Fluency
[Score 0 – 7]
☐

				≥ 22	7
				17-21	6
				14-16	5
				11-13	4
				9-10	3
				7-8	2
				5-6	1
				<5	0
				total	correct

Appendix D.3 The Mini-Addenbrooke's Cognitive Examination (M-ACE) (*continued*)

CLOCK DRAWING	
➢ Clock: Ask the subject to draw a clock face with numbers and the hands at ten past five. (For scoring see instruction guide: circle = 1, numbers = 2, hands = 2 if all correct).	**Visuospatial** [Score 0-5]

MEMORY RECALL		
➢ Ask "Now tell me what you remember about that name and address we were repeating at the beginning"		
Harry Barnes	....	**Memory** [Score 0-7]
73 Orchard Close	....	
Kingsbridge	....	
Devon	....	

TOTAL SCORE	**/ 30**

M-ACE: scoring ≤ 25/30 strongly suggests cognitive impairment; ≤ 21/30 almost certainly shows dementia, if other diagnoses have been excluded. (NB: If the clock-drawing test is done correctly, it almost certainly excludes dementia, due to the wide range of cognitive skills used.)

APPENDIX E

Mental health legislation

Anna M Burnside[1] & Penelope Brown[2], with thanks to Daniel M Bennett and Edward Noble

[1] *East London NHS Foundation Trust, London, England*
[2] *South London & Maudsley NHS Foundation Trust, London, England*

Table E.1 The Mental Health (Care and Treatment) (Scotland) Act 2003: common civil sections.

Detention/ Section (s)	Purpose	Who does it apply to?	Who authorises it?	Do consent to treatment provisions apply?	Duration
Short-term detention (s44)	Compulsory admission to hospital for assessment and/or treatment	Person suffering from a mental disorder where their ability to make decisions about medical treatment is significantly impaired *and* hospital admission is necessary for assessment/ treatment. If not detained, there'd be significant risk to the person's health, safety or welfare, or the safety of another person.	An approved medical practitioner and Mental health Officer (MHO)	Yes	Up to 28 days. Can be extended, pending a Compulsory Treatment Order
Emergency detention (s36)	Compulsory hospital admission/ detention for assessment. If used in the community, the patient must be transported to hospital within 72h.	As above, but arranging a short-term detention would involve undesirable delay	A medical practitioner, who should consult a MHO, unless 'impracticable'	No, treatment can't be given, unless in an emergency	Up to 72h from when the patient arrives at the hospital/ when the form is signed if already in hospital.
Nurse's Holding Power	To hold an informal patient who's trying to leave, enabling a doctor's assessment.	Informal patient the nurse believes to have a mental disorder and needs examination by a doctor to consider detention, due to risks to self/others.	A qualified mental health/LD nurse	No	2h. Can be extended by 1h to allow the doctor's examination

(continued overleaf)

Psychiatry: Breaking the ICE – Introductions, Common Tasks and Emergencies for Trainees, First Edition.
Edited by Sarah Stringer, Juliet Hurn and Anna M Burnside.
© 2016 John Wiley & Sons, Ltd. Published 2016 by John Wiley & Sons, Ltd.
Companion Website: www.psychiatryice.com

Table E.1 (*continued*)

Detention/ Section (s)	Purpose	Who does it apply to?	Who authorises it?	Do consent to treatment provisions apply?	Duration
Compulsory Treatment Order (CTO; s63)	Hospital *or community* treatment for mental disorder, following an agreed care plan	The patient has a mental disorder significantly impairing decision-making abilities about medical treatment. Medical treatment is available which will stop their condition worsening/treat symptoms. Without treatment, there'd be significant risk to self/others. The use of compulsory powers is necessary.	The Mental Health Tribunal. The MHO applies to the Tribunal, including their own report, reports from two doctors, and the proposed care plan by the Responsible Medical officer (RMO)	Yes	Up to 6 months. Can be extended for a further 6 months, then yearly.
Suspension certificate	Leave from hospital, e.g. for trips out, attending general hospital appointments, staying overnight at home. Leave is escorted/ unescorted, and other conditions may apply.	Someone under emergency or short-term detention. People on a CTO may also have their hospital detention suspended.	RMO	No	As long as the patient is detained in hospital.
s292	Warrant allowing a police constable, accompanied by a MHO ± medical practitioner/other person, to enter an address and remove a person to a place where they can be assessed/return them to hospital.	Concerns that someone is suffering from a mental disorder and may be a risk to self/others; patient liable to be detained.	Sheriff or Justice of the Peace (The MHO applies to the Sheriff's court)	No	–
s297	A police constable can remove someone from a public place to a place of safety for assessment	Someone who appears to be suffering from a mental disorder in a public place, appears to need immediate care/treatment and is thought to pose a risk to self/others.	A police officer	No	24 hours

Table E.2 The Mental Health (Northern Ireland) Order 1986: common sections (Part II).

Section	Purpose	Who does it apply to?	Who authorises it?	Do consent to treatment provisions apply?	Duration
Admission to Hospital for Assessment (Form 7, 8, 9)	Compulsory admission to hospital for assessment ± subsequent treatment	Person suffering from mental disorder of a nature/degree which warrants detention in hospital for assessment (±treatment). A failure to detain would create a substantial likelihood of serious physical harm to the patient/other persons. *Excludes* personality disorder, sexual deviance/promiscuity and substance misuse.	An approved social worker (ASW) or nearest relative, following a medical recommendation (preferably from the patient's GP/a doctor who knows the patient). At admission, a medical officer must immediately examine the patient to authorise the detention (by completing Form 7) The Responsible Medical Officer (RMO) must examine the patient within 48 hours, and send a further authorisation for detention (Form 8) unless *they* completed Form 7 (which then lasts the full 7 days). After 7 days, the RMO should re-examine the patient to authorise detention for a further 7 days (Form 9).	Yes (Once Form 7 is completed treatment for symptoms of mental disorder can be given without consent in some circumstances)	Up to 14 days
Detention for Treatment (Form 10)	Compulsory detention in hospital for treatment	Person suffering from mental *illness* (rather than mental disorder) plus the above criteria.	The RMO (preferably) or a Part II doctor must assess the patient during the second 7 days of the admission for assessment.	Yes	Up to 6 months. Can be renewed for a further 6 months, then yearly. A second opinion is sought from another part II doctor.
Nurse's Holding Power (Form 6)	To hold an informal patient who's trying to leave, enabling a doctor's assessment.	The nurse believes the informal patient requires an application for assessment. It's not possible to secure the immediate attendance of a doctor.	A qualified mental health or learning disability nurse	No	Up to 6h

Holding order (Form 5)	To hold an informal patient who's trying to leave, enabling assessment for detention to hospital.	The doctor believes the informal patient requires an application for assessment, and believes the criteria for detention (above) are met.	A doctor employed by the hospital	No (treatment can be given in certain circumstances)	Up to 48h
Guardianship	To ensure a patient receives the care and treatment they need. They can be compelled to *attend* but not to *receive medical* treatment. It can be used to compel them to live at a certain address (only if willing to go without resistance); to present themselves for treatment, occupation, education or training; and to allow access to a doctor/ASW/other named person. If the patient doesn't recognise the power of the guardian, there is no power to enforce guardianship and it should be discontinued.	Two criteria must be met: Medical & Welfare. The patient must be suffering from a mental illness/severe mental handicap of a nature/degree which warrants them being taken into guardianship. It must also be necessary for their welfare.	Guardianship requires two medical recommendations for the Medical grounds, and an ASW's recommendation for the Welfare grounds. The application itself is made by the nearest relative or an ASW who cannot be the same person making the Welfare recommendation).	Yes	Up to 6 months. Can be extended for a further 6 months, then yearly.

(continued overleaf)

Table E.2 (*continued*)

Section	Purpose	Who does it apply to?	Who authorises it?	Do consent to treatment provisions apply?	Duration
Leave of absence from hospital **Article 15(1)**	Leave from hospital, e.g. for trips out, attending general hospital appointments, staying overnight at home. Leave is escorted /unescorted, and other conditions may apply.	Person detained for assessment/treatment	RMO	No	As long as the patient is detained in hospital.
Article 129	Warrant allowing a police constable, accompanied by a medical practitioner, to force entry to a private address, and remove a person to a place where they can be assessed, or convey them to hospital if application for detention for assessment has been made or return them to hospital if they've absconded.	Concerns that someone suffers from a mental disorder and may be a risk to self/others; patients liable to be detained.	Justice of the Peace	No	–
Article 130	Police officer power to remove someone from a public place to a place of safety for assessment by a doctor and ASW.	Someone who appears to be suffering from a mental disorder in a public place, appears to be in need of immediate care and control in their own interest/for the protection of others.	A police officer	No	Up to 48h

NB: A new Capacity Bill is being drawn up to replace current legislation, combining consent to physical *and* mental health treatment. This aims to reduce stigma, as those with mental health diagnoses will no longer be managed under different legislation.

Table E.3 The Mental Health Act 1983, amended 2007 (England & Wales): forensic sections.

Section (s)	Purpose	Who does it apply to?	Who authorises it?	Do consent to treatment provisions apply?	Duration
s35	Remand of an accused person to hospital for a *report* to be prepared, prior to trial or sentencing. NB: If the patient absconds, they can be arrested without a warrant and returned to court. Patients on s35 can't receive s17 leave or appeal to a Tribunal.	A defendant charged with an imprisonable offence, in whom mental disorder is suspected. A report on their mental health is needed before trial or sentencing (and it's impossible to make this report if they were bailed).	Magistrates or Crown court, on recommendation of 1 RMP (s12 approved)	No If treatment is needed without the person's consent, it can be given under the MCA or a concurrent s2 or s3.	28 days, can be renewed for up to 12 weeks
s36	Remand of an accused person to hospital for *treatment* prior to trial or sentencing.	Same as s35, except that the mental disorder needs inpatient treatment. NB: admission isn't necessarily on the grounds of health or safety.	Crown court, on recommendation of 2 RMPs	Yes	As per s35
s37	Hospital order: admission for treatment. As for s3, but court-ordered. Patients can be granted s17 leave. Tribunals are available, after 6 months.	An offender *convicted of an* imprisonable offence who suffers from a mental disorder of a nature or degree requiring hospital admission for treatment (as an alternative to prison)	Crown or Magistrates' court, on recommendation of 2 RMPs	Yes	As for s3 (p99)
s37/41	Hospital order with restriction order Only the Secretary of State, via the Ministry of Justice (MoJ), can authorise leave and discharge from hospital. Tribunals are available, after 6 months.	As for s37, but a restriction order (41) means the offender is deemed at high risk of serious harm to the public	Crown court, on recommendation of 2 RMPs	Yes	Until the Secretary of State deems the patient is safe for absolute or conditional discharge. Conditional discharge means they can be recalled to hospital from the community if they breach certain rules.

(continued overleaf)

Table E.3 (*continued*)

Section (s)	Purpose	Who does it apply to?	Who authorises it?	Do consent to treatment provisions apply?	Duration
s38	Interim hospital order Allows the court to order a relatively brief period in hospital before sentencing, so the evaluating doctors can decide whether to recommend a hospital order (s37). Patients can't be granted s17 leave or appeal to a Tribunal.	An offender *convicted* of an imprisonable offence *before sentencing*	Crown or Magistrates' court, on recommendation of 2 RMPs	Yes	12 weeks. Can be renewed for 28 days at a time for up to a year
s45(A)	Hospital direction or "Hybrid order" Similar to a s37/41, except that when the patient no longer needs hospital treatment, they are returned to prison until the end of their sentence rather than being discharged into the community.	As for s37/41	Crown court, on recommendation of 2 RMPs	Yes	As for s37/41 or until the end of their prison sentence
s47/49	Transfer from prison to hospital for treatment S47 is usually given with s49, which is similar to a restriction order (s41). Leave and discharge can only be granted by the MoJ.	A *sentenced* prisoner suffering from a mental disorder of a nature or degree warranting treatment (i.e. as for s3, except the person is sentenced and in prison)	The Secretary of State, on the recommendation of 2 RMPs	Yes	As for s3. When the patient no longer requires hospital treatment they return to prison until the end of their sentence
s48/49	Transfer from prison to hospital for treatment.	A *non-sentenced* prisoner, usually remanded on bail awaiting trial or sentencing.	The Secretary of State, on the recommendation of 2 RMPs	Yes	As for s3, or until the patient is sentenced.

APPENDIX F
Useful contacts

Name	Contact details
Main switchboard	
My team	
Administrator	
Team manager	
Consultant	
Registrar	
Community services	
CMHTs:	
•	
•	
•	
•	
Home Treatment Team	
CAMHS	
Early Intervention Service	
Addictions	
Learning Disabilities	
Older Adults Team	
Forensic Team	
Perinatal Psychiatry	
Psychiatric Unit	
Bed manager	
Unit holder	
Duty doctor	
Emergency Response Team	
Wards	
•	
•	
•	
•	
•	
•	
•	
•	
•	
•	

Psychiatry: Breaking the ICE – Introductions, Common Tasks and Emergencies for Trainees, First Edition.
Edited by Sarah Stringer, Juliet Hurn and Anna M Burnside.
© 2016 John Wiley & Sons, Ltd. Published 2016 by John Wiley & Sons, Ltd.
Companion Website: www.psychiatryice.com

Name	Contact details
S136 suite	
Outpatients	
Pharmacy	
Clozapine clinic	
Depot clinic	
ECT coordinator	
IT services	
Psychotherapy	
MHA Office	
Safeguarding lead	
Patient advocacy	
Trust legal	
General Hospital	
Switchboard	
Liaison psychiatry	
Psychiatric Liaison Nurse	
Emergency Department	
Medical registrar	
Surgical registrar	
Biochemistry	
Haematology	
Pathology	
Radiology	
Security	
Social Services	
Main number	
AMHP service	
Duty social worker	
Child protection team	
Adult safeguarding	
Other	
Clozapine monitoring service	
Interpreting service	
Police liaison officer	

Index

Psychiatry: Breaking the ICE – Introductions, Common Tasks and Emergencies for Trainees, First Edition.
Edited by Sarah Stringer, Juliet Hurn and Anna M Burnside.
© 2016 John Wiley & Sons, Ltd. Published 2016 by John Wiley & Sons, Ltd.
Companion Website: www.psychiatryice.com

Printed and bound by CPI Group (UK) Ltd, Croydon, CR0 4YY

27/10/2024

14580221-0001